Cystoid Macular Edema

Shlomit Schaal • Henry J. Kaplan
Editors

Cystoid Macular Edema

Medical and Surgical Management

Springer

Editors
Shlomit Schaal, MD, PhD
Professor and Chair
Department of Ophthalmology
and Visual Sciences
University of Massachusetts
School of Medicine
Worcester, MA
USA

Henry J. Kaplan, MD
Evans Professor and Chair of
Ophthalmology and Visual Sciences
University of Louisville
Louisville, KY
USA

ISBN 978-3-319-39764-1 ISBN 978-3-319-39766-5 (eBook)
DOI 10.1007/978-3-319-39766-5

Library of Congress Control Number: 2016958301

Printed on acid-free paper

This Springer imprint is published by Springer Nature
The registered company is Springer International Publishing AG
The registered company address is Gewerbestrasse 11, 6330 Cham, Switzerland

This book is dedicated to my beloved mentor, Dr. Henry J. Kaplan, who is recognized around the world as one of the brightest and sharpest minds in retina and uveitis. For his wise guidance, admirable leadership, endless inspiration, and persistent support have produced generations of outstanding clinicians and scientists.
On behalf of all your grateful students,

Shlomit Schaal, M.D., Ph.D.

Acknowledgment

The authors would like to sincerely thank all the world renowned contributors to this book, who spent time and effort to write high quality state-of-the-art informative chapters.

Special thanks to Dr. Shivani Reddy, who helped proof reading the book.

This book was supported by an unrestricted institutional grant from Research to Prevent Blindness.

Contents

Part III Surgical Management of CME

Contributors

Motasem Al-latayfeh, MD Department of Opthalmology, Hashemite University, Zarqa, Jordan

Jorge L. Alió y Sanz, MD, PhD, FEBO Cataract and Refractive Surgery Unit, Vissum, Instituto Oftalmológico de Alicante, Alicante, Spain

Miguel Hernández University, Alicante, Spain

Pedro Amat-Peral, MD, PhD, FEBO Vitreous-Retina Unit, Vissum, Instituto Oftalmológico de Alicante, Alicante, Spain

J. Fernando Arevalo, MD, FACS Retina Division, Department of Ophthalmology, Wilmer Eye Institute, The Johns Hopkins University School of Medicine, Baltimore, MD, USA

Emerson Badaro, MD Vitreoretinal Sector, Department of Ophthalmology, Federal University of São Paulo, UNIFESP, Brazil, São Paulo, SP, Brazil

Francine Behar-Cohen, MD, PhD Department of Ophthalmology, University of Lausanne Jules Gonin Eye Hospital, Lausanne, Switzerland

Inserm U1138, Centre de Recherche des Cordeliers, Paris, France

Juliana Bottós, MD Vitreoretinal Sector, Department of Ophthalmology, Federal University of São Paulo, UNIFESP, Brazil, São Paulo, SP, Brazil

Wolf Buehl, MD Department of Ophthalmology, Medical University of Vienna, Vienna, Austria

Alejandra Daruich-Matet, MD, MS Department of Ophthalmology, University of Lausanne Jules Gonin Eye Hospital, Lausanne, Switzerland

Lucian V. Del Priore, MD, PhD Department of Ophthalmology, Yale University School of Medicine, New Haven, CT, USA

Dean Eliott, MD Retina Service, Department of Ophthalmology, Massachusetts Eye & Ear Infirmary, Harvard Medical School, Boston, MA, USA

Javier Elizalde, MD Vitreoretinal Surgery Unit, Institut Barraquer, Barcelona, Spain

Sarah M. Escott, MD Department of Ophthalmology, Feinberg School of Medicine, Northwestern University, Chicago, IL, USA

Debra A. Goldstein, MD Department of Ophthalmology, Feinberg School of Medicine, Northwestern University, Chicago, IL, USA

Dilraj S. Grewal, MD Duke Eye Center, Durham, NC, USA

Alexander L. Grigalunas, MD Department of Ophthalmology, Rush University Medical Center, Chicago, IL, USA

Ahmet M. Hondur, MD Department of Ophthalmology, School of Medicine, Gazi University, Ankara, Turkey

Glenn J. Jaffe, MD Duke Eye Center, Durham, NC, USA

Henry J. Kaplan, MD Ophthalmology and Visual Sciences, University of Louisville, Louisville, KY, USA

Matin Khoshnevis, MD VMR Institute for Vitreous Macula Retina, Huntington Beach, CA, USA

Temple University, Department of Ophthalmology, Philadelphia, PA, USA

Francisco L. Lugo-Quintás, MD, PhD Vitreous-Retina Unit, Vissum, Instituto Oftalmológico de Alicante, Alicante, Spain

Mauricio Maia, MD, PhD Vitreoretinal Surgery Unit, Universidade Federal de Sao Paulo, Brazilian Institute of Fight Against Blindness, Assis/Presidente Prudente, SP, Brazil

Alexandre Matet, MD, MSc Department of Ophthalmology, University of Lausanne Jules Gonin Eye Hospital, Lausanne, Switzerland

Pauline T. Merrill, MD Department of Ophthalmology, Rush University Medical Center, Chicago, IL, USA

Shlomit Schaal, MD, PhD Department of Ophthalmology and Visual Sciences, University of Massachusetts School of Medicine, Amherst, MA, USA

Ursula M. Schmidt-Erfurth, MD Department of Ophthalmology, Medical University of Vienna, Vienna, Austria

J. Sebag, MD, FACS, FRCOphth, FARVO VMR Institute for Vitreous Macula Retina, Huntington Beach, CA, USA

Katherine E. Talcott, MD Department of Ophthalmology, Massachusetts Eye & Ear Infirmary, Harvard Medical School, Boston, MA, USA

Tongalp H. Tezel, MD Department of Ophthalmology, Columbia University College of Physicians and Surgeons, Edward S. Harkness Eye Institute, Columbia University Medical Center, New York, NY, USA

Reid Turner, MD Department of Ophthalmology, Medical University of South Carolina, Storm Eye Institute, Charleston, SC, USA

Part I
Pathophysiology and Diagnosis of CME

Chapter 1
Introduction

Shlomit Schaal and Henry J. Kaplan

Macular edema is defined as swelling of the layers of the neurosensory retina within the macula. Although the classic presentation of macular edema is termed "cystoid macular edema" (CME), which represents the collection of excess fluid in "cysts" within the neurosensory retina, it is more broadly defined as extracellular accumulation of fluid within the outer plexiform layer of the retina. Thus, CME should be referred to as a subtype of macular edema with specific characteristics on imaging studies (e.g., fluorescein angiography and optical coherence tomography [OCT]). The most common clinical manifestation of macular edema is a reduction in central visual acuity. However, it is now recognized that macular edema may exist without impairing visual acuity but detectable on sophisticated retinal imaging. Thus, reliance on visual acuity to exclude the presence of macular edema is not sufficient, nor is it appropriate to rely on vision to suggest resolution of macular edema in response to treatment. Other clinical manifestations of macular edema include micropsia, in which objects appear smaller than they really are, as well as metamorphopsia. Although macular edema is reversible through both medical and surgical intervention, the development of chronic macular edema may eventually result in irreversible photoreceptor damage with a constant central scotoma. Other functional indications of the presence of macular edema include decreased reading speed, as well as reduced contrast sensitivity.

S. Schaal, MD, PhD
Professor and Chair, Department of Ophthalmology and Visual Sciences,
University of Massachusetts School of Medicine, Amherst, MA, USA
e-mail: S.Schaal@umassmed.edu

H.J. Kaplan, MD (✉)
Evans Professor and Chair of Ophthalmology and Visual Sciences,
University of Louisville, Louisville, KY, USA
e-mail: hank.kaplan@louisville.edu

S. Schaal, H.J. Kaplan (eds.), *Cystoid Macular Edema*,
DOI 10.1007/978-3-319-39766-5_1

The pathogenesis and etiology of macular edema is rather complex. Although the hallmark of this complication of many different diseases is the accumulation of intraretinal fluid, macular edema can occur as a result of multiple and diverse mechanisms: the breakdown of inner blood-retinal barrier (e.g., endothelial cell tight junctions), breakdown of the outer retinal barrier (e.g., tight junctions between RPE cells), and/or interference with the normal egress of retinal fluid by cells within the neurosensory retina (e.g., Mueller cell dysfunction or retinal pigment epithelium (RPE) dysfunction). Macular edema is the leading cause of central vision loss that accompanies many systemic diseases, including diabetes mellitus and systemic inflammatory conditions associated with uveitis. However, it is also a complication of many other retinal diseases including retinal vascular diseases (choroidal neovascularization in age-related macular degeneration, hypertensive retinopathy, central retinal vein occlusion, branch retinal vein occlusion), uveal inflammation (e.g., HLA-B27 acute anterior uveitis, pars planitis, birdshot chorioretinopathy), tractional forces on the retina (e.g., epiretinal membrane formation, vitreomacular traction syndrome), retinal dystrophies (e.g., retinitis pigmentosa, Goldman-Favre syndrome, juvenile x-linked retinoschisis), intraocular tumors (e.g., choroidal hemangioma, choroidal melanoma, retinal hemangioma), adverse effect of medications (e.g., niacin, tamoxifen), and idiopathic diseases.

Prior to the development of modern imaging techniques, funduscopy was the sole method to detect macular edema, in particular CME. The introduction of fluorescein angiography was a major imaging advancement that revolutionized our appreciation and quantification of CME, as well as the mechanisms leading to the development of macular edema. The more recent development of autofluorescence imaging and in particular the widespread use of spectral domain OCT have allowed us to obtain much greater insight into the anatomical alterations caused by macular edema. The application of these imaging technologies has allowed us to identify three different patterns of macular edema – (1) CME, characterized by clearly defined intraretinal cystic spaces within the neurosensory retina; (2) diffuse macular edema, characterized by increased retinal thickness and disturbance of the layered retinal structure; and (3) serous retinal detachment, characterized by separation of the neurosensory retina from the underlying RPE. It is also now apparent that the absence of macular edema on fluorescein angiography does not necessarily correlate with the results of other imaging techniques. Thus, multimodal imaging provides us with the most sophisticated tools to determine and document the presence of macular edema.

Since macular edema is associated with so many different causes, the response of macular edema to therapy is obviously quite variable. Multiple medications, as well as surgical intervention, have been used with reported success and CME resolution in several diseases. It is clear that the underlying pathogenesis of the disease must be clearly identified to obtain the best therapeutic response to intervention. However, it is recognized that response to treatment may vary between patients depending upon personal genetic makeup and exposure to environmental factors.

Since macular edema is a major cause of visual disability, we have been fortunate, as editors of this book, to have enlisted the expertise of several internationally respected clinicians and scientists to address three major areas in this text:

Part I – Pathophysiology and Diagnosis of CME
Part II – Medical Management of CME
Part III – Surgical Management of CME

It is our intent to provide a contemporary update into the cause of this major visual complication to allow a more accurate diagnosis, as well as therapeutic intervention for the reversal of this disease complication. The many advances that have been made in both diagnosis and in the understanding of the underlying pathophysiology of this disease have resulted in the development of novel medications that prevent the permanent loss of central vision. We are indebted to the many scholarly contributors to this text and personally thank them for their excellent contributions.

Chapter 2
Mechanisms of Macular Edema

Alejandra Daruich-Matet, Alexandre Matet, and Francine Behar-Cohen

Introduction

Macular edema (ME) can be defined as a collection of fluid within and/or under the retina in the macular region. ME can be identified by a diffuse increase in retinal thickness, the formation of intraretinal cysts, and the accumulation of subretinal fluid (Fig. 1). Whether distinct pathogenic mechanisms induce different types of fluid accumulation is unclear.

ME can manifest in nearly all retinal diseases at various phases of their development. Most frequently ME is associated with ischemia/hypoxia and/or inflammation. Systemic factors such as increased blood pressure (hypertension) or reduced plasma oncotic pressure (hypoalbuminemia) can aggravate ME.

In physiologic conditions, active mechanisms permanently maintain the retina in a transparent and relatively dehydrated state. Fluid can enter in the retina from the vitreous, from the retinal vessels, and from the subretinal space through the retinal pigment epithelium (RPE). Fluid entry from the circulation into the retina is controlled by the inner blood-retinal barrier, formed by endothelial tight junctions, pericytes, astrocytes, and retinal Müller glia (RMG) [1], and by the outer retinal barrier, formed by the tight junction of the retinal pigment epithelium (RPE) [2]. Fluid exit through the RPE is ensured by active ion and water channels

A. Daruich-Matet, MD, MS • A. Matet, MD, MSc
Department of Ophthalmology, University of Lausanne Jules Gonin Eye Hospital,
15 avenue de France, Lausanne 1004, Switzerland

F. Behar-Cohen, MD, PhD (✉)
Department of Ophthalmology, University of Lausanne Jules Gonin Eye Hospital,
15 avenue de France, Lausanne 1004, Switzerland

Inserm U1138, Centre de Recherche des Cordeliers,
15 rue de l'Ecole de Medecine, Paris 75006, France
e-mail: francine.behar@gmail.com

S. Schaal, H.J. Kaplan (eds.), *Cystoid Macular Edema*,
DOI 10.1007/978-3-319-39766-5_2

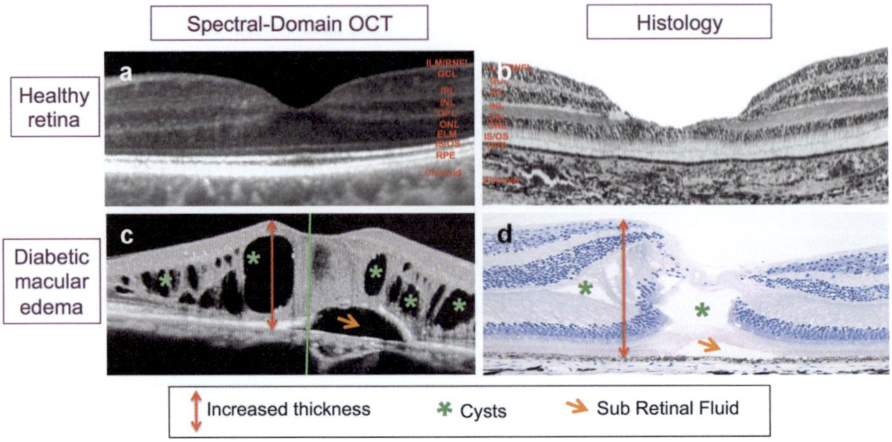

Fig. 1 Macular edema: fluid accumulation within and/or under the retina. Spectral-domain optical coherence tomography (SD-OCT) section (**a**) and histology (**b**) of a healthy human retina. Note the different retinal layers from the choroid to the vitreous cavity: *RPE* retinal pigment epithelium, *ELM* external limiting membrane, *IS/OS* photoreceptors inner segment/outer segment junction, *ONL* outer nuclear layer, *OPL* outer plexiform layer, *INL* inner nuclear layer, *IPL* inner plexiform layer, *GCL* ganglion cell layer, *ILM* internal limiting membrane, *RNFL* retinal nerve fiber layer. Diabetic macular edema imaged on SD-OCT (**c**) and histology of a human macula presenting macular edema (**d**), diplaying an increase in retinal thickness (*red arrows*), the formation of intra-retinal cysts (*green stars*), and the accumulation of subretinal fluid (*short red arrows*)

[3]. It is facilitated by the oncotic pressure-driven flow. Numerous ionic transports are strictly regulated in RPE cells and contribute to the outward flux from the subretinal space toward the choroid. RMG cells also play an important role in ion and water drainage from the inner retina toward the retinal vessels (Fig. 2). In physiologic conditions, potassium transport is associated with water drainage through Kir (inwardly rectifying potassium channels) and aquaporin (AQP) channels that are both expressed in RMG cells [4, 5]. The exact molecular partners of ion and water coupling are only partially known in the retina. It is accepted that Kir4.1 and AQP4, located in RMG cells around retinal vessels and in RMG end feet, are key players in this balance (Fig. 2). Moreover, tight-like junctions recently identified at the external limiting membrane (ELM) between RMG and photoreceptors control the passive movement of fluid in the outer retina (Fig. 3). Altogether, these different mechanisms act in a synchronized manner to control the retinal thickness.

The density of RMG cells is higher in the macula than in any other region of the retina. In addition, their morphology also differs, with a perifoveal portion orientated radially and almost parallel to the frontal plane [6, 7] which suggests that RMG cells exhibit different functions in the macula than in the periphery. Whether ion and water transport mechanisms also present specific features in the macula should be explored and could contribute to explain the specific location of edema in the macula.

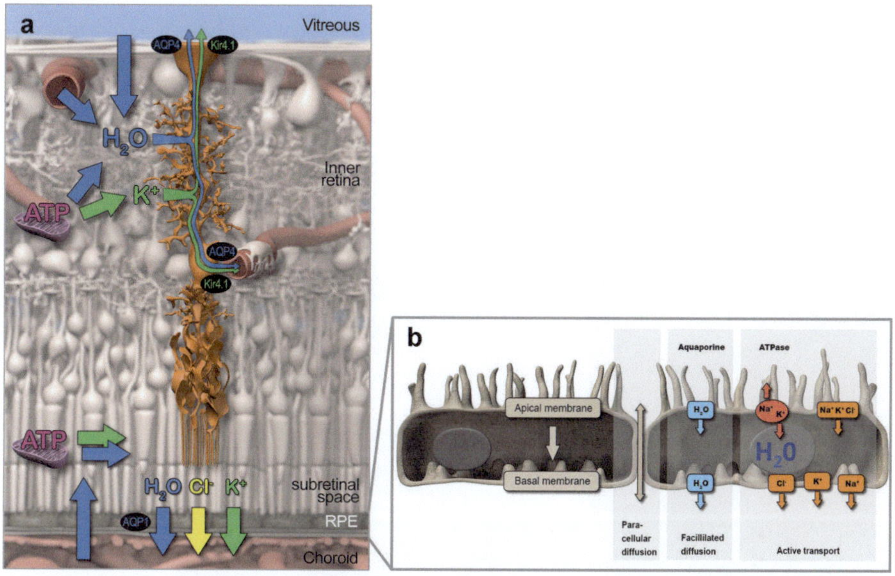

Fig. 2 (**a**) Schematic representation of a retinal Müller glial cell illustrating its roles in ion and water drainage from the inner retina toward the retinal vessels. Potassium transport is associated with water drainage through Kir4.1 (inwardly rectifying potassium channels) and AQP4 (aquaporin) channels, both located close to the interface of the retinal Müller glial cell with retinal vessels and in retinal Müller glial end feet at the level of the internal limiting membrane. (**b**) Schematic representation of RPE cells illustrating the drainage of water and electrolytes from the subretinal space to the choroid via paracellular diffusion, facilitated diffusion, and active transport

Mechanisms Leading to ME

ME results from an imbalance between fluid entry and fluid exit leading to an accumulation of fluid within and/or under the retina and in the extracellular and/or in the intracellular media (Fig. 4).

The pathogenic mechanisms of ME can be classified as "vasogenic," which reflects a vascular leakage with a volumetric influx of extracellular fluid or "cytotoxic" which reflects cell swelling induced by a volumetric increase in intracellular fluid.

Mechanisms Leading to Increased Retinal Fluid Entry or "Vasogenic" Mechanisms

Starling Equation

The Starling equation represents the movements of fluid in and out capillary vessels. It depends on capillary filtration, hydrostatic, and oncotic pressure – i.e., Starling forces.

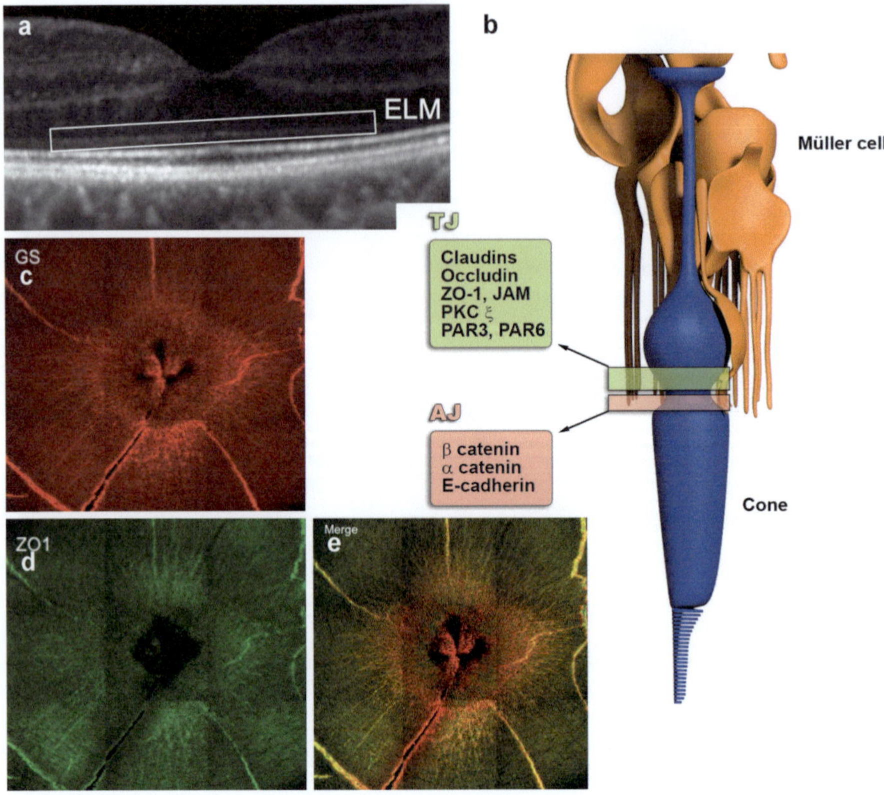

Fig. 3 The structure of the external limiting membrane and distribution of retinal Müller glial cells. (**a**) Spectral-domain optical coherence tomography of healthy macula highlighting the hyperreflective signal attributed to the external limiting membrane. (**b**) Tight-like junctions and adherens junctions are found at the level of the external limiting membrane between retinal Müller glia and photoreceptors and rely on specialized molecular families including zonula occludens-1. Macular flat mounts from healthy monkeys (*Macaca fascicularis*) after immunostaining of glutamine synthetase (**c**, *red*), marker of Müller cells, zonula occludens-1 (**d**, *green*), and fusion of both fluorescence images (**e**). The colocalization of both markers (appearing *yellow* in **e**) indicates a close relationship between tight junctions and retinal Müller glial cells

The Starling equation reads as follows:

$$J_v = K_f\left([P_c - P_i] - \sigma[\pi_c - \pi_i]\right)$$

where:

J_v is the net fluid movement between compartments
P_c is the capillary hydrostatic pressure
P_i is the interstitial hydrostatic pressure
π_c is the capillary oncotic pressure
π_i is the interstitial oncotic pressure
K_f is the filtration coefficient – a proportionality constant
σ is the reflection coefficient

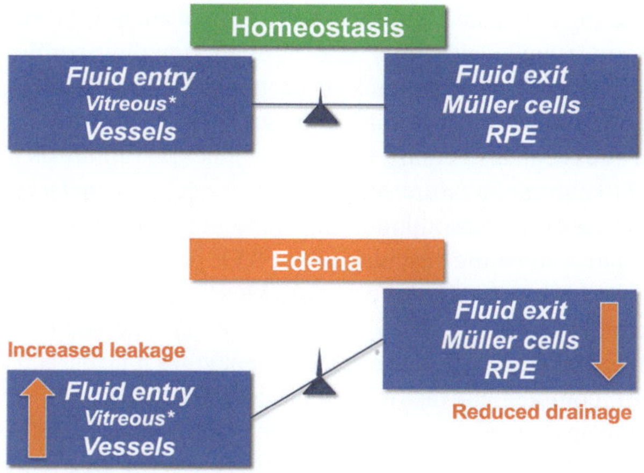

Fig. 4 Mechanisms of macular edema. Macular edema results from an imbalance between fluid entry and fluid exit leading to an abnormal accumulation of fluid within and/or under the retina (*the contribution of the vitreous on the retinal fluid entry is limited)

In conditions such as inflammation and elevated intracapillary pressure, the forces and membrane parameters governing transendothelial flux enhance filtration and increase the interstitial accumulation of albumin. The increased oncotic pressure in the neuroretina reduces fluid absorption and leads to retinal edema.

Rupture of Retinal Barriers

Barrier properties of retinal blood vessels and the RPE are due mainly to the presence of complex tight junction networks between cells. Tight junction and adherens junctions are integral membrane structures connected to the actin cytoskeleton via different adaptor molecules. Tight junctions are constituted by occludins, claudins (particularly claudin 5), and junction-associated molecules (JAM) connected to PDZ domain-containing proteins (among which is zonula occludens-1) and associated with an atypical protein kinase responsible for the tightly regulated phosphorylation of junction proteins (e.g., protein kinase C zeta, PKCζ). Junction proteins are transmembrane adhesive molecules closely linked to the cytoskeleton and with polarization proteins in the RPE. Tight junction destabilization can result from alteration of phosphorylation enzyme activity (e.g., PKCζ in diabetes), reduction of tight junction protein expression (e.g., occludin in diabetes), alteration of the cytoskeleton (e.g., secondary to oxidative damage or activation of RhoA/ROCK1 pathway), calcium dynamics [8], cell loss or severe cell damage (e.g., in case of severe inflammatory processes), and degradation of tight junction molecules by activation of proteases [9]. During inflammation, the exact molecular mechanisms that lead to tight junction disruption remain imperfectly understood. The cross talk between microglia and endothelial cells could contribute to tight junction expression regulation [10], while actin-binding molecules could also control vascular permeability via various signaling mechanisms such as activation of small GTPases [11]. Several extracellular signals could also intervene through signaling pathways leading to phosphorylation of actin and/or junction proteins, leading to their displacement from the membrane to other subcellular compartments.

Mechanical stress can also contribute to tight junction rupture as observed in the RPE submitted to chronic pressure secondary to vascular or melanocytic tumors in the choroid or to choroidal vasodilation in central serous chorioretinopathy.

Soluble mediators inducing vascular and/or RPE permeability include cytokines, such us monocyte chemoattractant protein-1 (MCP-1), tumor necrosis factor alpha (TNF-α), interleukins (IL-1b, IL-8, IL-6), vascular endothelial growth factor (VEGF) family members, acute phase proteins, enzymes, plasma activation systems (contact system, complement factor system, coagulation factors, fibrinolysis factors), arachidonic acid metabolites, biogenic or vasoactive amines (histamine, serotonin), eosinophil granular proteins, neuropeptides, oxygen free radicals, and nitric oxide.

Vascular Abnormalities Associated with Enhanced Permeability

Besides alteration of the tight and adherens junction complexes, other abnormal vascular changes can lead to increased fluid entry, visualized by "leakage" of dye during fluorescein angiography. This is the case for retinal neovascularization proliferating at the surface of the retina, with immature and low parietal stabilization, aneurysmal dilation of retinal capillaries (leaky microaneurysms in diabetic retinopathy), and vascular telangiectasia associated with intense protein leakage (as observed in Type 1 idiopathic macular telangiectasia and Coats' disease). Factors potentially increasing the vascular permeability include lower pericyte coverage, hemodynamic changes with focal occlusions and secondary endothelial alterations, and elevation of the intravascular pressure.

Factors inducing vascular abnormalization include ischemia through hypoxia-inducible factor 1-alpha (HIF-1a), VEGFA and placental growth factor (PGF), and oxidative stress through advanced glycation end products (AGE). In certain disorders, such as Type 2 idiopathic macular telangiectasia, they remain unknown. The role of microglial cells and RMG cells is now considered as important players in the development of retinal vascular diseases [12].

RPE Dysfunction

RPE dysfunction can contribute to fluid entry from the choroid into the subretinal space. This enhanced fluid entry does not strictly belong to the classical vasogenic mechanisms. Indeed, the RPE transports water from the subretinal space into the choroid without rupture of the RPE tight junctions. The important RPE absorption capacity is particularly obvious in case of retinal detachment. RPE transport of Cl^- and K^+ is thought to drive transepithelial water transport. But in physiologic basal conditions, the Cl^- conductance is up to 70% of the total basolateral conductance. The transport rate of water through RPE is estimated between 1.4 and 11 μl/cm²/h [13]. Fluid absorption involves complex mechanisms operating in the apical and basolateral membranes of the RPE cells that involve Cl^- transport, Na^{+}/K^{+}-ATPase activity, and $Ca2^+$-activated, volume-activated, and/or cAMP-activated ion channels. These mechanisms are differentially regulated under light or dark conditions and are influenced by the circadian rhythm. Ion absorption in the RPE is accompanied by water transport through aquaporins [5, 14–16]. Calcium channels in the RPE were shown to regulate VEGF expression, suggesting a potential link between RPE ion transport and VEGF-induced permeability [17].

In pathological conditions such as diabetic retinopathy, changes in aquaporin expression were shown at the level of RPE [18].

Subretinal fluid accumulation resulting from alteration of fluid and ion transport across the RPE has also been suggested in central serous chorioretinopathy (Fig. 10a), but whether such changes per se are able to induce subretinal fluid in the absence of RPE barrier disruption has not been demonstrated.

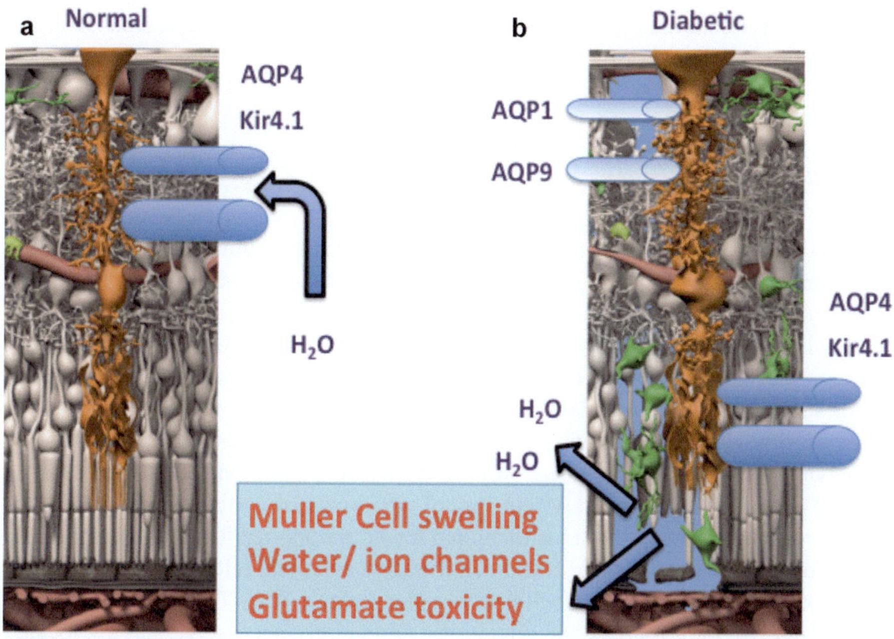

Fig. 5 (**a**) Normal retina; (**b**) Diabetic retina. Retinal Müller glial cells in normal and diabetic retina. Retinal Müller glial cells drive water flux in and out the vessels through AQP4 and Kir4.1 channels, which are altered in pathologic states provoking macular edema. In the diabetic retina, the drainage capability of the retinal Müller glial cell is overwhelmed, and AQP4 and Kir4.1 are displaced toward the outer portion of the retinal Müller glial cell. Additional channels (AQP1 and AQP9) are also expressed at the cell surface. As a consequence of macular edema, glutamate accumulates, and its cellular toxicity contributes to the persistence of the macular edema

Mechanisms Leading to Reduced Retinal Fluid Exit or "Cytotoxic" Mechanisms: Retinal Müller Glia Dysfunction

RMG drainage functions are altered in almost all retinal diseases associated with ischemia and inflammation, as well as in chronic hyperglycemia [19]. RMG cells play a central role in the hydro-ionic balance in the retina, absorbing water from the retinal tissue by water transport coupled to the potassium clearance function. Kir4.1 channels are localized in the RMG cells' membrane around the vessels in physiologic conditions but undergo a change in localization and/or levels of expression in pathologic conditions. This leads to potassium excess within RMG cells, subsequent cellular swelling, and enhanced potassium levels in the extracellular milieu with increased osmotic pressure. Retinal cysts can at least in part result from RMG swelling and necrotic death [4, 20]. RMG cells also drive water flux in and out the vessels through AQP4 channels, which are also altered in pathologic states (Fig. 5).

There are other evidences of the central role of RMG cells in ME formation such as pharmacotoxic ME induced by chemotherapy drugs, which presents with silent ME on fluorescein angiography. In these cases, drugs damaging the cytoskeleton can lead to pure cytotoxic edema without any clinically detectable vasogenic component.

Interestingly, studies have shown that potassium conductance decreases in the aging human retina favoring ME in elderly patients [21].

Mechanical Tractions

Any tractional force exerted at the vitreoretinal interface and/or under the retina can cause or aggravate ME (Fig. 6). Three hypotheses may explain the mechanical formation of ME: the deformations caused by traction on Müller cells, with subsequent metabolic impairment; the deformation of vessels with subsequent leakage from altered vascular walls; and the decreased interstitial hydrostatic pressure creating water, ion, and protein influx within the neuroretinal tissue.

In physiologic conditions, vitreous collagen fibers distribute tractional forces evenly to the vitreoretinal interface, where they are intertwined with RMG cell end feet at the internal limiting membrane (ILM). In case of vitreomacular traction exerted after partial vitreous detachment, the same tractional forces are applied locally to fewer RMG cells. This may lead to chronic RMG cell irritation and local release of inflammatory mediators, which in turn may facilitate vascular leakage [22]. The same mechanical process may account for vascular alterations, particularly because vessels are located in the inner retinal layers. Finally, persistent tractional forces applied to the vitreoretinal interface may lead to a decreased interstitial hydrostatic pressure within the neuroretinal tissue. By diminishing the interstitial pressure term in Starling's law, this traction results in an increased fluid influx from the vascular compartment [23, 24].

These processes probably occur simultaneously in the pathophysiology of mechanical ME. Epiretinal membranes, macular pucker, vitreomacular traction due to abnormal vitreous adhesion, and glial or glio-vascular proliferations observed in

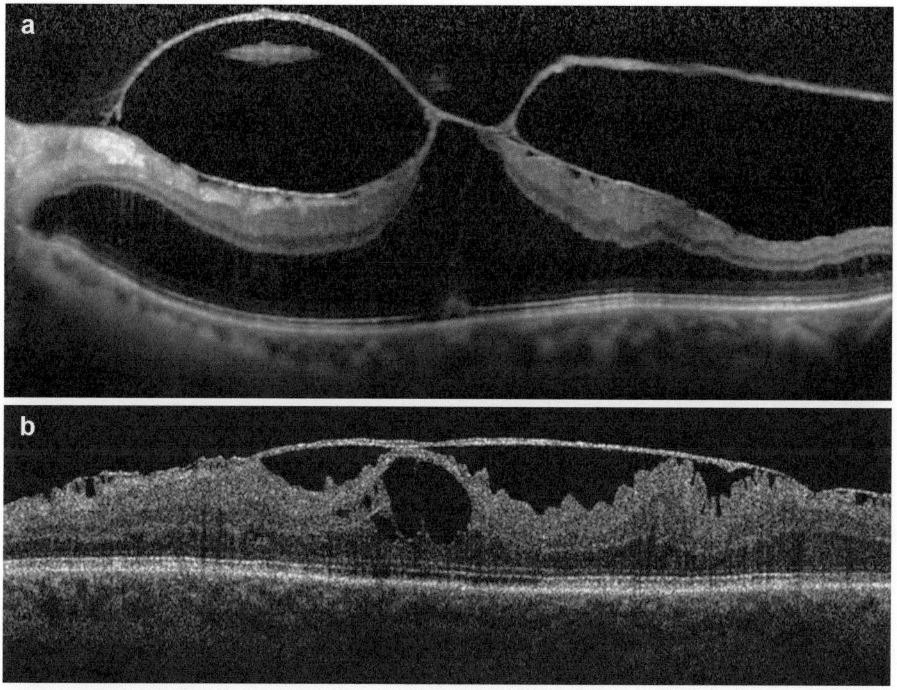

Fig. 6 Mechanical traction-induced macular edema. (**a**) Vitreomacular tractions leading to macular edema associated with an epiretinal membrane. (**b**) Epiretinal membrane and vitreomacular adhesion leading to cystoid macular edema and an irregular retinal surface

proliferative vitreoretinopathy following retinal detachment and proliferative diabetic retinopathy must be individually analyzed to understand their role in ME formation.

Causes of Macular Edema

ME can occur during the course of virtually every retinal disease at various phases of their evolution. The mechanisms of ME discussed above are intricate, but according to the causal disorder, certain mechanisms predominate.

Vasogenic Macular Edema

Retinal Vein Occlusion

Retinal vein occlusion leads to an increased intravascular pressure, blood-retinal barrier breakdown, and vascular leakage (Fig. 7a). Inner retinal hypoxia is associated with increased VEGF levels through HIF-1α, nitric oxide, and

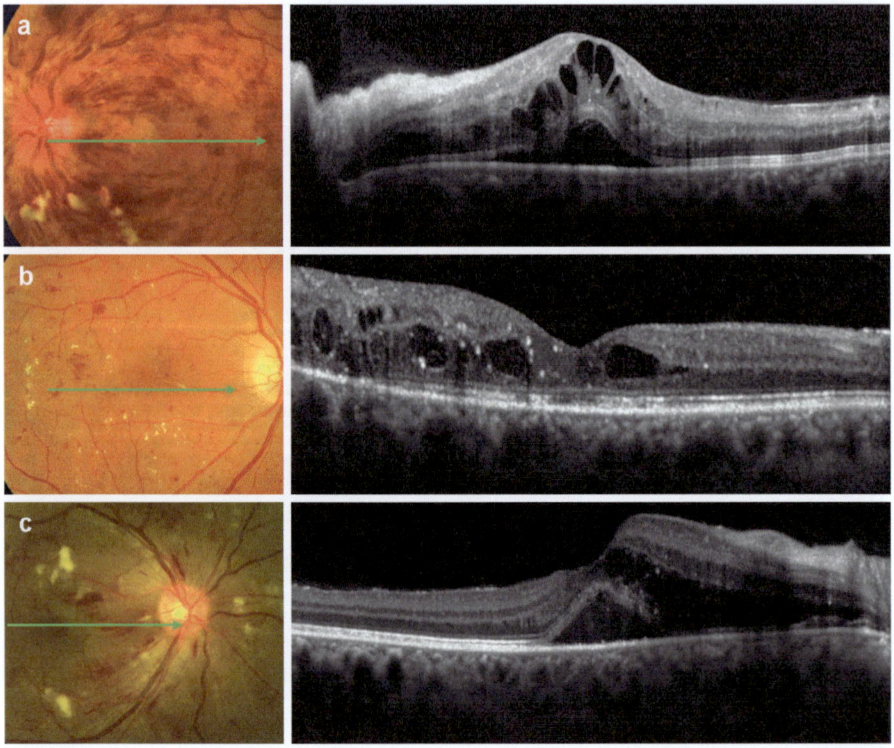

Fig. 7 Various causes of vasogenic macular edema imaged by color fundus photography and OCT. (**a**) Central retinal vein occlusion, characterized by flame-shaped hemorrhages, venous tortuosity, and few cotton-wool spots. Macular edema manifests by the intraretinal and subretinal accumulation of fluid. (**b**) Diabetic retinopathy and diabetic macular edema, displaying numerous dot-blot hemorrhages and lipid exudates. Optical coherence tomography shows diffuse cystoid macular edema and focal hyperreflective dots corresponding to the exudates. (**c**) Hypertensive retinopathy characterized by peripapillary distribution of cotton-wool spots, hemorrhages, and macular edema with subretinal fluid seen on optical coherence tomography

pro-inflammatory cytokines that contribute to the inner blood-retinal barrier rupture [25]. Hypertension, frequently associated with retinal vein occlusion, aggravates ME by further increasing the intracapillary hydrostatic pressure in the Starling equation. In addition, secondary hypoxic alterations of RMG cells may also lead to cytotoxic edema [26]. In cases of retinal vein occlusion with associated ischemia, excitotoxicity due to glutamate excess induces intracellular neuronal edema secondary to cellular energy failure [27]. Subretinal fluid is present in about half of central retinal vein occlusions and indicates that outer retinal barrier breakdown contributes to ME formation [28]. Indeed VEGF release also acts on the RPE barrier function through the VEGF receptor 1 (Flt-1), whose expression is under HIF-1α regulation [29].

Diabetic Macular Edema (DME)

The pathogenesis of DME is complex and multifactorial. Before any microangiopathy is clinically observed, intraretinal local inflammation (i.e., neuroinflammation) causes neuronal damage [30, 31]. Specifically, activation of microglial cells contributes to the local release of nitric oxide, TNF-α, interleukins, and VEGF [32]. In physiologic conditions, microglia trafficking contributes to retinal homeostasis. Active clearance of microglial cells through RPE transcytosis was demonstrated in the rodent retina, which prevents subretinal accumulation of activated cells. With aging, this active clearance increases in order to compensate for enhanced microglial activation to age-related debris, while it decreases in case of diabetic retinopathy as a consequence of alteration of cytoskeleton plasticity [32, 33]. Accumulation of microglia in the diabetic retina was also demonstrated to occur in humans [34, 35].

Besides microglia, RPE and RMG cells submitted to chronic hyperglycemia, as well as metabolic and oxidative stress, also release inflammatory mediators such as VEGF through the activating transcription factor 4 (ATF4), IL-6, IL-8, TNF-α, MCP-1, chemokines, thrombospondin-1, and many other soluble factors [31, 36].

Microangiopathy results from several mechanisms: neurodegeneration [37], activation of the polyol pathway, nonenzymatic glycation of proteins, glucose autooxidation and oxidative stress, hyperglycemic pseudohypoxia, activation of protein kinase C by de novo synthesis of diacyl glycerol, and others [38, 39]. These hyperglycemia-induced alterations of metabolic pathways affect endothelial cells and pericytes, leading to reduced pericyte coverage of retinal capillaries and microvascular degeneration [40–44]. Leukostasis, due to reduced deformability of leukocytes in diabetic patients; a reduced capillary lumen, due to basal membrane thickening and endothelial cell alterations; leukocyte activation by stromal cell-derived factor 1 (SDF-1); and increased adhesion all contribute to capillary occlusion [45]. Such vascular occlusion leads to increased levels of VEGF and other vascular permeability-inducing cytokines that contribute to vasogenic ME. Other vascular abnormalization processes such as the formation of microaneurysms contribute to focally enhanced fluid leakage and edema. The exact mechanisms leading to microaneurysms formation are not fully understood and involve VEGF, PGF [46], and pericyte alterations [47]. Activation of the renin-angiotensin system also contributes to the microvascular abnormalities in diabetic retinopathy, via the stimulation of growth factors such as VEGF, which induces vascular leakage, pericyte migration, angiogenesis, and fibrosis [48, 49]. The plasma kallikrein-kinin system (KKS) has also been related to diabetic ME. In advanced stages of diabetic retinopathy, the vitreous concentration of plasma kallikrein is increased. The intraocular activation of KKS induces retinal vascular permeability and ME, and it has been shown to be exacerbated in diabetic rats [50–52].

Compromised capillaries and leaky microaneurysms are the major vasogenic components in DME. But early alterations of the outer retinal barrier and the RMG drainage functions also contribute to DME [53–55].

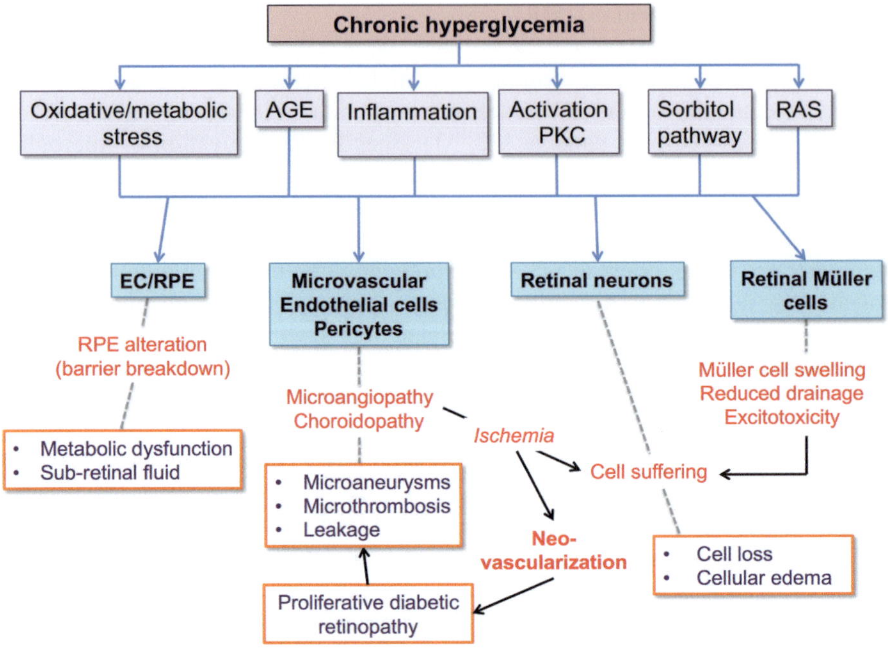

Fig. 8 Consequences of chronic hyperglycemia on the retina

Alteration of neuronal metabolism, glial cell death, and secondary ischemic cell suffering are also key players to DME through cytotoxic mechanisms. The role of insulin in DME remains disputed. Indeed, clinical trials and other studies have determined that initiation of acute intensive insulin therapy in patients with long-standing poor glycemic control results in a worsening of diabetic retinopathy [56]. A change in treatment from oral drugs to insulin in patients with non-insulin-dependent diabetes mellitus type 2 was associated with a significantly increased risk of retinopathy progression and visual impairment [57].

In summary, DME results from a combination of factors, whose contribution depends on the type of diabetes, the patient age, and their interaction with other systemic factors such as hypertension, vascular endothelial dysfunction, and lipid metabolism deregulation (Figs. 7b, 8, and 9).

Hypertensive Retinopathy

Acute arterial hypertension may provoke hypertensive retinopathy, hypertensive choroidopathy, and hypertensive optic neuropathy. Hypertensive retinopathy results from retinal capillary and precapillary occlusions, with a subsequent rupture of the inner blood-retinal barrier producing intraretinal edema. Hypertensive choroidopathy is characterized by focal areas of choriocapillaris occlusion resulting in RPE damage and rupture of the outer blood-retinal barrier leading to subretinal fluid accumulation and retinal edema (Fig. 7c) [58].

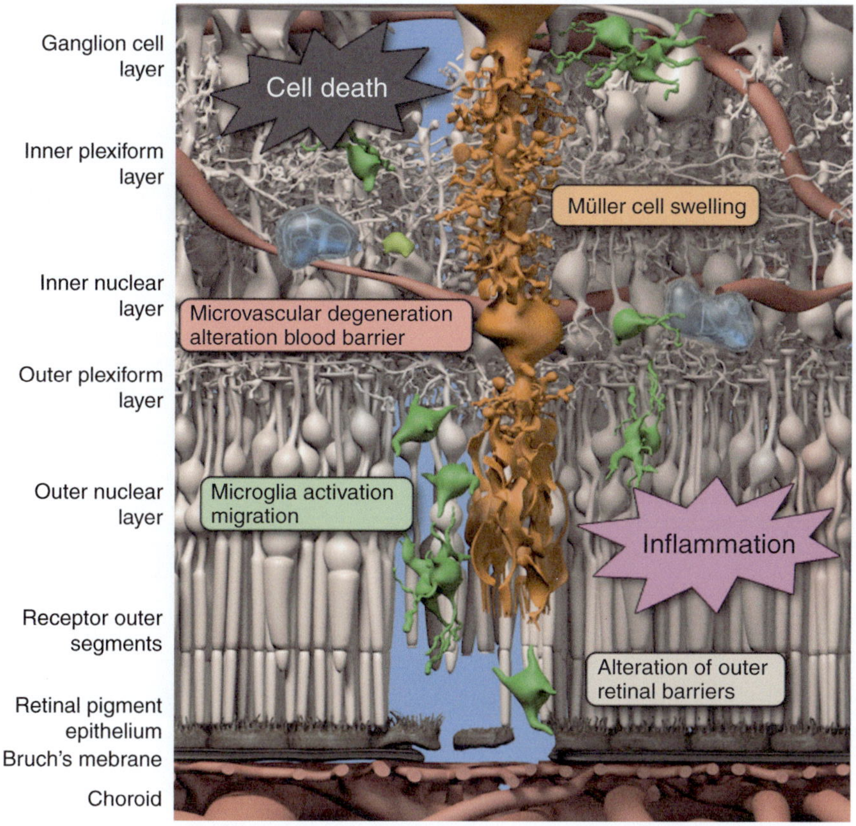

Fig. 9 The events leading to diabetic macular edema

Inflammatory Macular Edema

In the acute phases of an intraocular inflammatory process, ME is frequently not detected clinically. However, the rupture of the ocular barriers is obvious (as evidenced by the presence of aqueous or vitreous cells), supporting the idea that retinal barrier breakdown may not be sufficient to cause ME.

On the other hand, ME is a frequent manifestation in chronic uveitis (Fig. 10b) and results from enhanced fluid entry through compromised inner and outer retinal blood barriers and from diminished fluid exit secondary to inflammatory alterations of RPE and RMG cells. Vasopermeability-inducing cytokines such as VEGF, IL-1β, IL-6, IL-8, TNF-α, and nitric oxide are produced at high levels by ocular resident cells, immune cells, and infiltrating cells and contribute to vasogenic ME [59, 60].

Similarly, the delayed accumulation of fluid in the macula observed in postoperative cystoid ME (Irvine-Gass syndrome, Fig. 10c) is related to blood-aqueous barrier breakdown mechanisms [61, 62].

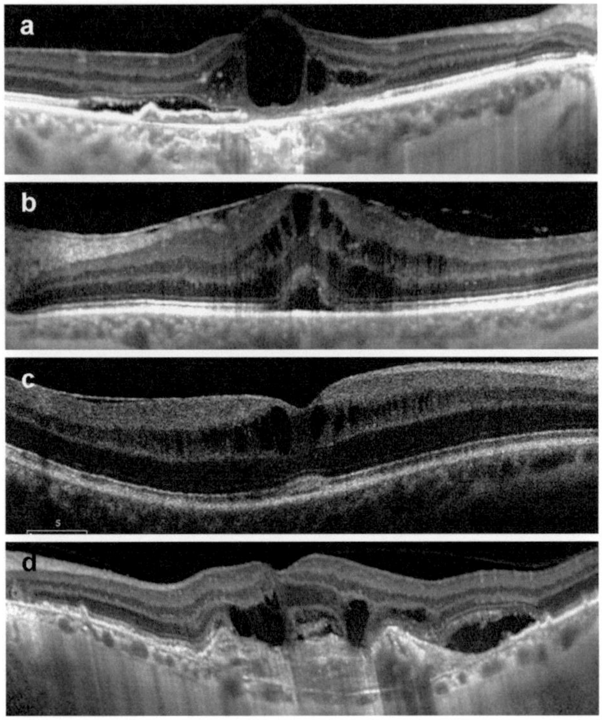

Fig. 10 Various causes of vasogenic macular edema seen on OCT. (**a**) Chronic central serous chorioretinopathy. (**b**) Extramacular toxoplasmic retinochoroiditis, with macular edema developing 4 months after onset of inflammation. Note the secondary epiretinal membrane that may aggravate the macular edema. (**c**) Irvine-Gass syndrome occurring 1 month after cataract surgery. (**d**) Active neovascular age-related macular degeneration with an advanced subretinal fibrotic complex

Macular Edema and Choroidal Neovascularization

Choroidal neovascularization, either idiopathic or secondary to AMD (Fig. 10d), pathologic myopia, or inflammation, induces the accumulation of subretinal and intraretinal fluid as a result of the enhanced permeability of the neovascular component itself and the secondary blood-retinal barrier breakdown. VEGF is not significantly elevated in the ocular media of patients with wet AMD as compared to control, but the efficacy of anti-VEGF drugs in choroidal neovascularization-induced ME gives evidence that VEGF is a major pathogenic player [63–65].

Cytotoxic Macular Edema

Pure cytotoxic ME is very rarely observed, and cytotoxic mechanisms are rather intricate and secondary to ME itself.

Chemotherapy-Induced Macular Edema

The best example of pure cytotoxic ME is caused by anti-microtubular agents, such us docetaxel and paclitaxel, used in the treatment of breast and ovarian cancers. Anti-microtubular agents have been reported to cause bilateral cystoid macular

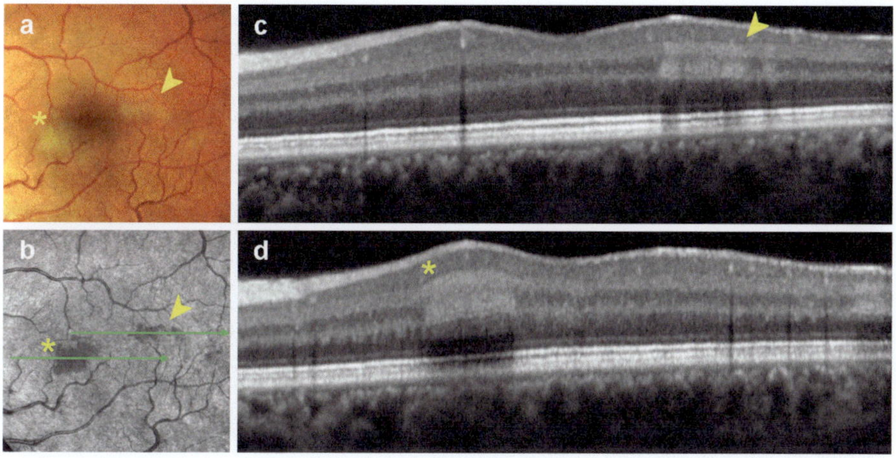

Fig. 11 An example of cytotoxic macular edema. Paracentral acute middle maculopathy with two ischemic lesions affecting mostly the inner nuclear and inner plexiform layers (*star and arrow*). The ischemic edema appears as focal whitish lesions on fundus examination (**a**), as hyporeflective lesions on near-infrared reflectance (**b**), and as focal hyperreflectivities on optical OCT (**c**, **d**)

edema without evidence of leakage in fluorescein angiography [66]. The targeting of cell microtubules alters molecular motors and subsequent membrane channel distribution, causing a dysfunction in drainage mechanisms and subsequent ME.

Retinal/Choroidal Ischemia and Macular Edema

Retinal arterial occlusions cause acute inner retinal edema secondary to intracellular swelling of neuronal and glial retinal cells, which manifests as an increased reflectivity on OCT, a well-known feature of central or branch retinal artery occlusions. In addition, localized retinal capillary ischemia also results in intracellular edema as recently described in paracentral acute middle maculopathy (Fig. 11) where no vascular angiographic leakage is present [67, 68]. Combined mechanisms may occur, as illustrated by the observation of paracentral acute middle maculopathy findings during the course of central retinal vein occlusions [69]. However, these alterations were not observed in areas of cystoid ME. In the majority of cystoid ME cases, the real contribution of pure cytotoxic ischemic mechanisms is difficult to evidence and has not been clearly demonstrated.

Conclusion

Mechanisms leading to ME are usually intricate and difficult to discriminate in the various clinical presentations of ME. The recent multimodal combination of fluorescein, indocyanine green angiography, and spectral-domain optical coherence tomography (SD-OCT) helps to better understand the exact alterations of retinal structures that cause fluid accumulation within or under the retina. It also contributes to guide more appropriate and targeted treatments. However, most of the molecular mechanisms described in this chapter result from experimental models in rodents that do not have a macula. Since in humans edema forms mostly, if not exclusively, in the macula, the extrapolation of such mechanisms remains approximate and hazardous. Basic research and human pathology is still required to identify molecular targets specific to the macula that could be regulated by pharmacological agents.

References

1. Hosoya K, Tachikawa M. The inner blood-retinal barrier: molecular structure and transport biology. Adv Exp Med Biol. 2012;763:85–104.
2. Rizzolo LJ, Peng S, Luo Y, Xiao W. Integration of tight junctions and claudins with the barrier functions of the retinal pigment epithelium. Prog Retin Eye Res. 2011;30:296–323.
3. Reichhart N, Strauss O. Ion channels and transporters of the retinal pigment epithelium. Exp Eye Res. 2014;126:27–37.
4. Bringmann A, Pannicke T, Grosche J, et al. Müller cells in the healthy and diseased retina. Prog Retin Eye Res. 2006;25:397–424.
5. Verkman AS, Ruiz-Ederra J, Levin MH. Functions of aquaporins in the eye. Prog Retin Eye Res. 2008;27:420–33.
6. Bringmann A, Reichenbach A, Wiedemann P. Pathomechanisms of cystoid macular edema. Ophthalmic Res. 2004;36:241–9.
7. Matet A, Savastano MC, Rispoli M, et al. En face optical coherence tomography of foveal microstructure in full-thickness macular hole: a model to study perifoveal Müller cells. Am J Ophthalmol. 2015;159(6):1142–1151.e3.
8. De Bock M, Wang N, Decrock E, et al. Endothelial calcium dynamics, connexin channels and blood-brain barrier function. Prog Neurobiol. 2013;108:1–20.
9. Alexander JS, Elrod JW. Extracellular matrix, junctional integrity and matrix metalloproteinase interactions in endothelial permeability regulation. J Anat. 2002;200:561–74.
10. Schoknecht K, David Y, Heinemann U. The blood-brain barrier-gatekeeper to neuronal homeostasis: clinical implications in the setting of stroke. Semin Cell Dev Biol. 2015;38:35–42.
11. García-Ponce A, Citalán-Madrid AF, Velázquez-Avila M, et al. The role of actin-binding proteins in the control of endothelial barrier integrity. Thromb Haemost. 2015;113:20–36.
12. Coorey NJ, Shen W, Chung SH, et al. The role of glia in retinal vascular disease. Clin Exp Optom J Aust Optom Assoc. 2012;95:266–81.
13. Wimmers S, Karl MO, Strauss O. Ion channels in the RPE. Prog Retin Eye Res. 2007;26:263–301.
14. Bialek S, Miller SS. K+ and Cl- transport mechanisms in bovine pigment epithelium that could modulate subretinal space volume and composition. J Physiol. 1994;475:401–17.
15. Tsuboi S, Pederson JE. Effect of plasma osmolality and intraocular pressure on fluid movement across the blood-retinal barrier. Invest Ophthalmol Vis Sci. 1988;29:1747–9.
16. Tsuboi S, Pederson JE. Volume flow across the isolated retinal pigment epithelium of cynomolgus monkey eyes. Invest Ophthalmol Vis Sci. 1988;29:1652–5.
17. Rosenthal R, Heimann H, Agostini H, et al. Ca2+ channels in retinal pigment epithelial cells regulate vascular endothelial growth factor secretion rates in health and disease. Mol Vis. 2007;13:443–56.
18. Hollborn M, Dukic-Stefanovic S, Pannicke T, et al. Expression of aquaporins in the retina of diabetic rats. Curr Eye Res. 2011;36:850–6.

19. Wang M, Wong WT. Microglia-Müller cell interactions in the retina. Adv Exp Med Biol. 2014;801:333–8.
20. Reichenbach A, Wurm A, Pannicke T, et al. Müller cells as players in retinal degeneration and edema. Graefes Arch Clin Exp Ophthalmol Albrecht Von Graefes Arch Für Klin Exp Ophthalmol. 2007;245:627–36.
21. Bringmann A, Kohen L, Wolf S, et al. Age-related decrease of potassium currents in glial (müller) cells of the human retina. Can J Ophthalmol J Can Ophthalmol. 2003;38:464–8.
22. Schubert HD. Cystoid macular edema: the apparent role of mechanical factors. Prog Clin Biol Res. 1989;312:277–91.
23. Simpson ARH, Petrarca R, Jackson TL. Vitreomacular adhesion and neovascular age-related macular degeneration. Surv Ophthalmol. 2012;57:498–509.
24. Steel DHW, Lotery AJ. Idiopathic vitreomacular traction and macular hole: a comprehensive review of pathophysiology, diagnosis, and treatment. Eye Lond Engl. 2013;27 Suppl 1:S1–21.
25. Kaur C, Foulds WS, Ling EA. Blood-retinal barrier in hypoxic ischaemic conditions: basic concepts, clinical features and management. Prog Retin Eye Res. 2008;27:622–47.
26. Jaulim A, Ahmed B, Khanam T, Chatziralli IP. Branch retinal vein occlusion: epidemiology, pathogenesis, risk factors, clinical features, diagnosis, and complications. An update of the literature. Retina Phila Pa. 2013;33:901–10.
27. Chen J, Chiang C-W, Zhang H, Song S-K. Cell swelling contributes to thickening of low-dose N-methyl-D-aspartate-induced retinal edema. Invest Ophthalmol Vis Sci. 2012;53:2777–85.
28. Catier A, Tadayoni R, Paques M, et al. Characterization of macular edema from various etiologies by optical coherence tomography. Am J Ophthalmol. 2005;140:200–6.
29. Miyamoto N, de Kozak Y, Normand N, et al. PlGF-1 and VEGFR-1 pathway regulation of the external epithelial hemato-ocular barrier. A model for retinal edema. Ophthalmic Res. 2008;40:203–7.
30. Scholl S, Augustin A, Loewenstein A, et al. General pathophysiology of macular edema. Eur J Ophthalmol. 2011;21 Suppl 6:S10–9.
31. Abcouwer SF. Angiogenic factors and cytokines in diabetic retinopathy. J Clin Cell Immunol. 2013;11 (Suppl 1):1–12.
32. Karlstetter M, Scholz R, Rutar M, et al. Retinal microglia: just bystander or target for therapy? Prog Retin Eye Res. 2015;45C:30–57.
33. Grigsby JG, Cardona SM, Pouw CE, et al. The role of microglia in diabetic retinopathy. J Ophthalmol. 2014;2014:705783.
34. Omri S, Behar-Cohen F, de Kozak Y, et al. Microglia/macrophages migrate through retinal epithelium barrier by a transcellular route in diabetic retinopathy: role of PKCζ in the Goto Kakizaki rat model. Am J Pathol. 2011;179:942–53.
35. Kaur C, Rathnasamy G, Ling E-A. Roles of activated microglia in hypoxia induced neuroinflammation in the developing brain and the retina. J Neuroimmune Pharmacol Off J Soc Neuro Immune Pharmacol. 2013;8:66–78.
36. Wang L-L, Chen H, Huang K, Zheng L. Elevated histone acetylations in Müller cells contribute to inflammation: a novel inhibitory effect of minocycline. Glia. 2012;60:1896–905.
37. Simó R, Hernández C, European Consortium for the Early Treatment of Diabetic Retinopathy (EUROCONDOR). Neurodegeneration in the diabetic eye: new insights and therapeutic perspectives. Trends Endocrinol Metab TEM. 2014;25:23–33.
38. Pfeiffer A, Schatz H. Diabetic microvascular complications and growth factors. Exp Clin Endocrinol Diabetes Off J Ger Soc Endocrinol Ger Diabetes Assoc. 1995;103:7–14.
39. Milne R, Brownstein S. Advanced glycation end products and diabetic retinopathy. Amino Acids. 2013;44:1397–407.
40. Lutty GA. Effects of diabetes on the eye. Invest Ophthalmol Vis Sci. 2013;54:ORSF81–7.
41. Ejaz S, Chekarova I, Ejaz A, et al. Importance of pericytes and mechanisms of pericyte loss during diabetes retinopathy. Diabetes Obes Metab. 2008;10:53–63.
42. Durham JT, Herman IM. Microvascular modifications in diabetic retinopathy. Curr Diab Rep. 2011;11:253–64.

43. Bharadwaj AS, Appukuttan B, Wilmarth PA, et al. Role of the retinal vascular endothelial cell in ocular disease. Prog Retin Eye Res. 2013;32:102–80.
44. Arboleda-Velasquez JF, Valdez CN, Marko CK, D'Amore PA. From pathobiology to the targeting of pericytes for the treatment of diabetic retinopathy. Curr Diab Rep. 2015;15:573.
45. Chibber R, Ben-Mahmud BM, Chibber S, Kohner EM. Leukocytes in diabetic retinopathy. Curr Diabetes Rev. 2007;3:3–14.
46. Kowalczuk L, Touchard E, Omri S, et al. Placental growth factor contributes to micro-vascular abnormalization and blood-retinal barrier breakdown in diabetic retinopathy. PLoS One. 2011;6:e17462.
47. Beltramo E, Porta M. Pericyte loss in diabetic retinopathy: mechanisms and consequences. Curr Med Chem. 2013;20:3218–25.
48. Wilkinson-Berka JL. Diabetes and retinal vascular disorders: role of the renin-angiotensin system. Expert Rev Mol Med. 2004;6:1–18.
49. Clermont A, Bursell S-E, Feener EP. Role of the angiotensin II type 1 receptor in the pathogenesis of diabetic retinopathy: effects of blood pressure control and beyond. J Hypertens Suppl Off J Int Soc Hypertens. 2006;24:S73–80.
50. Feener EP. Plasma kallikrein and diabetic macular edema. Curr Diab Rep. 2010;10:270–5.
51. Liu J, Feener EP. Plasma kallikrein-kinin system and diabetic retinopathy. Biol Chem. 2013;394:319–28.
52. Wilkinson-Berka JL, Fletcher EL. Angiotensin and bradykinin: targets for the treatment of vascular and neuro-glial pathology in diabetic retinopathy. Curr Pharm Des. 2004;10:3313–30.
53. Iandiev I, Pannicke T, Reichenbach A, et al. Diabetes alters the localization of glial aquaporins in rat retina. Neurosci Lett. 2007;421:132–6.
54. Omri S, Behar-Cohen F, Rothschild P-R, et al. PKCζ mediates breakdown of outer blood-retinal barriers in diabetic retinopathy. PLoS One. 2013;8:e81600.
55. Krügel K, Wurm A, Pannicke T, et al. Involvement of oxidative stress and mitochondrial dysfunction in the osmotic swelling of retinal glial cells from diabetic rats. Exp Eye Res. 2011;92:87–93.
56. Anon. Diabetic retinopathy after two years of intensified insulin treatment. Follow-up of the Kroc Collaborative Study. The Kroc Collaborative Study Group. JAMA. 1988;260:37–41.
57. Henricsson M, Janzon L, Groop L. Progression of retinopathy after change of treatment from oral antihyperglycemic agents to insulin in patients with NIDDM. Diabetes Care. 1995;18:1571–6.
58. Verougstraete C. Macular edema in arterial hypertension. Bull Société Belge Ophtalmol. 1991;240:23–33.
59. Klaassen I, Van Noorden CJF, Schlingemann RO. Molecular basis of the inner blood-retinal barrier and its breakdown in diabetic macular edema and other pathological conditions. Prog Retin Eye Res. 2013;34:19–48.
60. Bonfioli AA, Damico FM, Curi ALL, Orefice F. Intermediate uveitis. Semin Ophthalmol. 2005;20:147–54.
61. Ersoy L, Caramoy A, Ristau T, et al. Aqueous flare is increased in patients with clinically significant cystoid macular oedema after cataract surgery. Br J Ophthalmol. 2013;97:862–5.
62. Pande MV, Spalton DJ, Kerr-Muir MG, Marshall J. Postoperative inflammatory response to phacoemulsification and extracapsular cataract surgery: aqueous flare and cells. J Cataract Refract Surg. 1996;22 Suppl 1:770–4.
63. Solomon SD, Lindsley K, Vedula SS, et al. Anti-vascular endothelial growth factor for neovascular age-related macular degeneration. Cochrane Database Syst Rev. 2014;(8): CD005139.
64. Vedula SS, Krzystolik MG. Antiangiogenic therapy with anti-vascular endothelial growth factor modalities for neovascular age-related macular degeneration. Cochrane Database Syst Rev. 2008;(2):CD005139.
65. Wang E, Chen Y. Intravitreal anti-vascular endothelial growth factor for choroidal neovascularization secondary to pathologic myopia: systematic review and meta-analysis. Retina Phila Pa. 2013;33:1375–92.

66. Liu CY, Francis JH, Brodie SE, et al. Retinal toxicities of cancer therapy drugs: biologics, small molecule inhibitors, and chemotherapies. Retina Phila Pa. 2014;34:1261–80.
67. Yu S, Pang CE, Gong Y, et al. The spectrum of superficial and deep capillary ischemia in retinal artery occlusion. Am J Ophthalmol. 2015;159:53–63. e1–2.
68. Sarraf D, Rahimy E, Fawzi AA, et al. Paracentral acute middle maculopathy: a new variant of acute macular neuroretinopathy associated with retinal capillary ischemia. JAMA Ophthalmol. 2013;131:1275–87.
69. Rahimy E, Sarraf D, Dollin ML, et al. Paracentral acute middle maculopathy in nonischemic central retinal vein occlusion. Am J Ophthalmol. 2014;158:372–380.e1.

Chapter 3
Diagnosis of Cystoid Macular Edema: Imaging

Dilraj S. Grewal and Glenn J. Jaffe

Introduction

Early detection of cystoid macula edema (CME) is critical for diagnosis and management. Traditional methods of accessing macular edema include contact and noncontact slit lamp biomicroscopy, indirect ophthalmoscopy, fluorescein angiography (FA), and fundus stereo photography. However the interpretation of their results can be subjective, and subtle changes in retinal thickness in early CME may not be evident.

Optical coherence tomography (OCT) correlates well with retinal histology [1] and can be used to quantitatively and qualitatively monitor retinal thickness over time. Compared to biomicroscopy and FA, OCT is more sensitive in detection of macular edema and subretinal fluid, and subclinical macular edema is often only detected by OCT. In general, CME is visualized on OCT scans as multiple circular cystic spaces in the retina, indicating intraretinal edema. The cystic spaces are round or oval and originate around the outer plexiform layer (OPL) but can progress to involve the photoreceptor layer and the inner retinal layers. Occasionally, cystic retinal edema can enlarge and have the appearance of a foveal pseudocyst. OCT is highly effective to visualize CME because the cystoid fluid has less optical scattering than the surrounding retinal tissues.

Advancements in imaging technologies and resolution have improved our understanding of CME due to different pathologies and their differentiating characteristics. In this chapter, we discuss the imaging methods to diagnose CME of different etiologies.

D.S. Grewal, MD • G.J. Jaffe, MD (✉)
Duke Eye Center, Box 3802, Durham, NC 27705, USA
e-mail: Jaffe001@MC.duke.edu

S. Schaal, H.J. Kaplan (eds.), *Cystoid Macular Edema*,
DOI 10.1007/978-3-319-39766-5_3

CME Associated with Diabetes: Diabetic Macular Edema

Diabetic macular edema (DME) results from pathologic leakage from damaged retinal microvasculature and insufficient clearance of plasma by Müller and retinal pigment epithelial (RPE) cells. Vascular leakage and intraretinal fluid (IRF) accumulation can be imaged clinically using FA in eyes with DME. The classification of DME has evolved considerably since the Early Treatment Diabetic Retinopathy Study (ETDRS) characterization as focal or diffuse based on clinical examination and FA findings [2, 3].

OCT permits analysis of outer retinal layer integrity in DME, which is linked to the visual prognosis [4–10]. For example, disruption of the hyperreflective ellipsoid layer indicates macular photoreceptor damage and is associated with decreased visual acuity. Intraretinal fluid, increased retinal thickness, macular ischemia, and foveal exudates also contribute to the poor prognosis in DME [11]. Based on a 10 % test-retest variability of OCT retinal thickness measurements in diabetics, >10 % thickness change is often considered clinically relevant in DME [12]. Different patterns of fluid accumulation have now been described. Otani described three patterns of structural changes in DME: diffuse retinal thickening (DRT), CME, and serous retinal detachment (SRD) [13]. They reported that DRT (focal or diffuse edema) first appeared as a reduction in the tissue reflectivity and increased retinal thickness, followed by a "spongy" appearance of the retina. CME was defined as the accumulation of IRF in well-defined spaces. SRD was usually due to chronic edema and was characterized by coalescence of cystic cavities and sensory retinal elevation. Kim et al. similarly described five different morphologic patterns on OCT [14]: DRT, CME, SRD, posterior hyaloid traction (PHT) without macular tractional retinal detachment (TRD), and PHT with TRD. DRT was defined as increased retinal thickness with areas of reduced intraretinal reflectivity (Fig. 1). CME was characterized by intraretinal cystoid-like cavities defined as large ovoid hyporeflective areas

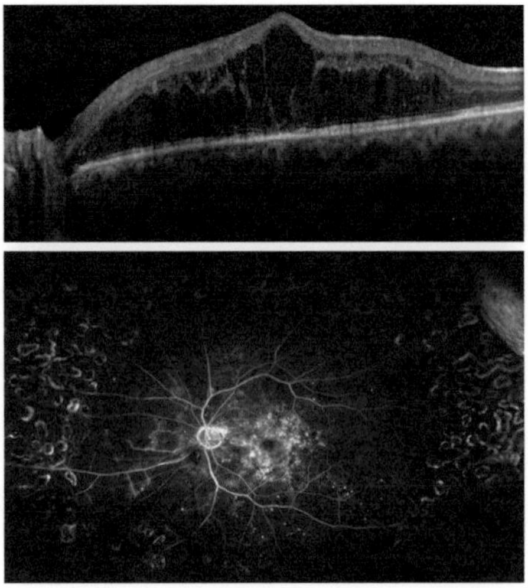

Fig. 1 Diffuse retinal thickening pattern of diabetic macular edema (DME) with increased retinal thickness and a "spongy" appearance of the retina. There is a reduction in the reflectivity of the outer retinal layers due to the overlying cystic spaces and intraretinal fluid (*top*). Fluorescein angiography (*bottom*) demonstrates generalized leakage prominent on late frames without a discretely identifiable source

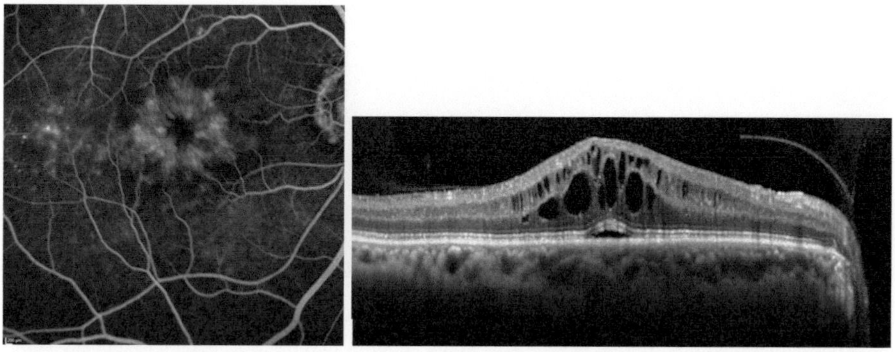

Fig. 2 Cystoid macular edema (CME) pattern of DME: Retinal thickening and hyporeflective cystic spaces in the inner retina separated by hyporeflective septae with subfoveal subretinal fluid (*right*). Fluorescein angiogram (*left*) shows paravoeal petaloid leakage corresponding to the CME and leakage temporally due to microaneurysms

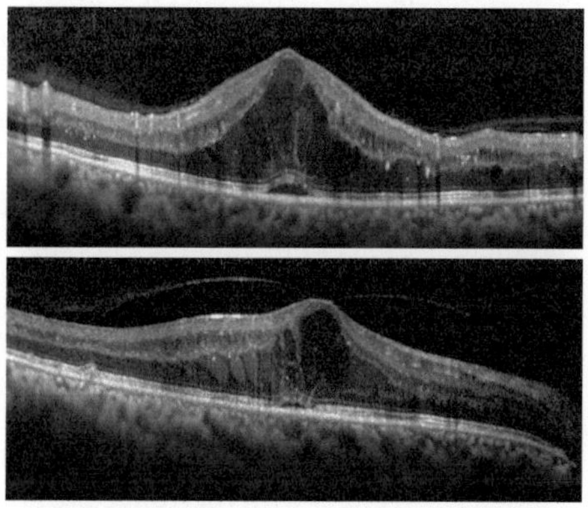

Fig. 3 DME with posterior hyaloid traction (PHT) without tractional retinal detachment. *Top figure* shows diffuse DME with large intraretinal cystic spaces and intraretinal fluid and an adherent posterior hyaloid. Following anti-vascular endothelial growth factor (VEGF) therapy, there is an improvement in intraretinal and subretinal fluid but a persistent foveal intraretinal cyst and posterior hyaloidal traction on the fovea (*bottom figure*)

separated by hyperreflective septae (Fig. 2). PHT was defined as a highly reflective band over the retinal surface and SRD appeared as a dark accumulation of subretinal fluid beneath the highly reflective and dome-like elevation of detached retina. They used the highly reflective band representing the outer surface of the detached retina to differentiate SRF from IRF (Fig. 3). TRD was identified as the area of low signal underlying the highly reflective border of the detached retina, often in a peaked configuration (Fig. 4). These TRDs may often be subclinical and visualized only on OCT [15].

In addition to these descriptive classifications, various intraretinal microstructural anatomical characteristics have been described in eyes with DME. These include hyperreflective foci (HRF), a morphologic sign of accumulation of IRF and lipid extravasation, suggested to be precursors of hard exudates before they become clinically visible [11, 16, 17]. Outer retinal HRF have been associated with disrupted ELM or ellipsoid layer and decreased VA, suggesting photoreceptor degeneration in DME. Pemp et al. [18] showed that DME reduction during anti-VEGF

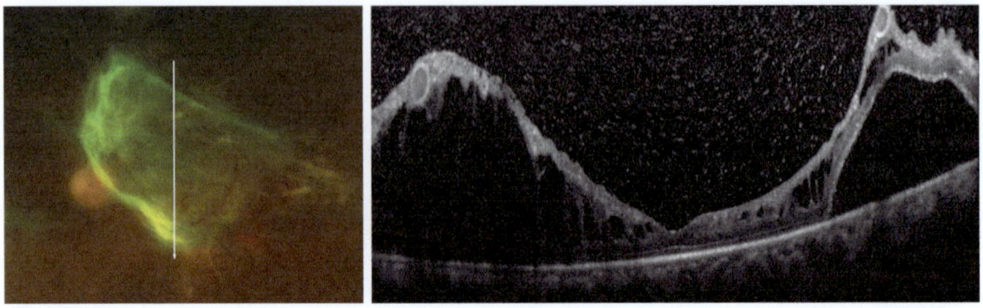

Fig. 4 DME with a tractional retinal detachment: Intraretinal cystic spaces superior and inferior to fovea with a tractional retinal detachment in the superior and inferior macula in a peaked configuration visualized on vertical OCT scan. Hyperreflective opacities in the vitreous represent a mild vitreous hemorrhage

therapy was accompanied by dynamic rearrangement of these intraretinal exudates. Type 1 diabetes patients have fewer HRF than with type 2 diabetes [19]. Gelman et al. [20] reported hyperreflective dots in a contiguous ring around the inner wall of cystoid spaces in the OPL, a pattern that they referred to as the "pearl necklace sign." This configuration was found adjacent to hard exudates in the OPL, and the hyperreflective material was speculated to be composed of lipoproteins or lipid-laden macrophages.

Microaneurysms (MAs) in DME have also been evaluated on OCT. The OCT parameters of leaking microaneurysms include outer and inner diameter of the microaneurysm and wall thickness [21, 22]. Hyperreflective spots on OCT in microaneurysm lumens have been suggested to be cellular components such as erythrocytes, leukocytes, and lipid deposits [22]. Lee et al. characterized microaneurysm closure following focal laser photocoagulation in DME using simultaneous FA and OCT [23]. Microaneurysm closure following focal laser photocoagulation was characterized either by hyperreflective spots or complete disappearance without any hyporeflectivity. Smaller microaneurysms with a heterogeneous lumen were more likely to close [23].

It is of critical importance to identify anatomical biomarkers of DME that predict visual outcome and guide the choice of candidate drugs for interventional trials. However, a reliable anatomical biomarker of VA in patients with DME has yet to be firmly established. OCT retinal thickness measurements, although an important clinical and anatomic evaluation tool, are not an ideal surrogate for VA as a primary outcome in DME studies. Although OCT-derived central retinal thickness is commonly utilized in DME evaluation and management, central foveal thickness (CFT) explains no more than 27 % of the variation in VA [24]. There have been attempts to identify various OCT-based biomarkers that better correlate anatomic microstructure with function and predict visual recovery in eyes with DME. These microstructures include the external limiting membrane (ELM), integrity of the ellipsoid layer (formerly described as the inner segment/outer segment photoreceptor junction) [6, 8, 25], thickness of the photoreceptor outer segments, status of the cone outer segment tips (COST) [7], presence of hyperreflective foci [11, 17, 26], and subretinal fluid (SRF) [27].

Horri et al. [28] showed that after triamcinolone acetonide treatment for DME, reduced reflectivity in foveal cystoid spaces was associated with a rebound in macular thickening and visual deterioration. Cystic macular changes have been associated with photoreceptor layer damage to a greater extent than diffuse edema and serous retinal detachment. ELM breakdown has been shown to lead to subfoveal SRF [16]. Foveal photoreceptor layer status has been closely related to visual acuity in patients with DME [9, 29]. However, the influence of the foveal avascular zone size on the photoreceptor layer integrity is yet to be clearly defined. Some of the changes evaluated on OCT persist even following DME treatment. Despite treatment and resolution of DME and restoration of macular thickness, the ganglion cell inner plexiform layer thickness in eyes with resolved DME is thinner than that in eyes without DME. This difference correlates with decreased visual acuity, suggesting that inner retinal alterations in DME may lead to visual deficiency that persists after treatment [30]. Lee et al. demonstrated that ischemia in eyes with DME caused photoreceptor outer segment shortening and ellipsoid layer disruption, resulting in outer retinal layer atrophic changes and subsequent visual loss [31]. Soliman et al. [32] found that cystoid spaces, especially in the INL, were associated with worse VA outcome after macular grid laser photocoagulation for DME. Areas beneath the OPL cystoid spaces have been shown to have longer spans of disrupted ellipsoid layer and ELM [29]. There is general consensus that a correlation exists between retinal thickness and visual acuity (VA) in patients with DME [14]. The OCT pattern that was found to be associated with worse VA was "CME"; eyes with CME had a 0.40 reduction in logMAR acuity compared with eyes that had DME without this pattern [14].

Retinal inner layer disorganization within the central 1 millimeter (mm) foveal area predict worse VA in eyes with center-involved DME [33, 34]. This anatomic feature had a higher correlation with VA than central retinal thickness, large intraretinal cysts, or current glycemic status. Disorganization of the retinal inner layers could identify eyes with a high likelihood of subsequent VA improvement or decline; disorganization of the retinal inner layers affecting 50 % or more of the central 1-mm-wide zone centered on the fovea had worse VA [33]. It has been proposed that this anatomic change represents disorganization or destruction of cells within the inner retinal layers, including bipolar, amacrine, or horizontal cells, and possibly indicates a disruption of pathways that transmit visual information from the photoreceptors to the ganglion cells. Histologic assessment of these changes would help confirm this hypothesis. If true, early-stage retinal inner layer disorganization could be used as a prognostic visual acuity marker in untreated eyes with DME.

Over recent years, in addition to improved resolution, the application of image processing to OCT image interpretation has mostly focused on the development of automated retinal layer segmentation methods [35, 36]. There have been several challenges in this effort. OCT images are often corrupted by speckle noise and need to undergo noise reduction to reduce its effect on the classification results. Speckle occurs in OCT due to the random interference of waves reflected from subresolution variances within the object. Maintaining edge-like features in the image after speckle denoising is particularly important for segmentation. It is easier to segment the retinal layers in early stages before the appearance of severe pathology [35, 37].

CME comprises a contiguous fluid-filled space containing columns of tissue; these spaces may falsely appear as separated cysts when viewed by OCT. It has been therefore suggested that retinal volume may be a better predictor of VA than central macular thickness in CME [38]. Automated segmentation of the cystoid fluid volume in CME has been described to identify regions of cystoid fluid within a three-dimensional retinal stack of images. However the correlation of this total cystoid volume with VA and its ability to distinguish intraretinal cysts from other features such as SRF or an epiretinal membrane (ERM) has yet to be established. Automated layer segmentation software allows detection of relatively few anatomical boundaries, which may limit its application in "real-world" clinical OCT images which are often not of the same quality as experimental images attained through study imaging sessions.

Imaging the Choroid in DME

There has been recent interest in the role of choroidal imaging in DME. The choroidal vasculature, especially the choriocapillaris layer, is critical to maintain the neurosensory retina as it nourishes the outer retina. Definitive changes in the choroid have been confirmed on histopathology [39]. New imaging techniques including long-wavelength OCT, polarization-sensitive OCT, and standard spectral-domain (SD) OCT with an enhanced depth-imaging mode allow assessment of choroidal thickness.

The choroid of patients with diabetic retinopathy and DME is thinner than that of age-matched healthy people as well as fellow eyes without DME [40, 41]. Subfoveal medium choroidal vessel layer and choriocapillaris layer thicknesses have also shown to be reduced in DME [42]. In contrast, Kim et al. showed that the subfoveal choroid was thicker in eyes with DME than in those without and was thickest in eyes with SRD-type DME [43]. Central choroidal thickness decreases 6 months after anti-vascular endothelial growth factor (VEGF) therapy for DME [44]. Eyes with thicker baseline subfoveal choroidal thickness may have better short-term anatomic and functional responses [45].

Fluorescein Angiography in DME

While OCT provides valuable morphologic information and is useful to monitor DME and its response to treatment [46], FA offers critical biological information such as location, intensity, and leakage source. Furthermore leakage area as measured by FA continues to be a relevant secondary endpoint in major studies of DME treatment [47].

Although FA provides additional information about DME that is complementary to OCT, change in FA leakage over time is considered by many to be a more valuable metric than the absolute leakage at a single timepoint. This is partly because quantification of features on FA is typically not as reproducible compared to other imaging modalities such as OCT. Identification of DME subtypes by FA has potential to guide therapy and monitor disease activity. Various subtypes of DME have been proposed based on differences in the pattern of fluorescein leakage [48]. Focal leakage manifests as discrete foci of leakage on early FA frames and corresponds to MAs. The diffuse subtype is characterized by generalized leakage prominent on late FA frames without a discretely identifiable source (Fig. 1). The angiographic appearance in eyes with DME can include either of these two leakage patterns, or a mixture of both [49].

Correlation between the FA macular leakage pattern and the edema morphology on OCT has been shown [21, 32, 50–52]. Variability of OCT reflectivity levels in the foveal cystoid spaces that corresponds to fluorescein pooling has been shown in DME. However the clinical relevance of this finding remains to be established [53].

While reproducible quantitative and qualitative analysis of FA is possible by experienced graders in the setting of a formal image reading center, its use for subtyping in the clinical setting is hindered by the subjective nature of FA interpretation. There has been long-standing interest in objective methods to quantify FA leakage. Segmentation of leakage on fluorescein angiograms obtained in the clinic is challenging, partly due to difficulties with FA sequence registration. There have been attempts to automate MA detection [54, 55], extraction of vessels [56], foveal avascular zone (FAZ) detection [57], and even automated leakage detection or quantification [58–61]. Rabbani et al. recently described a fully automated image segmentation algorithm without manual inputs to reproducibly and accurately quantify DME leakage area [62].

Using OCT and FA, Bolz et al. [21, 63] proposed the SAVE protocol for DME categorization. "S" stands for subretinal fluid, "A" for area, "V" for vitreoretinal interface abnormalities, and "E" for etiology. Based on etiology, DME leakage was categorized as focal or multifocal (FA with definable leakage source), non-focal capillary leakage (FA without definable leakage source), macular or peripheral ischemia (ischemia anywhere on FA associated with focal or non-focal edema on OCT), and atrophic edema (cystoid swelling on OCT). Newer technologies like en face OCT, OCT angiography, and retromode scanning laser ophthalmoscope (SLO) are also being investigated in DME.

Pseudophakic Cystoid Macular Edema

CME associated with cataract extraction was initially described by A. Ray and Irvine, Jr., in patients with unexplained visual loss following intracapsular cataract extraction. Subsequently, this phenomenon was identified by Gass and Norton as macular edema with a classic perifoveal petaloid FA staining pattern and late nerve leakage [64, 65].

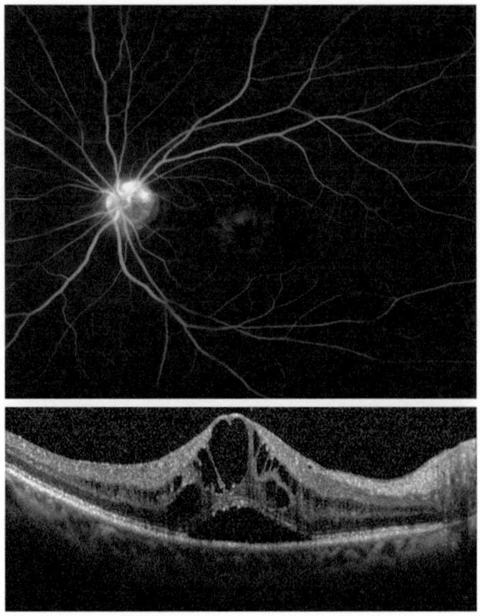

Fig. 5 Pseudophakic CME with cystic spaces and subfoveal subretinal fluid (*bottom*). There is parafoveal petaloid leakage on the fluorescein angiogram and mild leakage at the optic nerve (*top*)

More recently, OCT characteristics of pseudophakic CME have been described. These features include macular thickening and cystic spaces in the OPL, occasionally with subfoveal fluid (Fig. 5). An OCT-based automated statistical classification approach to differentiate DME from pseudophakic CME has been evaluated. Grading parameters included assessment of CME pattern, cyst distribution in ETDRS grid, morphologic features, and quantitative parameters such as individual layer thickness. Munk et al. [66] showed that higher central retinal thickness/volume ratio, the absence of ERM, and solely inner nuclear layer (INL) cysts indicated pseudophakic CME; a higher ONL/INL ratio, the absence of SRF, the presence of hard exudates, microaneurysms, and ganglion cell layer and/or retinal nerve fiber layer cysts favored DME. The optical density of subretinal fluid in DME and pseudophakic CME was similar [67].

Oh and associates reported the presence of vitreous hyperreflective dots following phacoemulsification. The number of hyperreflective dots detected 1 week following surgery predicted the development of CME at 1 month [68]. These vitreous hyperreflective dots were thought to correspond to lens fragments, denatured proteins, or clumps of intraocular cells. They were >20 μm in size which was larger than vitreous cavity cells seen as ~15 μm hyperreflective dots on OCT in uveitic eyes [69]. The authors concluded that despite the unclear nature of these dots, their association with pseudophakic CME suggested a relation to postoperative inflammation and vascular permeability.

Evaluation for previously undiagnosed photoreceptor disruption is important in assessment of eyes with unexplained vision loss despite resolution of pseudophakic CME. Using a 4 μm resolution OCT [70], persistent anatomic alteration of photoreceptors, described as a blurring of cone photoreceptor outer segment tips, correlated with reduced visual acuity in eyes with resolved pseudophakic CME that did not achieve 20/20 visual acuity compared with eyes that did.

Other OCT characteristics associated with pseudophakic CME include vitreomacular traction (VMT), extrafoveal vitreoretinal traction [71, 72], ERM, or ERM following prior ERM peeling [73, 74]. Odrobina et al. [75] recently suggested that a thinner choroid in eyes with pseudophakic CME compared to fellow eyes indicate that reduced choriocapillaris blood flow may be a possible CME etiologic factor. Others have reported, however, that eyes with pseudophakic CME had greater thickening of the subfoveal choroid, which preceded CME development by 1 month [76].

CME Associated with Retinal Vascular Occlusions

CME, a major cause of visual acuity loss in patients with retinal vascular occlusion (RVO) [77], is characterized by intraretinal fluid accumulation with diffuse retinal thickening or formation of cystoid spaces, SRF accumulation, or macular traction due to ERM formation (Figs. 6 and 7). OCT assessment of retinal thickness and structural changes provides useful information to determine treatment strategy for RVO-associated CME and to predict the long-term visual prognosis. OCT anatomic parameters such as foveal thickness, serous retinal detachment, central cystoid spaces, and pigment epithelial changes correlate with decreased visual recovery after RVO [78, 79].

Various RVO anatomic biomarkers have been evaluated with OCT. In eyes with central retinal vein occlusion (CRVO), foveal thickness >700 μm should raise suspicion for an ischemic form of CRVO [80]. In BRVO, cystoid spaces >600 μm in diameter have been associated with a longer occlusion of duration and poor visual

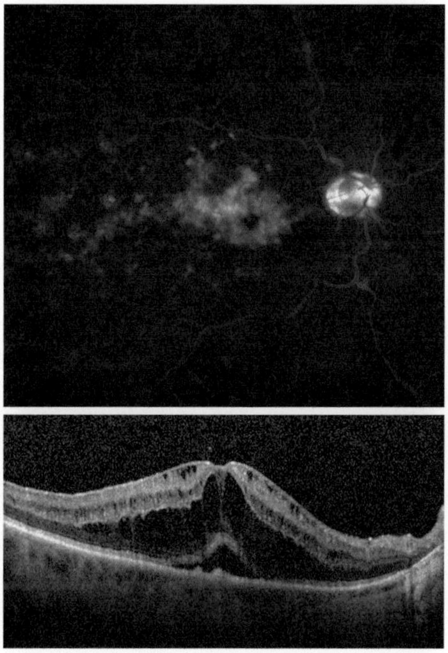

Fig. 6 CME in non-ischemic central retinal vein occlusion (CRVO) with diffuse retinal thickening, cystoid spaces, and accumulation of subretinal fluid (*top*). Fluorescein angiogram shows diffuse parafoveal leakage (*bottom*)

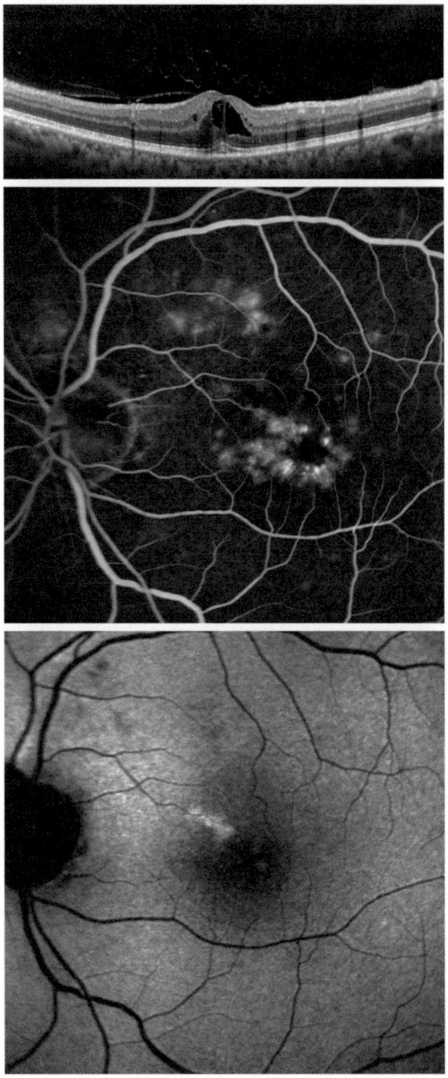

Fig. 7 CME in branch retinal vein occlusion (BRVO) with intraretinal cystoid spaces, no subretinal fluid (*top*), petaloid leakage on fluorescein angiogram (*middle*), and parafoveal hyper fundus autofluorescence (FAF) pattern on fundus autofluorescence (*bottom*)

improvement with bevacizumab therapy [81, 82]. Loss of the subfoveal ellipsoid layer and the absence of the inner retinal layers on OCT are correlated with poor visual outcomes in patients with CRVO [83] and branch retinal vein occlusion (BRVO) [79, 84, 85]. In addition, loss of the inner retinal layers correlates with macular ischemia diagnosed in early FA frames [78].

Tsujikawa and associates reported that a breakdown of the ELM barrier function caused movement of IRF into the subretinal space in RVO-associated CME [86]. They also reported highly reflective vertical lines beneath the cystoid spaces that were proposed to represent tracks through which the IRF within the cystoid spaces flowed into the subretinal space [16, 86, 87]. Hasegawa et al. also observed highly

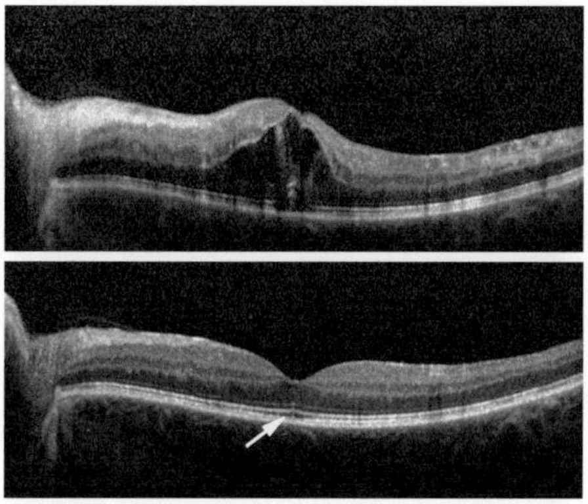

Fig. 8 CME in BRVO with subretinal fluid (*top*) and a hyperreflective track line (*below, white arrow*) at the fovea after resolution of CME

reflective vertical lines termed "track lines" beneath the cystoid spaces in the OCT images similar to those described by Tsujikawa et al., but note that the lines persisted despite resolution of CME [86, 88]. It has been suggested that the track lines probably developed when the CME resolved rapidly by the treatment. They observed these track lines at the fovea after resolution of CME associated with BRVO (Fig. 8). Track lines are thought to cause the localized damage of the photoreceptors. Hyperreflective foci are track line components, and it is thought that hyperreflective foci deposited in the outer retina causes the photoreceptor damage [11, 16, 89–91]. The specific mechanism that accounts for photoreceptor damage is unknown, but it has been proposed that macromolecules in IRF pass through small ELM disruptions and cause photoreceptor damage. Therefore, the track lines may be associated with localized rather than diffuse photoreceptor damage. Hasegawa et al. [88] suggested that the track lines are associated strongly with an initially disrupted ELM and thus might not be detected in eyes with spontaneous CME resolution. Track lines may thus be a useful marker of photoreceptor damage in eyes with resolved macular edema associated with BRVO.

Another biomarker that has been evaluated is an inward curvature of the foveal ellipsoid zone, seen in normal eyes, and termed the "foveal bulge" [92]. The foveal bulge is a good marker of visual functional in eyes with resolved BRVO-associated CME. The presence of the foveal bulge indicates better BCVA after resolution of the macular edema associated with BRVO [92]. In eyes with an intact foveal ellipsoid layer after resolution of BRVO-associated CME, the retinal thickness at the foveal center was thinner, and the photoreceptor OS length was shorter in the group without a foveal bulge than in the group with it [92]. The study suggested that CME damages foveal photoreceptor outer segments resulting in the absence of a foveal bulge.

Ellipsoid layer disruption at the central fovea has been shown in eyes with poor visual acuity despite complete resolution of CME (Fig. 9) [79, 83, 85]. It has also been shown that the integrity of the ellipsoid layer correlates with VA in eyes with resolved RVO-associated CME [92–94]. An association between the initial foveal thickness and final VA is somewhat controversial. While some have reported a correlation between the initial foveal thickness and final VA in eyes with RVO and persistent CME after treatment [82, 85], others have not observed this association [82, 94].

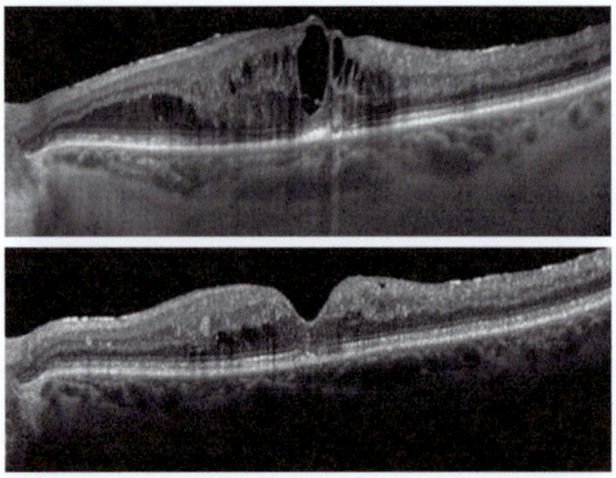

Fig. 9 Lack of visual acuity improvement in an eye (stable at 20/60) with CME associated with non-ischemic CRVO (*top*) despite near-complete resolution of CME following treatment with anti-vascular growth factor injections attributed to ellipsoid layer disruption at the central fovea (*bottom*)

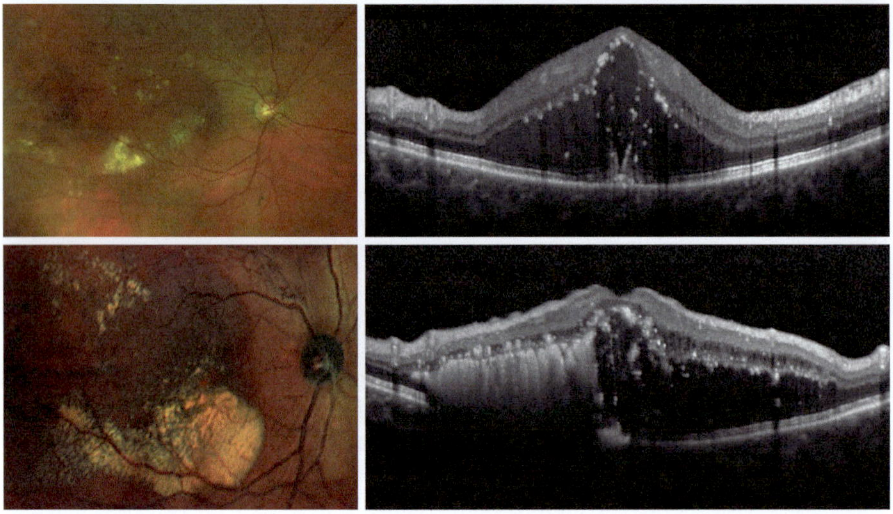

Fig. 10 Hyperreflective foci in an eye with BRVO and CME (*top*) with increased subretinal lipid exudates 8 weeks later (*bottom*). It has been suggested that these foci could be small intraretinal protein and/or lipid deposits and precursors of hard exudates

Various anatomical characteristics have been evaluated as potential prognostic indicators in RVO-associated CME. In CRVO-associated CME, the presence of SRF or the diameter of cystoid spaces has not been shown to be predictive for treatment outcome [82]. Ellipsoid layer integrity and ELM status at baseline correlate with better visual outcomes after anti-VEGF treatment for RVO- associated CME [94, 95]. Severe photoreceptor damage during the acute or chronic phase of RVO might lead to a substantial photoreceptor outer segment defect, resulting ellipsoid zone loss [79, 83]. Kang et al. suggested that hyperreflective foci detected on the baseline OCT were predictive of visual outcomes following anti-VEGF treatment [94]. Fine hyperreflective foci found on OCT, however, could not be found on fundus photographs taken simultaneously. In contrast, confluent hyperreflective foci on OCT were detected as hard exudates in the corresponding fundus photograph, and a previous study suggested that these fine foci, characterized by the same

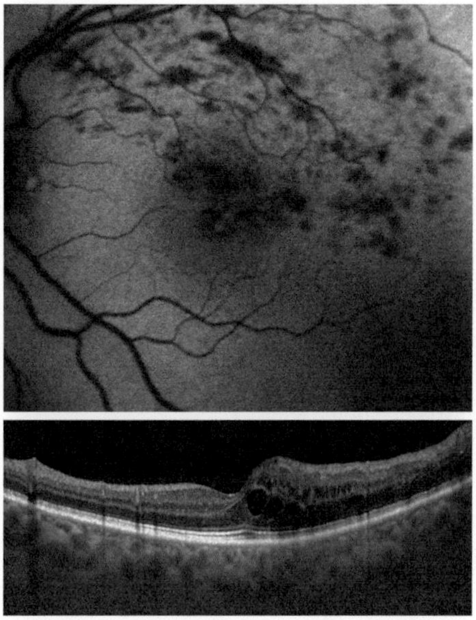

Fig. 11 CME associated with a superotemporal BRVO with intraretinal hemorrhages: fundus autofluorescence (FAF) demonstrates hyperautofluorescence in the fovea corresponding to the CME and hypoautofluorescence superiorly corresponding to the hemorrhages (*top*), vertical OCT scan shows a superior macular edema pattern (*bottom*)

hyperreflectivity as confluent dots, might be small intraretinal protein and/or lipid deposits which are precursors of hard exudates (Fig. 10) [16].

In eyes with BRVO, ELM and ellipsoid layer were significantly more disrupted in eyes that had hyperreflective foci as part of the track lines in the outer retinal layers [88]. These findings suggested that photoreceptor status, rather than foveal thickness, was more likely correlated with the final BCVA, after CME treatment in BRVO. Asymmetric CME distribution in the vertical scan is often pathognomonic for BRVO. Because of the higher prevalence of superotemporal vein occlusions [96], vertical line scans show a superior macular edema pattern in BRVO with a higher prevalence of cysts in the inner superior ETDRS subfield (Fig. 11).

Choroidal thickness has also been evaluated in RVO-associated CME. In both BRVO and CRVO, the choroidal thickness is greater than in the unaffected fellow eyes, and the choroidal volume is decreased following anti-VEGF treatment [97, 98].

CME Associated with Vitreoretinal Interface Abnormalities

An ERM results from proliferative change at the vitreoretinal interface. Tangential traction from ERM may cause macular thickening with or without fluorescein leakage. ERMs can also distort the underlying retina and create cystoid spaces.

On OCT the posterior hyaloid, a minimally reflective structure, can often be differentiated from an ERM, which is highly reflective [99]. Wilkins et al. described two patterns of ERM adherence [100]: a broadly attached ERM, which was most common (Fig. 12), and less frequently, ERM with focal attachments. OCT has also

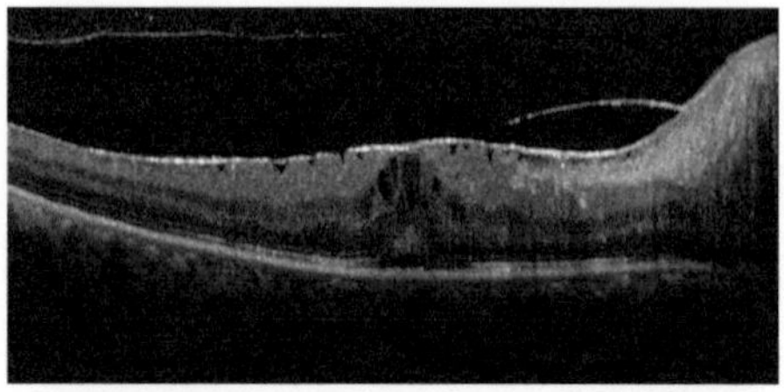

Fig. 12 CME with intraretinal cystoid spaces and subretinal fluid associated with a broad epiretinal membrane. The epiretinal membrane has caused distortion of the inner retina

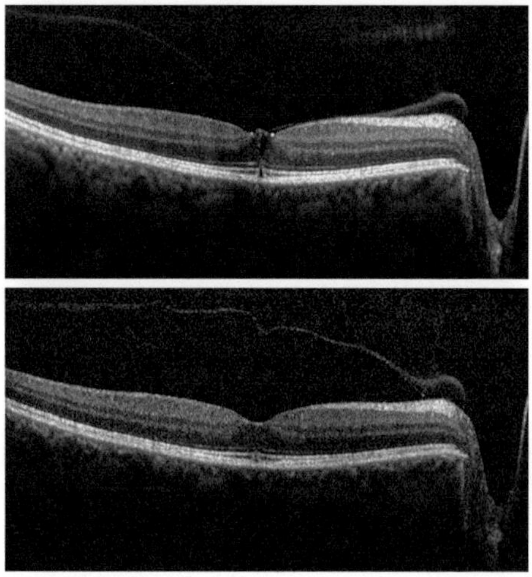

Fig. 13 Vitreomacular traction resulting in increased foveal thickness, intraretinal cysts and disruption of the ellipsoid layer (*top*), and restoration of normal foveal contour along with resolution of cystic spaces following spontaneous release of traction (*bottom*)

been helpful to confirm the relationship between a posterior vitreous detachment and ERM and is valuable to follow ERM natural history. Partial or complete PVD has been found in 80–95 % of eyes with idiopathic ERM [101–103].

VMT is an anomalous, posterior vitreous attachment that causes macular antero-posterior traction in areas of residual vitreous adhesion. The adherent vitreous cortex results in a broad, often dumbbell-shaped region, encompassing the macula and optic nerve [104]. This traction is associated with cystoid macular thickening (Fig. 13).

The phase III trials of Microplasmin Intravitreal Injection for Non-surgical Treatment of Focal Vitreomacular Adhesion (MIVI-TRUST) evaluated enzymatic vitreolysis with ocriplasmin. In these trials, OCT and clinical examination was used to assess retinal morphology; these investigations confirmed the superiority of OCT to clinical examination [105]. The study described two subclasses of VMT: focal (≤1500 μ) and broad (>1500 μ) adhesion [106–108]. Koizumi et al. [107] showed that eyes with focal VMT had a foveal cavitation, whereas eyes with broad VMT had more widespread CME. In VMT, the posterior hyaloid usually appears hyper-reflective and thickened on OCT. Yamada and Kishi [109] described two types of partial PVD patterns – incomplete vitreous detachment nasally and temporally causing a V-shaped pattern with attachment only at the fovea and the second type showing persistent nasal attachment and detachment temporal to the fovea. The first type of PVD had postoperatively better visual outcomes compared with the second type.

CME Associated with Uveitis

Hassenstein and colleagues were the first to describe the use of OCT in uveitis. This group found that OCT was useful in detection of early CME and monitoring of treatment efficacy, especially when vitreous cells were present [110, 111]. Specific OCT patterns have been identified in CME associated with uveitis, similar to those reported in DME: diffuse macular edema (characterized by increased retinal thickness, disturbance of the layered retinal structure or sponge-like low reflective areas) (Fig. 14), cystoid macular edema (characterized by clearly defined intraretinal cystoid spaces) (Fig. 15), and serous retinal detachment (characterized by a clean separation of the neurosensory retina from the RPE/choriocapillaris band) (Fig. 16) [13, 111, 112]. Iannetti et al. imaged 43 eyes and found that 58 % had cystoid macular edema, 42 % had diffuse macular edema, and 28 % of all cases had serous retinal detachment. The relative frequency of the three different patterns in uveitis varies depending on the patient selection criteria [111, 113, 114].

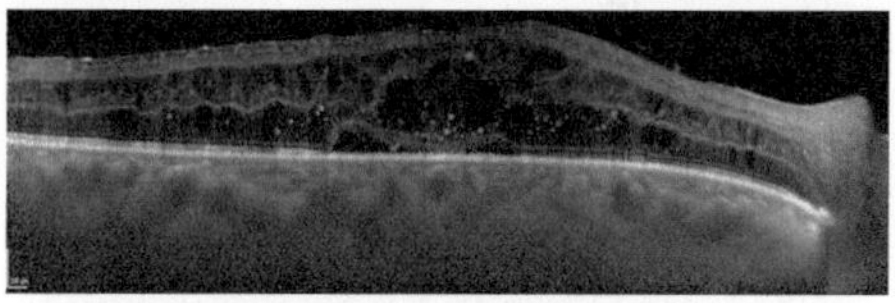

Fig. 14 Diffuse pattern of uveitic CME associated with sarcoid. The retina has inner and outer plexiform layer cystoid spaces, hyperreflective foci, and subretinal fluid

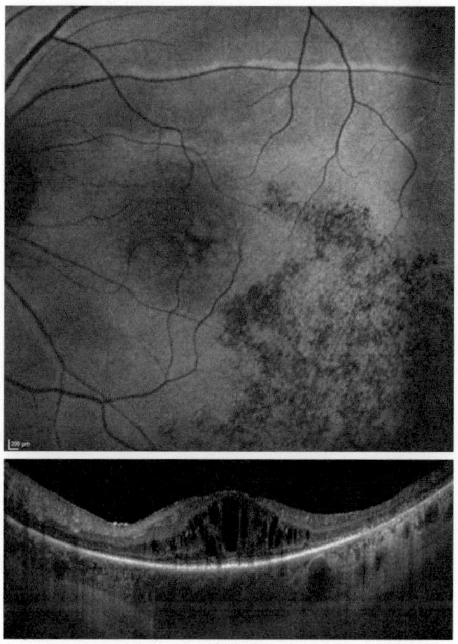

Fig. 15 CME associated with autoimmune retinopathy with parafoveal hyperautofluorescence on FAF (*top*). There is retinal thickening in the fovea with intraretinal cystoid spaces and diffuse retinal thinning with outer retinal loss in the surrounding temporal area without edema (*bottom*) and a corresponding hypo autofluorescent pattern on FAF

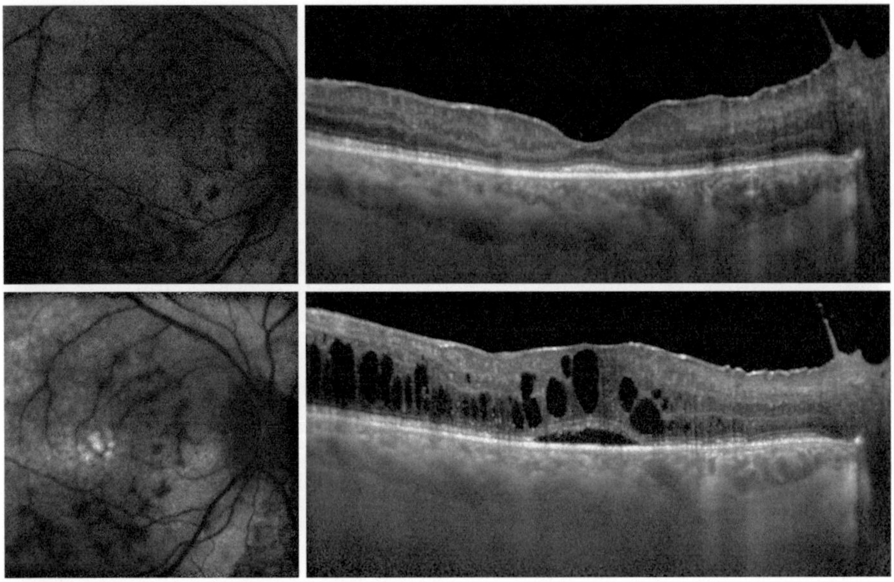

Fig. 16 Increased fundus hyperautofluorescence on FAF upon development of intraretinal cystoid spaces and subretinal fluid (*bottom*) in CME associated with birdshot chorioretinopathy

OCT also detects ERM, often with concurrent vitreoretinal traction in a higher percentage of uveitic CME eyes compared to ophthalmoscopy [112]. A tractional mechanism has also been hypothesized as a cause of or contributor to uveitic CME. The presence of an ERM is independent from the site of inflammation, type of edema, and macular thickness [112].

A ringlike non-cystic thickening that surrounds the foveal center has been seen in eyes with iridocyclitis. It has been theorized that the same pathophysiological mechanism that underlies this non-cystic ringlike thickening accounts for the CME in eyes with anterior uveitis. This thickening, lasting <6 months after an acute episode, has been reported in 45 % of acute anterior uveitis cases [115], and normal macular volumes are restored by 6 months after the uveitis flare-up [116].

A negative correlation between central subfield thickness and VA has been described in uveitic CME [111, 112, 114, 117, 118]. Microperimetry has also been shown to correlate with central subfield thickness and VA in eyes with uveitic CME [119]. Cystoid changes in OPL and INL and the presence of ERM were associated with poor VA. OCT has also been used to monitor the therapeutic response in uveitic CME [120–122]. Lehpamer et al. [123] demonstrated that SRF in uveitic CME was associated with increased central subfield thickness and worse VA at presentation. However, eyes with SRF responded well to treatment at 3 and 6 months, achieving greater rates of improvement than eyes without SRF and recovered to a similar level of final VA. An initial increase in SRF may occur during the process of macular edema absorption [124].

Markomichelakis et al. evaluated the prognostic significance of OCT patterns of macular edema. These coworkers found that eyes with a diffuse pattern of macular edema often have good visual acuity and do not need to be aggressively treated. This undertreatment, however, makes them prone to an increase in macular thickness and decreased VA during an inflammatory relapse [124]. They also found the presence of an ERM to be a poor prognostic factor in uveitic CME and associated with medical treatment failure [124]. IRF in uveitic CME may be dynamic; retinal thickness changes can be seen seconds after a change in patient position [125]. CME also has a diurnal variation with the main decrease in retinal thickness occurring before noon [125].

CME seen by OCT in patients with juvenile idiopathic arthritis (JIA)-associated uveitis has been reported in 84 % of eyes [126], a figure higher than that observed in previous ophthalmoscopy-based reports [127, 128]. JIA-associated uveitic OCT changes include perifoveal thickening, CME, foveal detachment, and atrophic changes. Duration of JIA-uveitis correlated with the development of CME [128].

Central subfield thickness is an important endpoint for various clinical trials and is an important parameter in the clinical management of uveitic CME. The Multicenter Uveitis Steroid Treatment (MUST) trial [129] evaluated a clinically meaningful OCT-determined thickness threshold in eyes with uveitic CME. A 20 % change in retinal thickness in eyes with uveitic CME (defined as retinal thickness at the central subfield >260 μm) was optimal to predict more than a 10-letter change in VA, with 77 % sensitivity and 75 % specificity. This threshold is important for uveitis trials wherein uveitic CME improvement is monitored through changes in central subfield thickness and associated with clinically meaningful VA changes. The MUST trial also showed that OCT and FA only agreed moderately to identify uveitic CME in eyes with intermediate, posterior, and panuveitis, probably because macular thickening on OCT (time domain) and macular leakage are related but nonidentical pathologic characteristics [130]. Fluorescein leakage indicates pathological leakage from blood vessels, which is often but not always associated with macular thickening. Reasons for lack of thickening when there is fluorescein vascular leakage include the following non-mutually exclusive mechanisms: severely damaged atrophic maculae, with superimposed ongoing inflammatory leakage, a macula with very recent leakage that has preceded retinal thickening, macular distortion secondary to ERM without associated thickening, or a steady state whereby macular leakage is balanced by physiologic fluid egress from the macular retina [130]. The MUST trial also showed that the presence of macular cysts on OCT was associated with increased retinal thickness by OCT, hyperfluorescent cystoid spaces on FA, and macular leakage on FA [130]. Small cysts and ERMs involving the center were common in intermediate and posterior/panuveitis and required systemic corticosteroid therapy [131]. The MUST reading center methodology defined ERM as a hyperreflective layer with a bridging effect over the inner retinal layers, thus potentially excluding broadly adherent ERMs if their reflectivity merged with the nerve fiber layer. Corrugation of inner retinal layers was also considered insufficient to identify an ERM [131]. These results suggest that in uveitic CME, FA and OCT offer related yet unique clinically important information on macular pathologic features.

Similar to DME, the relationship between VA and CME in uveitis is imperfect. Payne et al. [132] determined the utility of logarithmic transformation of OCT retinal thickness data to assess clinically meaningful changes in uveitic CME. Log scale OCT thickness correlated with logMAR visual acuity suggesting its use as an objective measure in uveitic CME [132]. These researchers also showed that in uveitic CME, the volume between the plexiform layers was the best indicator of visual function at baseline [38]. Brar et al. reviewed FA and OCT images of 87 patients with CME due to diabetes, ERM, uveitis, pseudophakia and vein occlusion. They concluded that while cystoid leakage on FA was always associated with cystic OCT changes, diffuse non-cystoid leakage on FA was associated with thickening and distortion of the retinal layers without cyst formation [133]. Diffuse uveitic CME has been associated with a poor visual prognosis and a poor prognosis for vision recovery [124]. SRF, however, is associated with a high probability of vision recovery in uveitic CME [134]. This is in contrast to SRF in DME that is associated with a poor prognosis for visual recovery [32].

FA is useful in differentiating active from inactive uveitis and also to confirm a CME diagnosis, choroidal neovascularization, and subtle retinal vasculitis, to monitor response to therapy, and to identify areas of capillary non-perfusion and retinal neovascularization. The small molecules of free, unbound fluorescein dye leak out even from minimally inflamed retinal vessels [135]. The characteristic appearance in eyes with uveitic CME is a "petaloid" pattern of parafoveal hyperfluorescence [135]. CME has been angiographically graded as [136] Grade 0, no sign of fluorescein leakage; Grade I, slight fluorescein leakage into cystic spaces but not enough to enclose the entire fovea centralis; Grade II, complete circular accumulation of the fluorescein in the cystic space but its diameter is smaller than 2 mm; and Grade III, the circular accumulation of fluorescein is larger than 2.0 mm in diameter.

There have been attempts to describe OCT anatomical characteristics that can identify CME of different etiologies. Microfoci, thought to be caused by lipid-rich and lipoprotein-rich deposits or lipid-laden macrophages [16], were found to be one such differentiating characteristic on OCT [137]. These foci are characteristic for DME and RVO, although they differ in location and presentation according to the underlying disease [16, 138]. Munk et al. reported that microfoci were found in 100 % of CME eyes with CRVO, in 98 % of the eyes with DME, and in 65 % of eyes with BRVO, but in no eye with pseudophakic CME or uveitic CME [137]. IRF accumulation occurs in CME irrespective of the disease entities and differences in morphologic and spatial presentation, although previous histologic reports indicate that IRF may vary according to its underlying pathology [26, 139, 140].

Posterior uveitis is accompanied by choroidal thickening especially in an acute phase [141, 142]. With this technique, macular choroidal changes in eyes with anterior and intermediate uveitis are less marked compared to posterior uveitis and panuveitis [143].

CME is related to the use of drugs like prostaglandin analogues, epinephrine and epinephrine-like drugs, nicotinic acid, pioglitazone, rosiglitazone, docetaxel, and paclitaxel presumably by inducing an inflammatory reaction that causes breakdown of the blood retinal barrier and can also be monitored using OCT [144–149].

Role of Fundus Autofluorescence Imaging in CME

Fundus autofluorescence (FAF) is determined by the lipofuscin distribution in the RPE and is also influenced by macular pigments in the INL, ONL, and OPL [150, 151]. RPE autofluorescence depends on outer segment renewal and can be affected by the RPE's ability to clear lipofuscin. Lipofuscin accumulation leads to reduced RPE phagocytic capacity which in turn can lead to RPE cell death and photoreceptor loss. Increased FAF is seen with RPE dysfunction and decreased FAF with loss of photoreceptors or the RPE [152].

CME is associated with increased FAF, thought to be due to macular neurosensory retinal tissue stretching that displaces macular pigments laterally thereby reducing the density of macular pigments, which increases the autofluorescence signal (Fig. 10) [153–155]. In eyes with CME, there have been attempts to correlate FAF with OCT parameters and VA and to predict restoration of photoreceptor integrity and subsequent visual recovery [156].

In DME, increased FAF is caused by the accumulation of oxidative products induced by activated microglia resulting in lipofuscin accumulation [157]. It has also been suggested that increased FAF in DME is not abnormal FAF. Rather, RPE autofluorescence is observed through a defect in the xanthophyll pigment [155]. At the foveola, blue-light FAF is very weak or almost absent in normal eyes because lutein and zeaxanthin are especially dense in the axons of the cone photoreceptors (Henle's fiber) at the foveola and absorb the incident blue light. Increased foveolar FAF in DME has been shown to be associated with low ONL thickness, larger ellipsoid layer defect, and poor vision [156].

Hyper-FAF has been associated with functional and structural macular impairment in DME; [156] FAF decreases with DME resolution [157]. VA in eyes with DME and increased FAF is worse than that in eyes without increased FAF [155]. However FAF correlates better with OCT patterns and central field microperimetry than with VA [157]. FAF changes are not uniform in all patients with DME. Chung el al. reported that not all patients with a significant DME had comparable levels of increased FAF, nor did all patients with improved DME exhibit a significant decrease in FAF [156]. Functional improvement after DME treatment can be quantified on FAF and correlated with OCT morphology, thereby demonstrating a role for FAF as a prognostic factor in DME.

Increased foveolar and perifoveolar petaloid FAF has been shown in uveitic CME (Fig. 15) [158, 159]. In some studies, however, the detection of pathologic FAF in patients with angiographically proven CME was only achieved in half the eyes, a limitation of FAF as compared to OCT [158]. Roesel et al. [158] focused on the correlation of FAF and OCT with visual acuity in eyes with uveitic CME. This group observed increased FAF and proposed that it arose from proteins such as retinoids in the extracellular fluid. Increased central FAF, the presence of cystoid changes, a disrupted ellipsoid layer, and ERM were associated with poor visual acuity. The FAF pattern found in uveitic CME may also reflect size, number, or fluorophore content of damaged RPE cells. Increased FAF has not been shown to be prominent in the diffuse type of uveitic CME [152]. There have also been attempts to classify abnormal FAF in CME with three main patterns described: cystoid hyper-FAF, single or multiple spot hyper-FAF, and irregular hypo-FAF [160].

En Face C-Scan Imaging in CME

En face imaging or C-scan OCT produces frontal sections of the retinal layers and can be used to highlight specific aspects of CME. Creating an en face section at the ILM will show ERM and macular surface alterations. A scan about 40 μm deeper will show INL cystoid cells and an even deeper scan will show ONL cystoid cells [161]. En face OCT scans 40 μm beneath and parallel to the ILM show petal-shaped central and peripheral cavities. Deeper en face scans in the ONL show ovoid polygonal flower-shaped cystoid cells converging toward the fovea. In cases with advanced CME, the cells merge vertically first, and cells in the INL grow toward the ONL forming large vertically ovoid cavities. In CME a reduced intensity in the inner and outer segment en face image in areas with increased retinal thickness has been shown [162]. En face OCT cannot, however, determine the exact extent of CME because of the different layer location of the cysts [163, 164].

Further Advances in Imaging CME

Several technologies are currently under development that could help visualize CME better. Already integrated in some platforms, Doppler OCT can measure blood flow in the retinal and choroidal vessels [165]. Swept-source OCT can achieve ultrahigh axial resolution by sweeping a narrow bandwidth light source through a broad optical range [166].

High-penetration posterior OCT (HP OCT) systems, which use a longer wavelength than standard penetration OCT (1060 vs. 830 nm), have higher choroidal penetration [167] allowing for better assessment of choroidal changes in CME.

Adaptive optics (AO) scanning laser ophthalmoscopy has been used to document microcystic macular edema from en face images in patients with autosomal-dominant optic atrophy [168]. On AO, after BRVO-associated CME resolution, there is decreased parafoveal cone density and disruption of the cone mosaic spatial arrangement [169]. Swelling of Müller cells due to disturbed fluid transport has been described in eyes with macular edema [170–172]. Ultrahigh resolution OCT has been combined with AO to increase image resolution and to demonstrate morphological changes of Müller cells, which could unveil new information on the pathogenesis of CME.

Other emerging technologies include optical coherence microangiography [173], phase variance imaging [174], and power or variance Doppler techniques [175] for noninvasive capillary level detection of the retinal vasculature. However the ability to acquire en face images of distinct capillary beds with current FA and OCT technology is limited. Prototype speckle variance OCT has been used for noninvasive real-time imaging the human retinal vasculature. This is complementary to FA and may provide superior capillary detail [176]. This method has the potential to noninvasively identify important pathological manifestations of CME [177]. Scattering OCT has the potential to visualize the choroidal vasculature of the macula and the optic nerve head without intravenous dye injection [166, 178].

Retromode scanning laser ophthalmoscopy (SLO) has been used to visualize cystoid spaces in DME without the appearance of a shadow to the silhouetted cystoid space due to light scattering [179, 180]. Retromode SLO showed good agreement with OCT, FA, and FAF in identifying both honeycomb and petaloid patterns of DME [179]. Cysts of different dimensions were comparable to FA and the extent of DME correlated with retinal sensitivity [179, 181].

The application of OCT to image CME in the pediatric retina is also promising. CME in very preterm infants usually manifests as cystoid structures in the INL and rarely involves the other retinal layers [182]. CME in very preterm infants screened for retinopathy of prematurity is a developmental biomarker associated with decreased language and motor skills at 18–24 months corrected age [183].

Conclusion

OCT, fluorescein angiography, and fundus autofluorescence have been demonstrated to be effective modalities to evaluate CME. While OCT allows evaluation of the location, extension, pattern, and microstructural anatomical features, FA allows identification of areas of leakage, thus providing complimentary yet distinct information for diagnosis of CME and monitoring its response to treatment. Future advances in imaging technology with higher acquisition speed and hardware motion tracking along with improved automated image segmentation analysis protocols will allow us to better characterize CME. Development of novel anatomical biomarkers can offer prognostic implications and monitor response to treatment. Newer imaging technologies including noninvasive OCT angiography hold promise to help better elucidate the pathology of CME.

Conflict of Interest Disclosures Dr. Jaffe is a consultant to Heidelberg Engineering. Dr. Grewal does not have any financial or proprietary interests in this manuscript. Grant Support: Heed Ophthalmic Foundation, San Francisco, CA (DSG).

References

1. Hee MR, Izatt JA, Swanson EA, Huang D, Schuman JS, et al. Optical coherence tomography of the human retina. Arch Ophthalmol. 1995;113:325–32.
2. Treatment techniques and clinical guidelines for photocoagulation of diabetic macular edema. Early Treatment Diabetic Retinopathy Study Report Number 2. Early Treatment Diabetic Retinopathy Study Research Group. Ophthalmology. 1987;94:761–74
3. Photocoagulation for diabetic macular edema. Early Treatment Diabetic Retinopathy Study report number 1. Early Treatment Diabetic Retinopathy Study research group. Arch Ophthalmol. 1985;103:1796–806
4. Baskin DE. Optical coherence tomography in diabetic macular edema. Curr Opin Ophthalmol. 2010;21:172–7.

5. Sakamoto A, Nishijima K, Kita M, Oh H, Tsujikawa A, et al. Association between foveal photoreceptor status and visual acuity after resolution of diabetic macular edema by pars plana vitrectomy. Graefes Arch Clin Exp Ophthalmol. 2009;247:1325–30.
6. Alasil T, Keane PA, Updike JF, Dustin L, Ouyang Y, et al. Relationship between optical coherence tomography retinal parameters and visual acuity in diabetic macular edema. Ophthalmology. 2010;117:2379–86.
7. Forooghian F, Stetson PF, Meyer SA, Chew EY, Wong WT, et al. Relationship between photoreceptor outer segment length and visual acuity in diabetic macular edema. Retina. 2010;30:63–70.
8. Maheshwary AS, Oster SF, Yuson RM, Cheng L, Mojana F, et al. The association between percent disruption of the photoreceptor inner segment-outer segment junction and visual acuity in diabetic macular edema. Am J Ophthalmol. 2010;150(63–67):e61.
9. Otani T, Yamaguchi Y, Kishi S. Correlation between visual acuity and foveal microstructural changes in diabetic macular edema. Retina. 2010;30:774–80.
10. Shin HJ, Lee SH, Chung H, Kim HC. Association between photoreceptor integrity and visual outcome in diabetic macular edema. Graefes Arch Clin Exp Ophthalmol. 2012;250:61–70.
11. Uji A, Murakami T, Nishijima K, Akagi T, Horii T, et al. Association between hyperreflective foci in the outer retina, status of photoreceptor layer, and visual acuity in diabetic macular edema. Am J Ophthalmol. 2012;153:710–7, 717.e711.
12. Browning DJ, Fraser CM, Propst BW. The variation in optical coherence tomography-measured macular thickness in diabetic eyes without clinical macular edema. Am J Ophthalmol. 2008;145:889–93.
13. Otani T, Kishi S, Maruyama Y. Patterns of diabetic macular edema with optical coherence tomography. Am J Ophthalmol. 1999;127:688–93.
14. Kim BY, Smith SD, Kaiser PK. Optical coherence tomographic patterns of diabetic macular edema. Am J Ophthalmol. 2006;142:405–12.
15. Kaiser PK, Riemann CD, Sears JE, Lewis H. Macular traction detachment and diabetic macular edema associated with posterior hyaloidal traction. Am J Ophthalmol. 2001;131:44–9.
16. Bolz M, Schmidt-Erfurth U, Deak G, Mylonas G, Kriechbaum K, et al. Optical coherence tomographic hyperreflective foci: a morphologic sign of lipid extravasation in diabetic macular edema. Ophthalmology. 2009;116:914–20.
17. Framme C, Schweizer P, Imesch M, Wolf S, Wolf-Schnurrbusch U. Behavior of SD-OCT-detected hyperreflective foci in the retina of anti-VEGF-treated patients with diabetic macular edema. Invest Ophthalmol Vis Sci. 2012;53:5814–8.
18. Pemp B, Deak G, Prager S, Mitsch C, Lammer J, et al. Distribution of intraretinal exudates in diabetic macular edema during anti-vascular endothelial growth factor therapy observed by spectral domain optical coherence tomography and fundus photography. Retina. 2014;34:2407–15.
19. De Benedetto U, Sacconi R, Pierro L, Lattanzio R, Bandello F. Optical coherence tomographic hyperreflective foci in early stages of diabetic retinopathy. Retina. 2015;35:449–53.
20. Gelman SK, Freund KB, Shah VP, Sarraf D. The pearl necklace sign: a novel spectral domain optical coherence tomography finding in exudative macular disease. Retina. 2014;34:2088–95.
21. Bolz M, Ritter M, Schneider M, Simader C, Scholda C, et al. A systematic correlation of angiography and high-resolution optical coherence tomography in diabetic macular edema. Ophthalmology. 2009;116:66–72.
22. Horii T, Murakami T, Nishijima K, Sakamoto A, Ota M, et al. Optical coherence tomographic characteristics of microaneurysms in diabetic retinopathy. Am J Ophthalmol. 2010;150:840–8.
23. Lee SN, Chhablani J, Chan CK, Wang H, Barteselli G, et al. Characterization of microaneurysm closure after focal laser photocoagulation in diabetic macular edema. Am J Ophthalmol. 2013;155:905–12.
24. Diabetic Retinopathy Clinical Research N, Browning DJ, Glassman AR, Aiello LP, Beck RW, et al. Relationship between optical coherence tomography-measured central retinal thickness and visual acuity in diabetic macular edema. Ophthalmology. 2007;114:525–36.

25. Ito S, Miyamoto N, Ishida K, Kurimoto Y. Association between external limiting membrane status and visual acuity in diabetic macular oedema. Br J Ophthalmol. 2013;97:228–32.
26. Deak GG, Bolz M, Kriechbaum K, Prager S, Mylonas G, et al. Effect of retinal photocoagulation on intraretinal lipid exudates in diabetic macular edema documented by optical coherence tomography. Ophthalmology. 2010;117:773–9.
27. Deak GG, Bolz M, Ritter M, Prager S, Benesch T, et al. A systematic correlation between morphology and functional alterations in diabetic macular edema. Invest Ophthalmol Vis Sci. 2010;51:6710–4.
28. Horii T, Murakami T, Akagi T, Uji A, Ueda-Arakawa N, et al. Optical coherence tomographic reflectivity of cystoid spaces is related to recurrent diabetic macular edema after triamcinolone. Retina. 2015;35:264–71.
29. Murakami T, Nishijima K, Sakamoto A, Ota M, Horii T, et al. Association of pathomorphology, photoreceptor status, and retinal thickness with visual acuity in diabetic retinopathy. Am J Ophthalmol. 2011;151:310–7.
30. Bonnin S, Tadayoni R, Erginay A, Massin P, Dupas B. Correlation between ganglion cell layer thinning and poor visual function after resolution of diabetic macular edema. Invest Ophthalmol Vis Sci. 2015;56:978–82.
31. Lee DH, Kim JT, Jung DW, Joe SG, Yoon YH. The relationship between foveal ischemia and spectral-domain optical coherence tomography findings in ischemic diabetic macular edema. Invest Ophthalmol Vis Sci. 2013;54:1080–5.
32. Soliman W, Sander B, Hasler PW, Larsen M. Correlation between intraretinal changes in diabetic macular oedema seen in fluorescein angiography and optical coherence tomography. Acta Ophthalmol. 2008;86:34–9.
33. Sun JK, Lin MM, Lammer J, Prager S, Sarangi R, et al. Disorganization of the retinal inner layers as a predictor of visual acuity in eyes with center-involved diabetic macular edema. JAMA Ophthalmol. 2014;132:1309–16.
34. Sun JK, Radwan S, Soliman AZ, Lammer J, Lin MM, et al. Neural retinal disorganization as a robust marker of visual acuity in current and resolved diabetic macular edema. Diabetes. 2015.
35. Lee JY, Chiu SJ, Srinivasan PP, Izatt JA, Toth CA, et al. Fully automatic software for retinal thickness in eyes with diabetic macular edema from images acquired by cirrus and spectralis systems. Invest Ophthalmol Vis Sci. 2013;54:7595–602.
36. Wilkins GR, Houghton OM, Oldenburg AL. Automated segmentation of intraretinal cystoid fluid in optical coherence tomography. IEEE Trans Biomed Eng. 2012;59:1109–14.
37. Srinivasan PP, Kim LA, Mettu PS, Cousins SW, Comer GM, et al. Fully automated detection of diabetic macular edema and dry age-related macular degeneration from optical coherence tomography images. Biomed Opt Express. 2014;5:3568–77.
38. Pelosini L, Hull CC, Boyce JF, McHugh D, Stanford MR, et al. Optical coherence tomography may be used to predict visual acuity in patients with macular edema. Invest Ophthalmol Vis Sci. 2011;52:2741–8.
39. Hidayat AA, Fine BS. Diabetic choroidopathy light and electron microscopic observations of seven cases. Ophthalmology. 1985;92:512–22.
40. Regatieri CV, Branchini L, Carmody J, Fujimoto JG, Duker JS. Choroidal thickness in patients with diabetic retinopathy analyzed by spectral-domain optical coherence tomography. Retina. 2012;32:563–8.
41. Gerendas BS, Waldstein SM, Simader C, Deak G, Hajnajeeb B, et al. Three-dimensional automated choroidal volume assessment on standard spectral-domain optical coherence tomography and correlation with the level of diabetic macular edema. Am J Ophthalmol. 2014;158:1039–48.
42. Adhi M, Brewer E, Waheed NK, Duker JS. Analysis of morphological features and vascular layers of choroid in diabetic retinopathy using spectral-domain optical coherence tomography. JAMA Ophthalmol. 2013;131:1267–74.
43. Kim JT, Lee DH, Joe SG, Kim JG, Yoon YH. Changes in choroidal thickness in relation to the severity of retinopathy and macular edema in type 2 diabetic patients. Invest Ophthalmol Vis Sci. 2013;54:3378–84.

44. Yiu G, Manjunath V, Chiu SJ, Farsiu S, Mahmoud TH. Effect of anti-vascular endothelial growth factor therapy on choroidal thickness in diabetic macular edema. Am J Ophthalmol. 2014;158(745–751):e742.
45. Rayess N, Rahimy E, Ying GS, Bagheri N, Ho AC, et al. Baseline choroidal thickness as a predictor for response to anti-vascular endothelial growth factor therapy in diabetic macular edema. Am J Ophthalmol. 2015;159(85–91):e81–3.
46. Schmidt-Erfurth U, Lang GE, Holz FG, Schlingemann RO, Lanzetta P, et al. Three-year outcomes of individualized ranibizumab treatment in patients with diabetic macular edema: the RESTORE extension study. Ophthalmology. 2014;121:1045–53.
47. Nguyen QD, Brown DM, Marcus DM, Boyer DS, Patel S, et al. Ranibizumab for diabetic macular edema: results from 2 phase III randomized trials: RISE and RIDE. Ophthalmology. 2012;119:789–801.
48. Browning DJ, Glassman AR, Aiello LP, Bressler NM, Bressler SB, et al. Optical coherence tomography measurements and analysis methods in optical coherence tomography studies of diabetic macular edema. Ophthalmology. 2008;115:1366–71, 1371.e1361.
49. Bhagat N, Grigorian RA, Tutela A, Zarbin MA. Diabetic macular edema: pathogenesis and treatment. Surv Ophthalmol. 2009;54:1–32.
50. Kang SW, Park CY, Ham DI. The correlation between fluorescein angiographic and optical coherence tomographic features in clinically significant diabetic macular edema. Am J Ophthalmol. 2004;137:313–22.
51. Hee MR, Puliafito CA, Duker JS, Reichel E, Coker JG, et al. Topography of diabetic macular edema with optical coherence tomography. Ophthalmology. 1998;105:360–70.
52. Goebel W, Kretzchmar-Gross T. Retinal thickness in diabetic retinopathy: a study using optical coherence tomography (OCT). Retina. 2002;22:759–67.
53. Horii T, Murakami T, Nishijima K, Akagi T, Uji A, et al. Relationship between fluorescein pooling and optical coherence tomographic reflectivity of cystoid spaces in diabetic macular edema. Ophthalmology. 2012;119:1047–55.
54. Frame AJ, Undrill PE, Cree MJ, Olson JA, McHardy KC, et al. A comparison of computer based classification methods applied to the detection of microaneurysms in ophthalmic fluorescein angiograms. Comput Biol Med. 1998;28:225–38.
55. Cree MJ, Olson JA, McHardy KC, Sharp PF, Forrester JV. A fully automated comparative microaneurysm digital detection system. Eye (Lond). 1997;11(Pt 5):622–8.
56. Koprowski R, Teper SJ, Weglarz B, Wylegala E, Krejca M, et al. Fully automatic algorithm for the analysis of vessels in the angiographic image of the eye fundus. Biomed Eng Online. 2012;11:35.
57. Zheng Y, Gandhi JS, Stangos AN, Campa C, Broadbent DM, et al. Automated segmentation of foveal avascular zone in fundus fluorescein angiography. Invest Ophthalmol Vis Sci. 2010;51:3653–9.
58. Phillips RP, Ross PG, Tyska M, Sharp PF, Forrester JV. Detection and quantification of hyperfluorescent leakage by computer analysis of fundus fluorescein angiograms. Graefes Arch Clin Exp Ophthalmol. 1991;229:329–35.
59. Cree MJ, Olson JA, McHardy KC, Sharp PF, Forrester JV. The preprocessing of retinal images for the detection of fluorescein leakage. Phys Med Biol. 1999;44:293–308.
60. Chen X, Zhang L, Sohn EH, Lee K, Niemeijer M, et al. Quantification of external limiting membrane disruption caused by diabetic macular edema from SD-OCT. Invest Ophthalmol Vis Sci. 2012;53:8042–8.
61. Smith RT, Lee CM, Charles HC, Farber M, Cunha-Vaz JG. Quantification of diabetic macular edema. Arch Ophthalmol. 1987;105:218–22.
62. Rabbani H, Allingham MJ, Mettu PS, Cousins SW, Farsiu S. Fully Automatic Segmentation of Fluorescein Leakage in Subjects with Diabetic Macular Edema. Invest Ophthalmol Vis Sci. 2015;56:1482–92.
63. Bolz M, Lammer J, Deak G, Pollreisz A, Mitsch C, et al. SAVE: a grading protocol for clinically significant diabetic macular oedema based on optical coherence tomography and fluorescein angiography. Br J Ophthalmol. 2014;98:1612–7.

64. Irvine SR. A newly defined vitreous syndrome following cataract surgery. Am J Ophthalmol. 1953;36:599–619.
65. Gass JD, Norton EW. Cystoid macular edema and papilledema following cataract extraction. A fluorescein fundoscopic and angiographic study. Arch Ophthalmol. 1966;76:646–61.
66. Munk MR Automated, software based differentiation of diabetic macular edema from pseudophakic cystoid macular edema using SD-OCT. 2015. IOVS 2015: ARVO E-Abstract 2020.
67. Neudorfer M, Weinberg A, Loewenstein A, Barak A. Differential optical density of subretinal spaces. Invest Ophthalmol Vis Sci. 2012;53:3104–10.
68. Oh JH, Chuck RS, Do JR, Park CY. Vitreous hyper-reflective dots in optical coherence tomography and cystoid macular edema after uneventful phacoemulsification surgery. PLoS One. 2014;9:e95066.
69. Saito M, Barbazetto IA, Spaide RF. Intravitreal cellular infiltrate imaged as punctate spots by spectral-domain optical coherence tomography in eyes with posterior segment inflammatory disease. Retina. 2013;33:559–65.
70. Hunter AA, Modjtahedi SP, Long K, Zawadzki R, Chin EK, et al. Improving visual outcomes by preserving outer retina morphology in eyes with resolved pseudophakic cystoid macular edema. J Cataract Refract Surg. 2014;40:626–31.
71. Schubert HD. Cystoid macular edema: the apparent role of mechanical factors. Prog Clin Biol Res. 1989;312:277–91.
72. Martinez MR, Ophir A. Pseudophakic cystoid macular edema associated with extrafoveal vitreoretinal traction. Open Ophthalmol J. 2011;5:35–41.
73. Henderson BA, Kim JY, Ament CS, Ferrufino-Ponce ZK, Grabowska A, et al. Clinical pseudophakic cystoid macular edema. Risk factors for development and duration after treatment. J Cataract Refract Surg. 2007;33:1550–8.
74. Huynh TH, Johnson MW. The behavior of surgically repaired idiopathic macular holes in the setting of subsequent cystoid macular edema. Retina. 2007;27:759–63.
75. Odrobina D, LaudaNska-Olszewska I. Choroidal thickness in clinically significant pseudophakic cystoid macular edema. Retina. 2015;35:136–40.
76. Pierru A, Carles M, Gastaud P, Baillif S. Measurement of subfoveal choroidal thickness after cataract surgery in enhanced depth imaging optical coherence tomography. Invest Ophthalmol Vis Sci. 2014;55:4967–74.
77. Hayreh SS. Classification of central retinal vein occlusion. Ophthalmology. 1983;90:458–74.
78. Lima VC, Yeung L, Castro LC, Landa G, Rosen RB. Correlation between spectral domain optical coherence tomography findings and visual outcomes in central retinal vein occlusion. Clin Ophthalmol. 2011;5:299–305.
79. Ota M, Tsujikawa A, Murakami T, Kita M, Miyamoto K, et al. Association between integrity of foveal photoreceptor layer and visual acuity in branch retinal vein occlusion. Br J Ophthalmol. 2007;91:1644–9.
80. Martinet V, Guigui B, Glacet-Bernard A, Zourdani A, Coscas G, et al. Macular edema in central retinal vein occlusion: correlation between optical coherence tomography, angiography and visual acuity. Int Ophthalmol. 2012;32:369–77.
81. Kim M, Lee JH, Lee SJ. Diabetic papillopathy with macular edema treated with intravitreal ranibizumab. Clin Ophthalmol. 2013;7:2257–60.
82. Hoeh AE, Ruppenstein M, Ach T, Dithmar S. OCT patterns of macular edema and response to bevacizumab therapy in retinal vein occlusion. Graefes Arch Clin Exp Ophthalmol. 2010;248:1567–72.
83. Ota M, Tsujikawa A, Kita M, Miyamoto K, Sakamoto A, et al. Integrity of foveal photoreceptor layer in central retinal vein occlusion. Retina. 2008;28:1502–8.
84. Murakami T, Tsujikawa A, Ohta M, Miyamoto K, Kita M, et al. Photoreceptor status after resolved macular edema in branch retinal vein occlusion treated with tissue plasminogen activator. Am J Ophthalmol. 2007;143:171–3.
85. Ota M, Tsujikawa A, Murakami T, Yamaike N, Sakamoto A, et al. Foveal photoreceptor layer in eyes with persistent cystoid macular edema associated with branch retinal vein occlusion. Am J Ophthalmol. 2008;145:273–80.

86. Tsujikawa A, Sakamoto A, Ota M, Kotera Y, Oh H, et al. Serous retinal detachment associated with retinal vein occlusion. Am J Ophthalmol. 2010;149(291–301):e295.
87. Marmor MF. Mechanisms of fluid accumulation in retinal edema. Doc Ophthalmol. 1999;97:239–49.
88. Hasegawa T, Masuda N, Ogata N. Highly reflective line in optical coherence tomography images of eyes with macular edema associated with branch retinal vein occlusion. Am J Ophthalmol. 2015;159(5):925–33.e1.
89. Kang JW, Lee H, Chung H, Kim HC. Correlation between optical coherence tomographic hyperreflective foci and visual outcomes after intravitreal bevacizumab for macular edema in branch retinal vein occlusion. Graefes Arch Clin Exp Ophthalmol. 2014;252:1413–21.
90. Nishijima K, Murakami T, Hirashima T, Uji A, Akagi T, et al. Hyperreflective foci in outer retina predictive of photoreceptor damage and poor vision after vitrectomy for diabetic macular edema. Retina. 2014;34:732–40.
91. Akagi-Kurashige Y, Tsujikawa A, Oishi A, Ooto S, Yamashiro K, et al. Relationship between retinal morphological findings and visual function in age-related macular degeneration. Graefes Arch Clin Exp Ophthalmol. 2012;250:1129–36.
92. Hasegawa T, Ueda T, Okamoto M, Ogata N. Presence of foveal bulge in optical coherence tomographic images in eyes with macular edema associated with branch retinal vein occlusion. Am J Ophthalmol. 2014;157(390–396):e391.
93. Yamaike N, Tsujikawa A, Ota M, Sakamoto A, Kotera Y, et al. Three-dimensional imaging of cystoid macular edema in retinal vein occlusion. Ophthalmology. 2008;115(355–362):e352.
94. Kang HM, Chung EJ, Kim YM, Koh HJ. Spectral-domain optical coherence tomography (SD-OCT) patterns and response to intravitreal bevacizumab therapy in macular edema associated with branch retinal vein occlusion. Graefes Arch Clin Exp Ophthalmol. 2013;251:501–8.
95. Shin HJ, Chung H, Kim HC. Association between integrity of foveal photoreceptor layer and visual outcome in retinal vein occlusion. Acta Ophthalmol. 2011;89:e35–40.
96. Haymore JG, Mejico LJ. Retinal vascular occlusion syndromes. Int Ophthalmol Clin. 2009;49:63–79.
97. Chung YK, Shin JA, Park YH. Choroidal volume in branch retinal vein occlusion before and after intravitreal anti-vegf injection. Retina. 2015;35(6):1234–9.
98. Tsuiki E, Suzuma K, Ueki R, Maekawa Y, Kitaoka T. Enhanced depth imaging optical coherence tomography of the choroid in central retinal vein occlusion. Am J Ophthalmol. 2013;156(543–547):e541.
99. Mirza RG, Johnson MW, Jampol LM. Optical coherence tomography use in evaluation of the vitreoretinal interface: a review. Surv Ophthalmol. 2007;52:397–421.
100. Wilkins JR, Puliafito CA, Hee MR, Duker JS, Reichel E, et al. Characterization of epiretinal membranes using optical coherence tomography. Ophthalmology. 1996;103:2142–51.
101. Sebag J. Oval defect in detached posterior hyaloid membrane in idiopathic preretinal macular fibrosis. Am J Ophthalmol. 1995;119:814–5.
102. Kishi S, Shimizu K. Oval defect in detached posterior hyaloid membrane in idiopathic preretinal macular fibrosis. Am J Ophthalmol. 1994;118:451–6.
103. Johnson MW. Perifoveal vitreous detachment and its macular complications. Trans Am Ophthalmol Soc. 2005;103:537–67.
104. Jaffe NS. Vitreous traction at the posterior pole of the fundus due to alterations in the vitreous posterior. Trans Am Acad Ophthalmol Otolaryngol. 1967;71:642–52.
105. Gandorfer A, Benz MS, Haller JA, Stalmans P, Pakola SJ, et al. Association between anatomical resolution and functional outcomes in the mivi-trust studies using ocriplasmin to treat symptomatic vitreomacular adhesion/vitreomacular traction, including when associated with macular hole. Retina. 2015;35(6):1151–7.
106. Chang LK, Fine HF, Spaide RF, Koizumi H, Grossniklaus HE. Ultrastructural correlation of spectral-domain optical coherence tomographic findings in vitreomacular traction syndrome. Am J Ophthalmol. 2008;146:121–7.

107. Koizumi H, Spaide RF, Fisher YL, Freund KB, Klancnik Jr JM, et al. Three-dimensional evaluation of vitreomacular traction and epiretinal membrane using spectral-domain optical coherence tomography. Am J Ophthalmol. 2008;145:509–17.
108. Sonmez K, Capone Jr A, Trese MT, Williams GA. Vitreomacular traction syndrome: impact of anatomical configuration on anatomical and visual outcomes. Retina. 2008;28:1207–14.
109. Yamada N, Kishi S. Tomographic features and surgical outcomes of vitreomacular traction syndrome. Am J Ophthalmol. 2005;139:112–7.
110. Hassenstein A, Bialasiewicz AA, Richard G. Optical coherence tomography in uveitis patients. Am J Ophthalmol. 2000;130:669–70.
111. Markomichelakis NN, Halkiadakis I, Pantelia E, Peponis V, Patelis A, et al. Patterns of macular edema in patients with uveitis: qualitative and quantitative assessment using optical coherence tomography. Ophthalmology. 2004;111:946–53.
112. Iannetti L, Accorinti M, Liverani M, Caggiano C, Abdulaziz R, et al. Optical coherence tomography for classification and clinical evaluation of macular edema in patients with uveitis. Ocul Immunol Inflamm. 2008;16:155–60.
113. Estafanous MF, Lowder CY, Kaiser PK. Patterns of macular edema in uveitis patients. Ophthalmology. 2005;112:360; author reply 360–1.
114. Sivaprasad S, Ikeji F, Xing W, Lightman S. Tomographic assessment of therapeutic response to uveitic macular oedema. Clin Experiment Ophthalmol. 2007;35:719–23.
115. Castellano CG, Stinnett SS, Mettu PS, McCallum RM, Jaffe GJ. Retinal thickening in iridocyclitis. Am J Ophthalmol. 2009;148:341–9.
116. Moreno-Arrones JP, Gorrono-Echebarria MB, Teus-Guezala MA. Macular thickening in acute anterior uveitis with a 6-month remission period. Can J Ophthalmol. 2010;45:91–2.
117. Al-Mezaine HS, Al-Muammar A, Kangave D, Abu El-Asrar AM. Clinical and optical coherence tomographic findings and outcome of treatment in patients with presumed tuberculous uveitis. Int Ophthalmol. 2008;28:413–23.
118. Iannetti L, Spinucci G, Abbouda A, De Geronimo D, Tortorella P, et al. Spectral-domain optical coherence tomography in uveitic macular edema: morphological features and prognostic factors. Ophthalmologica. 2012;228:13–8.
119. Roesel M, Heimes B, Heinz C, Henschel A, Spital G, et al. Comparison of retinal thickness and fundus-related microperimetry with visual acuity in uveitic macular oedema. Acta Ophthalmol. 2011;89:533–7.
120. Belair ML, Kim SJ, Thorne JE, Dunn JP, Kedhar SR, et al. Incidence of cystoid macular edema after cataract surgery in patients with and without uveitis using optical coherence tomography. Am J Ophthalmol. 2009;148(128–135):e122.
121. Faia LJ, Sen HN, Li Z, Yeh S, Wroblewski KJ, et al. Treatment of inflammatory macular edema with humanized anti-CD11a antibody therapy. Invest Ophthalmol Vis Sci. 2011;52:6919–24.
122. Androudi S, Tsironi E, Kalogeropoulos C, Theodoridou A, Brazitikos P. Intravitreal adalimumab for refractory uveitis-related macular edema. Ophthalmology. 2010;117:1612–6.
123. Lehpamer B, Moshier E, Goldberg N, Ackert J, Godbold J, et al. Subretinal fluid in uveitic macular edema: effect on vision and response to therapy. Am J Ophthalmol. 2013;155:143–9.
124. Markomichelakis NN, Halkiadakis I, Pantelia E, Georgalas I, Chrysanthi K, et al. Course of macular edema in uveitis under medical treatment. Ocul Immunol Inflamm. 2007;15:71–9.
125. Munk MR, Kiss CG, Ekmekcioglu C, Huf W, Sulzbacher F, et al. Influence of orthostasis and daytime on retinal thickness in uveitis-associated cystoid macular edema. Curr Eye Res. 2014;39:395–402.
126. Ducos de Lahitte G, Terrada C, Tran TH, Cassoux N, LeHoang P, et al. Maculopathy in uveitis of juvenile idiopathic arthritis: an optical coherence tomography study. Br J Ophthalmol. 2008;92:64–9.
127. Kalinina Ayuso V, Makhotkina N, van Tent-Hoeve M, de Groot-Mijnes JD, Wulffraat NM, et al. Pathogenesis of juvenile idiopathic arthritis associated uveitis: the known and unknown. Surv Ophthalmol. 2014;59:517–31.

128. de Boer J, Steijaert A, van den Bor R, Stellato R, Ossewaarde-van Norel J. Development of macular edema and impact on visual acuity in uveitis associated with juvenile idiopathic arthritis. Ocul Immunol Inflamm. 2015;23:67–73.
129. Sugar EA, Jabs DA, Altaweel MM, Lightman S, Acharya N, et al. Identifying a clinically meaningful threshold for change in uveitic macular edema evaluated by optical coherence tomography. Am J Ophthalmol. 2011;152(1044–1052):e1045.
130. Kempen JH, Sugar EA, Jaffe GJ, Acharya NR, Dunn JP, et al. Fluorescein angiography versus optical coherence tomography for diagnosis of uveitic macular edema. Ophthalmology. 2013;120:1852–9.
131. Domalpally A, Altaweel MM, Kempen JH, Myers D, Davis JL, et al. Optical coherence tomography evaluation in the Multicenter Uveitis Steroid Treatment (MUST) trial. Ocul Immunol Inflamm. 2012;20:443–7.
132. Payne JF, Bruce BB, Lee LB, Yeh S. Logarithmic transformation of spectral-domain optical coherence tomography data in uveitis-associated macular edema. Invest Ophthalmol Vis Sci. 2011;52:8939–43.
133. Brar M, Yuson R, Kozak I, Mojana F, Cheng L, et al. Correlation between morphologic features on spectral-domain optical coherence tomography and angiographic leakage patterns in macular edema. Retina. 2010;30:383–9.
134. Tran TH, de Smet MD, Bodaghi B, Fardeau C, Cassoux N, et al. Uveitic macular oedema: correlation between optical coherence tomography patterns with visual acuity and fluorescein angiography. Br J Ophthalmol. 2008;92:922–7.
135. De Laey JJ. Fluorescein angiography in posterior uveitis. Int Ophthalmol Clin. 1995;35: 33–58.
136. Miyake K. Prevention of cystoid macular edema after lens extraction by topical indomethacin (I). A preliminary report. Albrecht Von Graefes Arch Klin Exp Ophthalmol. 1977;203: 81–8.
137. Munk MR, Sacu S, Huf W, Sulzbacher F, Mittermuller TJ, et al. Differential diagnosis of macular edema of different pathophysiologic origins by spectral domain optical coherence tomography. Retina. 2014;34:2218–32.
138. Ogino K, Murakami T, Tsujikawa A, Miyamoto K, Sakamoto A, et al. Characteristics of optical coherence tomographic hyperreflective foci in retinal vein occlusion. Retina. 2012;32: 77–85.
139. Tso MO. Animal modeling of cystoid macular edema. Surv Ophthalmol. 1984;28(Suppl): 512–9.
140. Ossewaarde-van Norel J, Berg EM, Sijssens KM, Rothova A. Subfoveal serous retinal detachment in patients with uveitic macular edema. Arch Ophthalmol. 2011;129:158–62.
141. Nakayama M, Keino H, Okada AA, Watanabe T, Taki W, et al. Enhanced depth imaging optical coherence tomography of the choroid in Vogt-Koyanagi-Harada disease. Retina. 2012;32: 2061–9.
142. Kim M, Kim H, Kwon HJ, Kim SS, Koh HJ, et al. Choroidal thickness in Behcet's uveitis: an enhanced depth imaging-optical coherence tomography and its association with angiographic changes. Invest Ophthalmol Vis Sci. 2013;54:6033–9.
143. Gehl Z, Kulcsar K, Kiss HJ, Nemeth J, Maneschg OA, et al. Retinal and choroidal thickness measurements using spectral domain optical coherence tomography in anterior and intermediate uveitis. BMC Ophthalmol. 2014;14:103.
144. Moroi SE, Gottfredsdottir MS, Schteingart MT, Elner SG, Lee CM, et al. Cystoid macular edema associated with latanoprost therapy in a case series of patients with glaucoma and ocular hypertension. Ophthalmology. 1999;106:1024–9.
145. Telander DG, Sarraf D. Cystoid macular edema with docetaxel chemotherapy and the fluid retention syndrome. Semin Ophthalmol. 2007;22:151–3.
146. Modi D, Dubovy SR. Non-leaking cystoid maculopathy secondary to systemic paclitaxel. Ophthalmic Surg Lasers Imaging Retina. 2013;44:183–6.
147. Koo NK, Kim YC. A case of paclitaxel-induced maculopathy treated with methazolamide. Korean J Ophthalmol. 2012;26:394–7.

148. Joshi MM, Garretson BR. Paclitaxel maculopathy. Arch Ophthalmol. 2007;125:709–10.
149. Ryan Jr EH, Han DP, Ramsay RC, Cantrill HL, Bennett SR, et al. Diabetic macular edema associated with glitazone use. Retina. 2006;26:562–70.
150. Schmitz-Valckenberg S, Holz FG, Bird AC, Spaide RF. Fundus autofluorescence imaging: review and perspectives. Retina. 2008;28:385–409.
151. Trieschmann M, van Kuijk FJ, Alexander R, Hermans P, Luthert P, et al. Macular pigment in the human retina: histological evaluation of localization and distribution. Eye (Lond). 2008;22: 132–7.
152. Meleth AD, Sen HN. Use of fundus autofluorescence in the diagnosis and management of uveitis. Int Ophthalmol Clin. 2012;52:45–54.
153. McBain VA, Forrester JV, Lois N. Fundus autofluorescence in the diagnosis of cystoid macular oedema. Br J Ophthalmol. 2008;92:946–9.
154. Bessho K, Gomi F, Harino S, Sawa M, Sayanagi K, et al. Macular autofluorescence in eyes with cystoid macula edema, detected with 488 nm-excitation but not with 580 nm-excitation. Graefes Arch Clin Exp Ophthalmol. 2009;247:729–34.
155. Pece A, Isola V, Holz F, Milani P, Brancato R. Autofluorescence imaging of cystoid macular edema in diabetic retinopathy. Ophthalmologica. 2010;224:230–5.
156. Chung H, Park B, Shin HJ, Kim HC. Correlation of fundus autofluorescence with spectral-domain optical coherence tomography and vision in diabetic macular edema. Ophthalmology. 2012;119:1056–65.
157. Vujosevic S, Casciano M, Pilotto E, Boccassini B, Varano M, et al. Diabetic macular edema: fundus autofluorescence and functional correlations. Invest Ophthalmol Vis Sci. 2011;52: 442–8.
158. Roesel M, Henschel A, Heinz C, Dietzel M, Spital G, et al. Fundus autofluorescence and spectral domain optical coherence tomography in uveitic macular edema. Graefes Arch Clin Exp Ophthalmol. 2009;247:1685–9.
159. Bindewald A, Jorzik JJ, Roth F, Holz FG. cSLO digital fundus autofluorescence imaging. Ophthalmologe. 2005;102:259–64.
160. Shen Y, Xu X, Liu K. Fundus autofluorescence characteristics in patients with diabetic macular edema. Chin Med J (Engl). 2014;127:1423–8.
161. Lumbroso B, Huang D, Romano A, Rispoli M, Coscas G. Clinical en face OCT atlas. New Delhi: Jaypee Brother Medical Publishers; 2013.
162. Wanek J, Zelkha R, Lim JI, Shahidi M. Feasibility of a method for en face imaging of photoreceptor cell integrity. Am J Ophthalmol. 2011;152(807–814):e801.
163. Ohkoshi K, Tsuiki E, Kitaoka T, Yamaguchi T. Visualization of subthreshold micropulse diode laser photocoagulation by scanning laser ophthalmoscopy in the retro mode. Am J Ophthalmol. 2010;150:856–62.
164. Yamamoto M, Mizukami S, Tsujikawa A, Miyoshi N, Yoshimura N. Visualization of cystoid macular oedema using a scanning laser ophthalmoscope in the retro-mode. Clin Experiment Ophthalmol. 2010;38:27–36.
165. Michaely R, Bachmann AH, Villiger ML, Blatter C, Lasser T, et al. Vectorial reconstruction of retinal blood flow in three dimensions measured with high resolution resonant Doppler Fourier domain optical coherence tomography. J Biomed Opt. 2007;12: 041213.
166. Yasuno Y, Hong Y, Makita S, Yamanari M, Akiba M, et al. In vivo high-contrast imaging of deep posterior eye by 1-microm swept source optical coherence tomography and scattering optical coherence angiography. Opt Express. 2007;15:6121–39.
167. Povazay B, Hermann B, Unterhuber A, Hofer B, Sattmann H, et al. Three-dimensional optical coherence tomography at 1050 nm versus 800 nm in retinal pathologies: enhanced performance and choroidal penetration in cataract patients. J Biomed Opt. 2007;12: 041211.
168. Gocho K, Kikuchi S, Kabuto T, Kameya S, Shinoda K, et al. High-resolution en face images of microcystic macular edema in patients with autosomal dominant optic atrophy. Biomed Res Int. 2013;2013:676803.

169. Akagi-Kurashige Y, Tsujikawa A, Ooto S, Makiyama Y, Muraoka Y, et al. Retinal microstructural changes in eyes with resolved branch retinal vein occlusion: an adaptive optics scanning laser ophthalmoscopy study. Am J Ophthalmol. 2014;157(1239–1249):e1233.
170. Scholl S, Kirchhof J, Augustin AJ. Pathophysiology of macular edema. Ophthalmologica. 2010;224 Suppl 1:8–15.
171. Augustin A, Loewenstein A, Kuppermann BD. Macular edema. General pathophysiology. Dev Ophthalmol. 2010;47:10–26.
172. Reichenbach A, Wurm A, Pannicke T, Iandiev I, Wiedemann P, et al. Muller cells as players in retinal degeneration and edema. Graefes Arch Clin Exp Ophthalmol. 2007;245:627–36.
173. Wang RK. Optical microangiography: a label free 3D imaging technology to visualize and quantify blood circulations within tissue beds in vivo. IEEE J Sel Top Quantum Electron. 2010;16:545–54.
174. Kim DY, Fingler J, Werner JS, Schwartz DM, Fraser SE, et al. In vivo volumetric imaging of human retinal circulation with phase-variance optical coherence tomography. Biomed Opt Express. 2011;2:1504–13.
175. Makita S, Hong Y, Yamanari M, Yatagai T, Yasuno Y. Optical coherence angiography. Opt Express. 2006;14:7821–40.
176. Xu J, Han S, Balaratnasingam C, Mammo Z, Wong KS, et al. Retinal angiography with real-time speckle variance optical coherence tomography. Br J Ophthalmol. 2015;99(10):1315–9.
177. Hendargo HC, Estrada R, Chiu SJ, Tomasi C, Farsiu S, et al. Automated non-rigid registration and mosaicing for robust imaging of distinct retinal capillary beds using speckle variance optical coherence tomography. Biomed Opt Express. 2013;4:803–21.
178. Hong Y, Makita S, Yamanari M, Miura M, Kim S, et al. Three-dimensional visualization of choroidal vessels by using standard and ultra-high resolution scattering optical coherence angiography. Opt Express. 2007;15:7538–50.
179. Vujosevic S, Trento B, Bottega E, Urban F, Pilotto E, et al. Scanning laser ophthalmoscopy in the retromode in diabetic macular oedema. Acta Ophthalmol. 2012;90:e374–80.
180. Vujosevic S, Pucci P, Daniele AR, Convento E, Pilotto E, et al. Extent of diabetic macular edema by scanning laser ophthalmoscope in the retromode and its functional correlations. Retina. 2014;34:2416–22.
181. Murakami T, Nishijima K, Sakamoto A, Ota M, Horii T, et al. Foveal cystoid spaces are associated with enlarged foveal avascular zone and microaneurysms in diabetic macular edema. Ophthalmology. 2011;118:359–67.
182. Maldonado RS, O'Connell R, Ascher SB, Sarin N, Freedman SF, et al. Spectral-domain optical coherence tomographic assessment of severity of cystoid macular edema in retinopathy of prematurity. Arch Ophthalmol. 2012;130:569–78.
183. Rothman AL, Tran-Viet D, Gustafson KE, Goldstein RF, Maguire MG, et al. Poorer neurodevelopmental outcomes associated with cystoid macular edema identified in preterm infants in the intensive care nursery. Ophthalmology. 2015;122:610–9.

Part II
Medical Management of CME

Chapter 4
Medical Management of CME Associated with Uveitis

Sarah M. Escott and Debra A. Goldstein

Introduction

Cystoid macular edema (CME) develops following disruption to the blood-retinal barrier (BRB) and is the most common cause of vision loss in patients with uveitis [1]. Intraocular inflammation causes cellular damage resulting in activation of the arachidonic acid cascade and release of prostaglandins (PGE), nitric oxide (NO), interleukin 6 (IL-6), and vascular endothelial growth factor (VEGF) [2, 3]. These inflammatory mediators have been identified in the aqueous humor of patients with active uveitis leading to a pathologic hyperpermeability of the retinal vessel walls and causing damage to the RPE, resulting in fluid and protein extravasation into the retinal interstitium [4, 5]. Smoking and coexistent vascular disease also play a role in the pathogenesis of inflammatory macular edema [4, 6, 7].

The overall reported prevalence of visual impairment associated with uveitic CME is 33–42 % and is influenced by the location, severity, and duration of retinal edema [1, 8, 9]. Uveitic macular edema does not correlate with degree of active inflammation and may be diagnosed in up to 29 % of patients despite an overall inactivity of their uveitis [10]. Vision loss resulting from CME is more commonly reported in cases of intermediate and panuveitis as compared to anterior uveitis [8]. Poor visual prognostic indicators include advanced age, prolonged duration of uveitis, prolonged presence of edema, enlarged foveal avascular zone, and incomplete vitreous detachment [11]. Visual improvement occurs more often when CME has been present for ≤12 months compared to longer than 24 months [12, 13]. Chronic edema can lead to permanent photoreceptor damage, retinal atrophy, and fibrosis, such that normal vision may not return even with resolution of edema [14]. Further, restoring normal retinal architecture, even without restoration of normal vision, has

S.M. Escott, MD • D.A. Goldstein, MD (✉)
Department of Ophthalmology, Feinberg School of Medicine, Northwestern University, Chicago, IL, USA
e-mail: debrgold@yahoo.com

S. Schaal, H.J. Kaplan (eds.), *Cystoid Macular Edema*,
DOI 10.1007/978-3-319-39766-5_4

a better prognosis for maintaining visual acuity [8]. For these reasons, the presence of any amount of CME warrants treatment.

Medical treatment options include nonsteroidal anti-inflammatory medications (NSAIDs), corticosteroids, anti-VEGF agents, and systemic immunomodulatory therapies. Steroids can be given topically, orally, via periocular or intravitreal injection, and by administration of depot preparations. The use of carbonic anhydrase inhibitors and octreotide has been suggested, but are not routinely used to treat uveitic ME [15, 16].

Nonsteroidal Anti-inflammatory Medications

Topical NSAIDs block cyclooxygenase enzymes and inhibit prostaglandin synthesis thereby reducing inflammation, and have been shown to be effective at reestablishing the blood-aqueous barrier [17]. While the use of topical nonsteroidal anti-inflammatory medications has been proven efficacious for pseudophakic macular edema following cataract extraction, its use in uveitic ME has been disappointing [18]. Although not available in the USA, 3 months of topical 0.5 % indomethacin (INDOM) was shown to statistically improve acute inflammatory ME related to uveitis as compared to placebo in a randomized prospective trial [19].

Corticosteroids

Corticosteroids possess anti-inflammatory and antiangiogenic properties due to their ability to suppress the production of inflammatory mediators (IL-6, PGE, VEGF) in a dose-dependent manner making them a good therapeutic option; they have been the mainstay of treatment for decades. More importantly, they have been shown to stabilize the endothelial and RPE tight junctions [20]. During the acute phase of inflammation, corticosteroids are highly effective due to their quick onset of action; however, side effects limit their long-term use [21].

Topical Corticosteroids

Most topical treatments are inadequate for posterior segment disease due to pharmacokinetic limitations [22]. Recently, however, data suggest that topical difluprednate 0.05 % (Durezol; Alcon Laboratories) may have superior intraocular penetration as compared to other topical steroids. In addition, it does not contain the preservative benzalkonium chloride, an agent known to cause immunoallergic reactions, disrupt tear film stability, and cause toxic effects to the corneal epithelium [23]. Its high potency and limited systemic absorption make it an attractive therapeutic option [24]. It has been FDA approved for the treatment of postoperative inflammation and pain as well as anterior uveitis [25, 26].

Slabaugh et al. demonstrated a dramatic improvement in uveitic CME with difluprednate as both monotherapy and an adjuvant to immunomodulatory therapy in children with uveitis and macular edema; however, its benefit must be weighed against the heightened risk of cataract development (38 %) and clinically significant intraocular pressure elevation in this age group [27, 28]. Peak intraocular pressures of more than 30 mmHg were demonstrated to occur in 20 % of all eyes treated with difluprednate in one study, with 80 % of children experiencing a rise of more than 15 mmHg [28]. These studies emphasize the unpredictable, rapid, and dramatic IOP response to difluprednate in patients with uveitis and the need for close monitoring of IOP at every visit, especially in children. There are currently no randomized controlled trials comparing the efficacy of topical difluprednate to other steroid therapies for the treatment of uveitic CME.

Systemic Corticosteroids

Oral corticosteroids are indicated for the treatment of vision-threatening uveitis. Oral prednisone is most often used, starting at a dosage of 0.75–2 mg/kg/day until inflammation responds, and then tapered gradually [29]. High doses of systemic corticosteroids can achieve rapid anatomical recovery of CME; however, their long-term use is not recommended due to serious potential side effects including peptic ulceration, Cushing syndrome, adrenal suppression, aseptic necrosis of the hip, systemic hypertension, and hyperglycemia [21, 30]. The Standardization of Uveitis Nomenclature (SUN) Working group has recommended consideration of alternate therapy if intraocular inflammation cannot be controlled with less than 7.5–10 mg per day of oral prednisone, or its equivalent, by 3 months [31].

Periocular Corticosteroids

Periocular injection of corticosteroids has the ability to deliver a high concentration of drug within close proximity to the macula, making it an effective treatment for uveitic CME [32]. These injections are a useful adjunct to systemic treatment for uveitis when persistent or refractory macular edema is present; however, the effects can be temporary and serial injections are often necessary [33, 34]. Posterior subtenon (PSTK) or orbital floor injections of 40 mg of triamcinolone acetonide are the most commonly used methods of administration [34–36]. The effect on active inflammation has been observed to occur within days, and improvement in CME occurs within weeks to months [35, 36]. Resolution of macular edema occurs in approximately 50 % of patients 1–3 months following a single periocular injection, and the effect can last between 3 and 7 months [33–35]. In patients whose edema does not respond to one injection, resolution of edema has been demonstrated in 50–78 % of patients following serial injections, suggesting that there is added benefit with repeated treatments [33, 34].

Periocular triamcinolone injections have also been proven effective at controlling inflammation and reducing uveitic CME in children. In one combined prospective study, all eyes experienced improvement in anterior chamber inflammation following a single injection; however, relapse occurred after a mean of 4 months in 50 % of eyes. Of those eyes with uveitic CME at the time of treatment, resolution of the edema was observed in 55 % of eyes [37].

Common complications from periocular injections include ptosis, elevated IOP, and cataract progression. Elevation of IOP >24 mmHg is reported to occur in 22–34 % of eyes following periocular steroid injection, with a progression to requiring glaucoma surgery in 0.9–2.4 % within a year. The incidence of cataract progression is between fifteen and twenty percent [38, 39]. In children, visually significant cataract developed in 21 % of eyes at 5 months in one series, and was more common in eyes with mild posterior subcapsular opacities at the time of injection [37]. Rare but potentially devastating complications of periocular injections include globe perforation, optic nerve injuries, retinal detachment, and vascular occlusion [34, 40].

Intravitreal Corticosteroids

Intravitreal corticosteroids have been used to treat various types of macular edema. Because other corticosteroids disappear in the vitreal cavity within a few days, triamcinolone acetonide (TA), which is largely water insoluble, is most commonly administered [41]. One study demonstrated the elimination half-life following a single injection of triamcinolone (4 mg/0.1 ml) to be approximately 18.7 (+/- 5) days for nonvitrecomized eyes and 2.3 days for one vitrecomized eye [41].

Intravitreal TA leads to a better response in resolving inflammatory macular edema when compared to periocular administration; however, the benefits are also transient, and they carry similar rates of posterior subcapsular cataract and IOP elevation, with the added risk of endophthalmitis [42]. Studies suggest improvement in macular edema can be detected as early as 1 week, with a peak response in 4–6 weeks and duration of effect between 6 weeks and 6 months. Many patients require more than one injection, and similar improvements in visual acuity and inflammatory edema may be achieved with repeat injections [43–45]. The greatest improvement in visual acuity was achieved in patients less than 60 years of age and in eyes with CME present for less than 12 months duration in one series. CME present for longer than 24 months was associated with the least improvement in visual acuity, even with improvement in macular thickness on OCT [13].

Elevation of intraocular pressure >10 mmHg has been reported in 25–34 % of eyes at a mean duration of 4–5 weeks following intravitreal triamcinolone injection. Antiglaucoma treatment was necessary in nearly 50 % of eyes in two large case series with no eyes requiring filtration surgery [13, 45]. Kok et al. observed a more profound IOP effect in eyes of patients younger than 40 years [13].

Cataract development has been observed in 15–30 % of patients receiving intravitreal triamcinolone injections; the risk increases following repeated injections [45]. In addition to elevated IOP and cataract, intravitreal triamcinolone carries a 0.05–0.1 % risk of endophthalmitis [46, 47].

Intravitreal Corticosteroid Depot Preparations

Implantable long-acting corticosteroid therapies allow for delivery of a higher concentration of medication to the posterior segment over a sustained period while avoiding systemic side effects. These are beneficial options for treating patients with moderate to severe disease and for whom systemic immunosuppression medications are contraindicated, intolerable, or not able to completely control inflammation.

Ozurdex

Dexamethasone is five times more potent than triamcinolone acetonide and more hydrophilic, allowing for higher vitreous concentrations; however, the clinical utility of single intravitreal injection is limited due to its short half-life of only 3 h [48].

The biodegradable dexamethasone intravitreal implant (Ozurdex, Allergan) is designed to deliver 700 μg of preservative-free dexamethasone in a sustained-release manner over 3–6 months. The implant is made of a solid polymer which enables dual-phase pharmacokinetics, initially releasing a burst of dexamethasone to rapidly achieve a therapeutic concentration, followed by a slower sustained release [49]. The implant is administered as an office-based intravitreal injection using a 22-gauge injecting applicator through the pars plana under a sterile biplanar technique [49] (Fig. 1). The biodegradable design allows repeat implantation to be performed without need for surgical removal [9].

Ozudex was approved by the US FDA in 2010 as first-line therapy in the treatment of macular edema associated with noninfectious intermediate and posterior uveitis [50]. Drug diffusion and clearance from the vitreous cavity is more rapid in vitrectomized eyes; studies show the effect at 3 months is only maintained in a third of vitrectomized eyes which had improvement in CME at 1 month. Due to risk of migration into the anterior chamber and subsequent corneal decompensation, the implant should not be used in aphakic vitrectomized eyes [51].

A randomized clinical trial demonstrated excellent results in the reduction of vitreous haze for patients with noninfectious intermediate uveitis; however, the mean improvement in macular edema dissipated before 26 weeks, suggesting the need for reinjection to treat CME [52]. Other reports suggest the implant is effective at treating refractory uveitic ME refractory for a period of 3–4 months with most patients requiring repeat implants within 6 months for recurrent CME [51, 53].

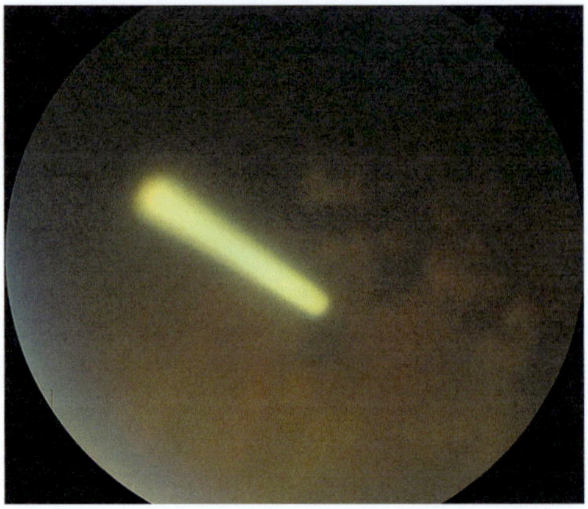

Fig. 1 Ozurdex implant imaged in the vitreous immediately following injection in a patient with multifocal choroiditis

Multiple implants were required in 63 % of eyes in one retrospective observational study of patients with active noninfectious uveitis, 91 % of which had CME, over a 17-month period [54]. The response to repeat Ozurdex implantation mirrors that seen after a single injection; improvement in visual acuity and macular edema is observed after 1 month. The effects of repeated injections have shown to be cumulative, with long-term improvement in best-corrected visual acuity and stabilization of central retinal thickness over 24 months [54].

Although studies suggest no statistically significant increase in the rate of cataract formation between treatment and sham patients following one dexamethasone implant [52], one study did report development of posterior subcapsular opacity following a third injection [54]. Lowder et al. described <5 % incidence of IOP ≥ 30 mg Hg following a single Ozurdex implantation, with no eyes requiring surgical intervention [52]. However, there is some evidence that, in clinical practice, IOP elevation secondary to the dexamethasone implant may be greater than that reported in the registration trials [55, 56].

Retisert

In 2005, the FDA approved a nonbiodegradable intraocular sustained-release implant containing fluocinolone acetonide (Retisert, Bausch and Lomb) for use in the treatment of noninfectious intermediate, posterior, and panuveitis [57] (Fig. 2). The implant is designed to deliver 590 μg of fluocinolone acetonide over a 2–3-year period with minimal systemic absorption [58, 59]. The device is surgically anchored to the pars plana in the operating room under sterile conditions and can be monitored in the office through the dilated pupil (Fig. 3).

A large multicenter trial has demonstrated a reduction in uveitis recurrences from 51 to 6 % over 34 weeks with improvement in visual acuity [60]. Further, the proportion of eyes with a reduction in CME was greater for implanted eyes (86 %) compared to nonimplanted eyes (28 %) at 1 year, and this effect was maintained at 3 years [58].

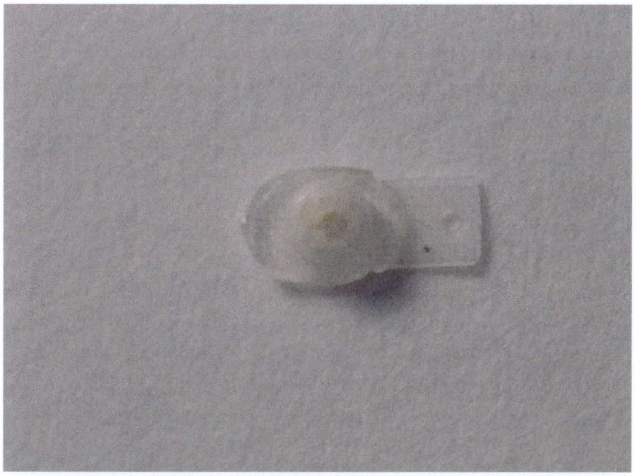

Fig. 2 Retisert pellet and strut before implantation. This is the currently available implant

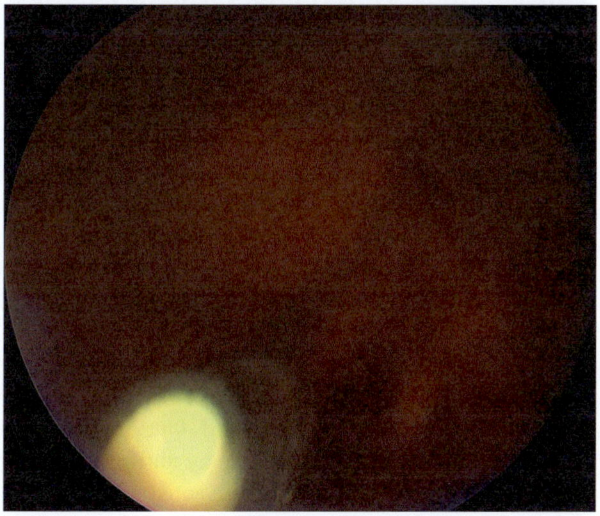

Fig. 3 Retisert imaged in position. Note the ability to see the pellet properly positioned on the strut. This is the model of implant that is no longer available, because of issues with pellet strut separation

In another report, 92 % of patients using systemic medications to control intraocular inflammation were able to reduce their dose following implantation, and all eyes with preoperative CME had statistically significant reduced retinal thickness at 6 and 12 months [61]. In a randomized controlled parallel superiority study comparing the fluocinolone implant with systemic therapy, 46 % of the patients in the implant group with macular edema experienced resolution of CME compared to only 23 % of systemically treated patients [62].

Data from three large registration trials revealed that, over a 3-year treatment period, 74.8 % of eyes receiving a fluocinolone acetonide implant required intraocular pressure lowering therapy. Approximately 50 % of eyes experienced an IOP >30 mmHg, commonly occurring within the first year following implantation. Surgical intervention was required in one-third of patients based on uncontrolled

IOP, visual field, or disk changes [60, 63, 64]. Baseline visual field testing and optic nerve imaging are therefore recommended for patients undergoing fluocinolone implant surgery [63]. The fluocinolone acetonide implant carries a nearly 100 % incidence of cataract progression [60, 64]. Studies have demonstrated the feasibility and success of combined cataract extraction with IOL insertion at the time of fluocinolone acetonide implantation [61].

Additional risks of implant surgery include vitreous hemorrhage, hyphema, retinal detachment, and endophthalmitis [61]. Spontaneous separation of the medication pellet from its attachment is a rare but potential complication that may require surgery [65–67]. Complications such as retinal commotio, retinal tear, and endothelial failure due to dislocation of the pellet into the anterior chamber have also been reported [66, 67].

Anti-vascular Endothelial Growth Factor Medications

Vascular endothelial growth factor (VEGF) has been found in the aqueous humor of patients with uveitis and plays a role in the loss of vascular integrity which ultimately causes CME [4, 68, 69]. VEGF expression is induced by inflammatory mediators and cytokines which are produced and abundantly present in the eyes of patients with uveitis [4, 68]. Further, VEGF concentrations have been shown to be higher in patients who had CME associated with uveitis as compared to those without CME [69].

The use of intravitreal anti-VEGF therapies bevacizumab and ranibizumab has recently been described as off-label treatment for inflammatory CME; however, their effects in this setting are not well established and results have been inconsistent [12, 70–76]. Numerous studies have observed statistically significant decrease in central retina thickness on optical coherence tomography [71–74], while others report limited to no change [75, 76]. One reason for this may be that anti-VEGF agents have not been shown to display anti-inflammatory properties, and therefore, studies which included patients with active uveitis at the time of treatment may have underestimated their effect on CME [75, 76].

Mackensen et al. showed statistically significant reduction in macular thickness beginning as early as 2 weeks following a single bevacizumab injection for patients with controlled uveitis but breakthrough CME refractory to steroid therapies. These effects, however, were sustained for only 6–8 weeks, and repeat injections were required [73]. Lott et al. observed a 40 % worsening of vision and no improvement in central retinal thickness for eyes treated with intravitreal bevacizumab only; however, most of the patients in this series had active uveitis at the time of treatment [75].

Acharya et al. demonstrated a positive effect of monthly ranibizumab injection in eyes with controlled uveitis and persistent CME in a small prospective, noncomparative, interventional case series [71]. Improvement in macular edema occurred as early as 1 week and was maintained at 3 months in all eyes. Approximately 60 % of eyes required repeat injection, and these results were preserved 3 months after cessation of treatment [71].

The ideal dosing and sequence for intravitreal anti-VEGF agents in the treatment of inflammatory CME has yet to be determined; however, their length of effect is shorter than for periocular or intravitreal steroid therapies [77]. These agents are much less likely to cause glaucoma or cataract progression compared to steroid therapies; however, serial injections (every 5 weeks) in patients with macular degeneration were shown to lead to sustained elevation of IOP in 3.5–4.5 % of patients following a mean of 20 injections [78]. Mild anterior uveitis has been reported as an adverse side effect following 0.14–1.57 % of bevacizumab injections and 1.38 % with ranibizumab [79, 80].

Intravitreal Methotrexate

Methotrexate (MTX) is a folate antagonist designed to competitively inhibit dihydrofolate reductase which is required for cellular proliferation [81]. It has long been used as a systemic immunomodulatory therapy. MTX has been increasingly used to treat various ophthalmic conditions both locally and systemically.

The off-label use of intravitreal methotrexate to treat uveitic cystoid macular edema was examined in a few small studies [82–84]. In one prospective case series, patients with unilateral active, noninfectious uveitis or inflammatory CME were given intravitreal injections of MTX (400 μg/0.1 ml). A rapid reduction in inflammation and macular thickness was observed within 1 week. Visual acuity improvement of at least two Snellen lines was achieved in 87 % of patients at 3 months. While the inflammation tended to relapse after 4 months, the reduction in macular thickness was maintained at 6 months in all patients where OCT was able to be performed [82].

Other reports have described promising results of intravitreal methotrexate on the control of uveitis with or without CME [84, 85]. One study describes its use for the treatment of refractory unilateral retinal vasculitis due to Behçet disease in patients intolerant of corticosteroids or in whom they were contraindicated [84]. Study eyes underwent monthly intravitreal injections of MTX until remission of intraocular inflammation and/or stable visual acuity was achieved. Increase in visual acuity by three or more Snellen lines was observed in 85 % of study eyes following an average of four injections. Intravitreal MTX therapy resulted in a decrease in aqueous humor levels of IL-6 and IL-8 in treatment eyes [84]. IL-6 has been associated with breakdown of the blood-retinal barrier in uveitic disease, while IL-8 is a mediator of the innate immune response and is thought to play a role in altered vascular permeability [86, 87]. Significant reduction in the levels of these cytokines was associated with clinical improvement in 87 % of eyes [84].

A larger, multicenter, international retrospective case series evaluated eyes with active uveitis or uveitic CME treated with intravitreal MTX. Following one injection, 79 % of eyes entered a period of remission averaging 17 months. Of those who relapsed after one injection, 87 % entered a period of extended remission following a second injection. There was an overall average reduction in macular thickness maintained over a range of 10–30 months. Half of the patients receiving oral corticosteroids at the time of TX injection were able to successfully reduce steroid doses following intravitreal MTX [85].

Based on limited available data, intravitreal MTX may be a reasonable and effective option for patients with active unilateral uveitis and/or inflammatory CME who are known steroid responders or those in whom an elevation of IOP could be immediately detrimental.

Subcutaneous Interferon Alpha

Interferon alpha (IFN) is a cytokine belonging to the subgroup of type I interferons that exert strong antiviral, antiproliferative, and various immunomodulatory effects [88]. The interferons influence both innate and adaptive immune responses and have been successful at treating Behçet disease and multiple sclerosis [89]. They are approved for the treatment of viral hepatitis and myeloproliferative syndromes. In recent years, systemic interferon alpha has been reported to be very successful in the treatment of Behçet disease and other cases of refractory uveitis [90, 91].

Dueter et al. reported resolution of chronic macular edema in a small series of patients treated with systemic interferon-α. All patients had otherwise inactive uveitis with CME that had been persistent for an average of 36 months and had failed to respond to corticosteroids. All patients were treated with an initial dose of three to six million IU subcutaneously based on body weight which was tapered in a stepwise fashion. Stable complete remission of CME was achieved in more than half of patients [92].

Common side effects of interferons are dose dependent and include flu-like illness, nausea, fatigue, diarrhea, rash, anemia, elevated liver transaminases, leucopenia, alopecia, dermatitis, and mild depression [93]. Some patients will develop neutralizing antibodies which render them unresponsive to this treatment. Interferon therapy, like all other systemic therapies except the recently approved TNF inhibitor, adalimumab, has not been US FDA approved for the treatment of uveitis.

Antitumor Necrosis Factor Alpha Medications

Tumor necrosis factor alpha (TNF α), one of the proinflammatory cytokines found to occur at high levels in eyes with uveitis, activates T cells and macrophages, thereby increasing the expression of endothelial adhesion molecules and other proinflammatory cytokines [94, 95]. Inhibition of TNF α provides an attractive opportunity for more targeted anti-inflammatory therapy.

Murphy et al. were the first to demonstrate efficacy of TNF inhibition in the treatment of refractory noninfectious posterior uveitis [96]. Several case series have reported resolution of coexisting CME following TNF-alpha treatment for noninfectious uveitis; however, their use must be weighed against the risk of possible side effects [97–101]. TNF inhibitors are increasingly used for the therapy of posterior uveitis and retinal vasculitis, and more data will likely be available regarding their effects on uveitic macular edema. As well, other biologic therapies are being used in the treatment of uveitis, and data on their efficacy is gradually becoming available. Adalimumab received US FDA approval for the treatment of adults with noninfectious intermediate, posterior, or panuveitis in June, 2016, making it the first FDA-approved non-corticosteroid therapy for uveitis. Data regarding its effects on CME in patients in the registration trials is not yet available.

Choosing the Right Treatment

The decision regarding how to approach the treatment of inflammatory CME should include a careful assessment of individual clinical factors. The first priority must always be to quiet the inflammation, followed by restoration of normal structural integrity. Therapy differs depending upon laterality, severity, coexisting conditions such as cataract and glaucoma, history of steroid response, systemic comorbidities, and patient age. Local therapy may be more appropriate for unilateral disease, while systemic medications are often favored for bilateral conditions. Pseudophakic patients with mild disease and normal intraocular pressure may be treated with topical or periocular steroids; phakic patients should be counseled on their risk of cataract progression. Refractory cases or those who develop a steroid response should be considered for alternate therapy. For patients with moderate to severe disease who would like to avoid systemic immunosuppression or in whom such therapy is contraindicated, steroid implants may be the preferred option. For patients on systemic therapy in whom intraocular inflammation is active at the time of CME diagnosis, adjustments to dosing or frequency of immunomodulatory therapy may be all that is required. In some patients, systemic therapy may need to be initiated.

Care must be taken when treating children with steroid therapy. The risks of developing cataract and glaucoma with topical or local steroid therapy may be higher in children, and the significance of these diagnoses also carries more weight in children. Intraocular pressure and optic disk health must always be monitored in children with uveitis, especially those treated with steroid therapy. Alternative treatment measures should be sought if signs of glaucoma are observed.

Finally, the clinician should also be alert to the presence of structural abnormalities such as vitreomacular traction, epiretinal membrane, and gliosis of the internal limiting membrane (ILM) which can contribute to chronic macular edema that is refractory to medical therapies and which may require surgery.

Our expanding knowledge regarding the pathophysiology of uveitis and the advent of enhanced imaging modalities have improved our ability to diagnose and develop novel therapeutic approaches to manage inflammatory CME. Despite this, the treatment continues to be challenging. There is no single preferred approach, and therapy should be tailored to the individual. Early and aggressive treatment is recommended to give the best potential for visual recovery.

References

1. Rothova A, Suttorp-van Schlten MSA, Treffers WF, Kijlstra A. Causes and frequency of blindness in patients with intraocular inflammatory disease. Br J Ophthalmol. 1996;80(4):332–6.
2. Johnson MW. Etiology and treatment of macular edema. Am J Ophthalmol. 2009;147(1):11–21.
3. Saishin Y, Takahashi K, Melia M, Vinores SA, Campochiaro PA. Inhibition of protein kinase C decreases prostaglandin-induced breakdown of the blood-retinal barrier. J Cell Physiol. 2003;195(2):210–9.
4. van Kooij B, Rothova A, Rijkers GT, de Groot-Mijnes JDF. Distinct cytokine and chemokine profiles in the aqueous of patients with uveitis and cystoid macular edema. Am J Ophthalmol. 2006;142(1):192–4.
5. Lightman S, Greenwood J. Effect of lymphocytic infiltration on the blood-retinal barrier in experimental autoimmune uveoretinitis. Clin Exp Immunol. 1992;88(3):473–7.
6. Thorne JE, Daniel E, Jabs DA, Kedhar SR, Peters GB, Dunn JP. Smoking as a risk factor for cystoid macular edema complicating intermediate uveitis. Am J Ophthalmol. 2008;145(5):841–6.
7. Lin P, Loh AR, Margolis TP, Acharya NR. Cigarette smoking as a risk factor for uveitis. Ophthalmology. 2010;117(3):585–90.
8. Lardenoye CW, van Kooij B, Rothova A. Impact of macular edema on visual acuity in uveitis. Ophthalmology. 2006;113(8):1446–9.
9. Ossewaarde-van Norel A, Rothova A. Clinical review: update on treatment of inflammatory macular edema. Ocul Immunol Inflamm. 2011;19(1):75–83.
10. Levin MH, Pistilli M, Daniel E, Gangaputra SS, Nuseenblatt RB, Rosenbaum JT, Suhler EB, Thorne JE, Foster CS, Jabs DA, Levy-Clarke GA, Kempen JH. Incidence of visual improvement in uveitis cases with visual impairment caused by macular edema. Ophthalmology. 2014;121(2):588–95.
11. Rothova A. Inflammatory cystoid macular edema. Curr Opin Ophthalmol. 2007;18(6):487–92.
12. Lasave AF, Zeballos DG, El-Haig WM, Diaz-Llopis M, Salom D, Arevalo JF. Short-term results of a single intravitreal bevacizumab (Avastin) injection versus a single intravitreal triamcinolone acetonide (Kenacort) injection for the management of refractory noninfectious uveitic cystoid macular edema. Ocular Immunol Inflam. 2009;17(6):423–30.
13. Kok H, Lau C, Maycock N, Mccluskey P, Lightman S. Outcomes of intravitreal triamcinolone in uveitis. Ophthalmology. 2005;112(11):1916–21.
14. Guex-Crosier Y. The pathogenesis and clinical presentation of macular edema in inflammatory diseases. Doc Ophthalmol. 1999;97(3–4):297–309.
15. Cox SN, Hay E, Bird AC. Treatment of chronic macular edema with acetazolamide. Arch Ophthalmol. 1988;106(9):1190–5.
16. Missotten T, Van Laar JAM, Van Der Loos TL, Van Daele LA, Kuijpers RWAM, Baarsma GS, Van Hagen PM. Octreotide long-acting repeatable for the treatment of chronic macular edema in uveitis. Am J Ophthalmol. 2007;144(6):838–43.
17. Simone JN, Pendelton RA, Jenkins JE. Comparison of the efficacy and safety of ketorolac tromethamine 0.5% and prednisolone acetate 1% after cataract surgery. J Cat Ref Surg. 1999;25(5):699–704.
18. van Kooij B, De Boer J, Ten Dam N, Fijnheer R, Rothova A. The effect of non-steroidal anti-inflammatory drugs on inflammatory macular edema. Am J Ophthalmol. 2005;140(3):563–4.
19. Allegri P, Murialdo U, Peri S, Carniglia R, Crivelli MG, Compiano S, Autuori S, Mastromarino A, Zurria M, Marrazzo G. Randomized, double-blind, placebo-controlled clinical trial on the efficacy of 0.5% indomethacin eye drops in uveitic macular edema. Invest Ophthalmol Vis Sci. 2014;55(3):1463–70.

20. Singer KL, Stevenson BR, Woo PL, Firestone GL. Relationship of serine/threonine phosphorylation/dephosphorylation signaling to glucocorticoid regulation of tight junction permeability and ZO-1 distribution in nontransformed mammary epithelial cells. J Biol Chem. 1994; 269(23):16108–15.
21. Tamesis RR, Rodriguez A, Christen WG, Akova YA, Messmer E, Foster CS. Systemic drug toxicity trends inimmunosuppressive therapy of immune and inflammatory ocular disease. Ophthalmology. 1996;103(5):768–75.
22. Weijtens O, Schoemaker RC, Romijn FP, Cohen AF, Lentjes EG, van Meurs JC. Intraocular penetration and systemic absorption after topical application of dexamethasone disodium phosphate. Ophthalmology. 2002;109(10):1887–91.
23. Yee RW. The effect of drop vehicle on the efficacy and side effects of topical glaucoma therapy: a review. Curr Opin Ophthalmol. 2007;18(2):134–9.
24. Jamal KN, Callanan DG. The role of difluprednate ophthalmic emulsion in clinical practice. Clin Ophthalmol. 2009;3:381–90.
25. Sheppard JD, Toyos MM, Kempen JH, Kaur P, Foster CS. Difluprednate 0.05% versus prednisolone acetate 1% for endogenous anterior uveitis, a phase III, multicenter, randomized study. Invest Ophthalmol Vis Sci. 2014;55(5):2993–3002.
26. Korenfeld MS, Silverstein SM, Cooke DL, Vogel R, Crockett RS, Difluprednate Ophthalmic Emulsion 0.05% (Durezol) Study Group. Difluprednate ophthalmic emulsion 0.05% for postoperative inflammation and pain. J Cat Refract Surg. 2009;35(1):26–34.
27. Slabaugh MA, Herlihy E, Ongchin S, Van Gelder RN. Efficacy and potential complications of difluprednate use for pediatric uveitis. Am J Ophthalmol. 2012;153(5):932–8.
28. Birnbaum AD, Jiang Y, Tessler HH, Goldstein DA. Elevation of intraocular pressure in patients with uveitis treated with topical difluprednate. Arch Ophthalmol. 2011;129(5): 667–8.
29. Jabs DA, Akpek EK. Immunosuppression for posterior uveitis. Retina. 2005;25(1):1–18.
30. Jabs DA, Rosenbaum JT, Foster CS, Holland GN, Jaffe GJ, Louie JS, Nussenblatt RB, Stiehm ER, Tessler H, Van Gelder RN, Whitcup SM, Yocum D. Guidelines for the use of immunosuppressive drugs in patients with ocular inflammatory disorders: recommendations of an expert panel. Am J Ophthalmol. 2000;130(4):492–513.
31. Jabs DA, Nussenblatt RB, Rosenbaum JT, Standardization of Uveitis Nomenclature (SUN) Working Group. Standardization of uveitis nomenclature for reporting clinical data: results of the first international workshop. Am J Ophthalmol. 2005;140(3):509–16.
32. Taylor SR, Isa H, Joshi L, Lightman S. New developments in corticosteroid therapy for uveitis. Ophthalmologica. 2010;224 Suppl 1:46–53.
33. Salek SS, Leder HA, Butler NJ, Gan TJ, Dunn JP, Thorne JE. Periocular triamcinolone acetonide injections for control of intraocular inflammation associated with uveitis. Ocul Immunol Inflamm. 2013;21(4):257–63.
34. Leder HA, Jabs DA, Galor A, Dunn JP, Thorne JE. Periocular traimcinolone acetonide injections for cystoid macular edema complicating noninfectious uveitis. Am J Ophthalmol. 2011;152(3):441–8.
35. Tanner V, Kanski JJ, Frith PA. Posterior sub-Tenon's triamcinolone injection in the treatment of uveitis. Eye (Lond). 1998;12(Part 4):679–85.
36. Jermack CM, Dellacroce JT, Heffez J, Peyman GA. Triamcinolone acetonide in ocular therapeutics. Surv Ophthalmol. 2007;52(5):503–22.
37. Habot-Wilner Z, Sallam A, Roufas A, Kabasele PMB, Grigg JR, McCluskey P, Lightman S. Periocular corticosteroid injection in the management of uveitis in children. Acta Ophthalmol. 2010;88(8):e299–304.
38. Sen HN, Vitale S, Gangaputra SS, Nussenblatt RB, Liesagang TL, Levy-Clarke GA, Rosenbaum JT, Suhler EB, Thorne JE, Foster CS, Jabs DA, Kempen JH. Periocular corticosteroids injections in uveitis: effects and complications. Ophthalmology. 2014;121(11): 2275–86.

39. Iwao K, Inatani M, Kawaji T, Koga T, Mawatari Y, Tanihara H. Frequency and risk factors for intraocular pressure elevation after posterior sub-tenon capsule triamcinolone acetonide injection. J Glaucoma. 2007;16(2):251–6.
40. Venkatesh P, Kumar CS, Abbas Z, Garq S. Comparison of the efficacy and safety of different methods of posterior sub-tenon injection. Ocul Immunol Inflamm. 2008;16(5):217–23.
41. Beer PM, Bakri SJ, Singh RJ, Liu W, Peters GB, Miller M. Intraocular concentration and pharmacokinetics of triamcinolone acetonide after a single intravitreal injection. Ophthalmology. 2003;110(4):681–6.
42. Cunningam MA, Edelman JL, Kaushal S. Intravitreal steroids for macular edema: the past, the present, and the future. Surv Ophthalmol. 2008;53(2):139–49.
43. Antcliff RJ, Spalton DJ, Stanford MR, Graham EM, Ffytche TJ, Marshall J. Intravitreal triamcinolone for uveitic macular edema: an optical coherence tomography study. Ophthalmology. 2001;108(4):765–72.
44. Androudi S, Letko E, Meniconi M, Papadaki T, Ahmed M, Foster CS. Safety and efficacy of intravitreal triamcinolone acetonide for uveitic macular edema. Ocul Immunol Inflamm. 2005;13(2–3):205–12.
45. Sallam A, Taylor SRJ, Habot-Wilner Z, Elgohary M, Do HH, McCluskey P, Lightman S. Repeat intravitreal triamcinolone acetonide injections in uveitic macular edema. Acta Ophthalmol. 2012;90(4):e323–5.
46. Bhavsar AR, Ip MS, Glassman AR, DRCRnet and the SCORE Study Groups. The risk of endophthalmitis following intravitreal triamcinolone injection in the DRCRnet and SCORE clinical trials. Am J Ophthalmol. 2007;144(3):454–6.
47. Jonas JB, Kreissig I, Spandau UH, Harder B. Infectious and noninfectious endophthalmitis after intravitreal high-dosage triamcinolone acetonide. Am J Ophthalmol. 2006;141(3):579–80.
48. Graham RO, Peyman GA. Intravitreal injection of dexamethasone. Treatment of experimentally induced endophthalmitis. Arch Ophthalmol. 1974;92(2):149–54.
49. London NJ, Chiang A, Haller JA. The dexamethasone drug delivery system: indications and evidence. Adv Ther. 2011;28(5):351–66.
50. Hunter RS, Lobo AM. Dexamethasone intravitreal implant for the treatment of noninfectious uveitis. Clin Ophthalmol. 2011;5:1613–21.
51. Adan A, Pelegrin L, Rey A, Llorenc V, Mesquida M, Molins B, Rios J, Keller J. Dexamethasone intravitreal implant for treatment of uveitis persistent cystoid macular edema in vitrectomized patients. Retina. 2013;33(7):1435–40.
52. Lowder C, Belfort Jr R, Lightman S, Foster CS, Robinson MR, Schiffman RM, Li XY, Cui H, Whitcup SM, Ozurdex HURON Study Group. Dexamethasone intravitreal implant for noninfectious intermediate or posterior uveitis. Arch Ophthalmol. 2011;129(5):545–53.
53. Cao JH, Mulvahill M, Zhang L, Joondeph BC, Dacey MS. Dexamethasone intravitreal implant in the treatment of persistent uveitic macular edema in the absence of active inflammation. Ophthalmology. 2014;121(10):1871–6.
54. Tomkins-Netzer O, Taylor SRJ, Bar A, Lula A, Yaganti S, Talat L, Lightman S. Treatment with repeat Dexamethasone implants results in long-term disease control in eyes with noninfectious uveitis. Ophthalmology. 2014;121(8):1649–54.
55. Saraiya NV, Patel SS, Goldstein DA. A report of high intraocular pressure with the dexamethasone intraocular implant. Arch Ophthalmol. 2011;129(12):1638–9.
56. Meyer LM, Schõnfeld CL. Secondary glaucoma after Intravitreal dexamethason 0.7 mg implant in patients with retinal vein occlusion: a one-year follow-Up. J Ocul Pharmacol Ther. 2013;29(6):560–5.
57. Brumm MV, Nguyen QD. Fluocinolone acetonide intravitreal sustained release device-a new addition to the armamentarium of uveitic management. Int J Nanomedicine. 2007;2(1):55–64.
58. Callanan DG, Jaffe GJ, Martin DF, Pearson PA, Comstock TL. Treatment of posterior uveitis with a fluocinolone acetonide implant: three-year clinical trial results. Arch Ophthalmol. 2008;126(9):1191–201.

59. Jaffe GJ, Ben-Nun J, Guo H, Dunn JP, Ashton P. Fluocinolone acetonide sustained drug delivery device to treat severe uveitis. Ophthalmology. 2000;107(11):2024–33.
60. Jaffe GJ, Martin D, Callanan D, Pearson PA, Levy B, Comstock T, Fluocinolone Acetonide Uveitis Study Group. Fluocinolone acetonide implant (Retisert) for noninfectious posterior uveitis: thirty-four week results of a multicenter randomized clinical study. Ophthalmology. 2006;113(6):1020–7.
61. Cheih JJ, Carlson AN, Jaffe GJ. Combined fluocinolone acetonide intraocular delivery system insertion, phacoemulsification, and intraocular lens implantation for severe uveitis. Am J Ophthalmol. 2008;146(4):589–94.
62. Kempen JH, Altaweel MM, Holbrook JT, Jabs DA, Louis TA, Sugar EA, Thorne JE, Multicenter Uveitis Steroid Treatment (MUST) Trial Research Group. Randomized comparison of systemic anti-inflammatory therapy versus fluocinolone acetonide implant for intermediate, posterior, and panuveitis: the multicenter uveitis steroid treatment trial. Ophthalmol. 2011;118(10):1916–26.
63. Goldstein DA, Godfrey DG, Hall A, Callanan DG, Jaffe GJ, Pearson A, Usner DW, Comstock TL. Intraocular pressure in patients with uveitis treated with fluocinolone acetonide implants. Arch Ophthalmol. 2007;125(11):1478–85.
64. Taban M, Lowder CY, Kaiser PK. Outcome of fluocinolone acetonide implant (Retisert) reimplantation for chronic noninfectious posterior uveitis. Retina. 2008;28(9):1280–8.
65. Yeh S, Cebulla CM, Witherspoon SR, Emerson GG, Emerson MV, Suhler EB, Albini TA, Flaxel CJ. Management of fluocinolone implant dissociation during implant exchange. Arch Ophthalmol. 2009;127(9):1218–21.
66. Rofahga S, Preschanond T, Stewart JM. Late spontaneous dissociation of a fluocinolone acetonide implant (Retisert). Ocul Immunol Inflamm. 2013;21(3):255.
67. Akduman L, Cetin EN, Levy J, Becker MD, Mackensen F, Lim LL. Spontaneous dissociation and dislocation of Retisert pellet. Ocul Immunol Inflamm. 2013;21(1):87–9.
68. Cohen T, Nahari D, Cerem LW, Neufeld G, Levi BZ. Interleukin 6 induces the expression of vascular endothelial growth factor. J Biol Chem. 1996;271(2):736–41.
69. Fine HF, Baffi J, Reed GF, Csaky KG, Nussenblatt RB. Aqueous humor and plasma vascular endothelial growth factor in uveitis-associated cystoid macular edema. Am J Ophthalmol. 2001;132(5):794–6.
70. Gulati N, Forooghian F, Lieberman R, Jabs DA. Vascular endothelial growth factor inhibition in uveitis: a systematic review. Br J Ophthalmol. 2011;95(2):162–5.
71. Acharya NR, Hong KC, Lee SM. Ranibizumab for refractory uveitis-related macular edema. Am J Ophthalmol. 2009;148(2):303–9.
72. Coma MC, Sobrin L, Onal S, Christen W, Foster CS. Intravitreal bevacizumab for treatment of uveitic macular edema. Ophthalmology. 2007;114(8):1574–9.
73. Soheilian M, Rabbanikhah Z, Ramezani A, Kiavash V, Yaseri M, Peyman GA. Intravitreal bevacizumab versus triamcinolone acetonide for refractory uveitic cystoid macular edema: a randomized pilot study. Jnl Ocul Pharmacol Thera. 2010;26(2):199–205.
74. Mackensen F, Heinz C, Becker MD, Heiligenhaus A. Intravitreal bevacizumab (Avastin) as a treatment for refractory macular edema in patients with uveitis: a pilot study. Retina. 2008;28(1):41–5.
75. Lott MN, Schiffman JC, Davis JL. Bevacizumab in Inflammatory eye disease. Am J Ophthalmol. 2009;148(5):711–7.
76. Weiss K, Steinbrugger I, Weger M, Ardjomand N, Maier R, Wegscheider BJ, Wedrich A, El-Shabrawi Y. Intravitreal VEGF levels in uveitis patients and treatment of uveitic macular edema. Eye (Lond). 2009;23(9):1812–8.
77. Bea JH, Lee CS, Lee SC. Efficacy and safety of intravitreal bevacizumab compared with intravitreal and posterior sub-tenon triamcinolone acetonide for treatment of uveitic cystoid macular edema. Retina. 2011;31(1):111–8.
78. Tseng JJ, Vance SK, Torre KED, Mendonca LS, Cooney MJ, Klancnik JM, Sorenson JA, Freund KB. Sustained increased intraocular pressure related to intravitreal antivascular endothelial growth factor therapy for neovascular age-related macular degeneration. J Glaucoma. 2012;21(4):241–7.

79. Ladas ID, Karagiannis DA, Rouvas AA, Kotsolis AI, Liotsou A, Vergados I. Safety of repeat intravitreal injections of bevacizumab versus ranibizumab. Retina. 2009;29(3):313–8.
80. Fung AE, Rosenfeld PJ, Reichel E. The international l intravitreal bevacizumab safety survey: using the internet to assess drug safety worldwide. Br J Ophthalmol. 2006;90(11):1344–9.
81. Cronstein BN. The mechanism of action of methotrexate. Rheum Dis Clin North Am. 1997;23(4):739–55.
82. Taylor SR, Habot-Wilner Z, Pacheco P, Lightman SL. Intraocular methotrexate in the treatment of uveitis and uveitic cystoid macular edema. Ophthalmology. 2009;116(4):797–801.
83. Hardwig PW, Pulido JS, Erie JC, Baratz KH, Buettner H. Intraocular methotrexate in ocular diseases other than primary central nervous system lymphoma. Am J Ophthalmol. 2006;142(5):883–5.
84. Bea JH, Lee SC. Effect of intravitreal methotrexate and aqueous humor cytokine levels in refractory retinal vasculitis in Behcet disease. Retina. 2012;32(7):1395–402.
85. Taylor SRJ, Banker A, Schlaen A, Couto C, Matthe E, Joshi L, Menezo V, Nguyen E, Tokinsnetzer O, Bar A, Morarji J, McCluskey P, Lightman S. Intraocular methotrexate can induce extended remission in some patients in noninfectious uveitis. Retina. 2013;33(10):2149–54.
86. Hoekzema R, Verhagen C, van Haren M, Kijlstra A. Endotoxin-induced uveitis in the rat. The significance of interleukin-6. Invest Ophthalmol Vis Sci. 1992;33(3):532–9.
87. Yoshida A, Yoshida S, Khalil AK, et al. Role of NF-kappaB mediated interleukin-8 expression in intraocular neovascularization. Invest Ophthalmol Vis Sci. 1998;39(7):1097–106.
88. Dueter CM, Koetter I, Guenaydin I, Stuebiger N, Zierhut M. Interferon alfa-2a: a new treatment option for long lasting refractory cystoid macular edema in uveitis? A pilot study. Retina. 2006;26(7):786–91.
89. Mackensen F, Max R, Becker MD. Interferons and their potential in the treatment of ocular inflammation. Clin Ophthalmol. 2009;3:559–66.
90. Bodaghi B, Gendron G, Wechsler TC, Cassoux N, du Huong LT, Lemitre C, Fradeau C, LeHoang P, Piette JC. Efficacy of interferon alpha in the treatment of refractory and sight threatening uveitis: a retrospective monocentric study of 45 patients. Br J Ophthalmol. 2007;91(3):335–9.
91. Kotter I, Zierhut M, Eckstein AK, Vonthein R, Ness T, Gunaydin I, Grimbacher B, Blaschke S, Meyer-Riemann W, Peter HH, Stubiger N. Human recombinant interferon alpha-2a for the treatment of Behcet's disease with sight threatening posterior or panuveitis. Br J Ophthalmol. 2003;87(4):423–31.
92. Deuter CM, Kotter I, Gunaydin I, Stubiger N, Doycheva DG, Zierhut M. Efficacy and tolerability of interferon alpha treatment in patients with chronic cystoid macular edema due to noninfectious uveitis. Br J Ophthalmol. 2009;93(7):906–13.
93. Sleijfer S, Bannink M, Van Gool AR, Kruit WH, Stoter G. Side effects of interferon-alpha therapy. Pharm World Sci. 2005;27(6):423–31.
94. Dick AD, Forrester JV, Liversidge J, Cope AP. The role of tumor necrosis factor (TNF-alpha) in experimental autoimmune uveoretinitis (EAU). Prog Retin Eye Res. 2004;23(6):617–37.
95. Santos LM, Marcos MC, Gallardo GJM, Gomez VMA, Collantes EE, Ramirez CR, Omar M. Aqueous humor and serum tumor necrosis factor-alpha in clinical uveitis. Ophthalmic Res. 2001;33(5):251–5.
96. Murphy CC, Ayliffe WH, Booth A, Makanjuola D, Andrews PA, Jayne D. Tumor necrosis factor alpha blockage with infliximab for refractory uveitis and scleritis. Ophthalmology. 2004;111(2):352–6.
97. Murphy CC, Greiner K, Plskova J, Duncan L, Frost A, Isaacs JD, REbello P, Waldmann H, Hale G, Forrester JV, Dick AD. Neutralizing tumor necrosis factor activity leads to remission in patients with refractor noninfectious posterior uveitis. Arch Ophthalmol. 2004;122(6):845–51.
98. Markomichelakis NN, Theodossiadis PG, Pantelia E, Papaefthimiou S, Theodossiadis GP, Sfikakis PP. Infliximab for chronic cystoid macular edema associated with uveitis. Am J Ophthalmol. 2004;138(4):648–50.

99. Erckens RJ, MOstard RL, Wijnen PA, Schouten JS, Drent M. Adalimumab successful in sarcoidosis patients with refractory chronic noninfectious uveitis. Graefes Arch Clin Exp Ophthalmol. 2012;250(5):713–20.
100. Hale S, LIghtman S. Anti-TNF therapies in the management of acute and chronic uveitis. Cytokine. 2006;33(4):231–7.
101. Schaap-Fogler M, Amer R, Friling R, Priel E, Kramer M. Anti-TNF agents for refractory cystoid macular edema associated with noninfectious uveitis. Graefes Arch Clin Exp Ophthalmol. 2014;252(4):633–40.

Chapter 5
Medical Management of CME Associated with Diabetes

Reid Turner and Lucian V. Del Priore

Introduction

The World Health Organization reported in 2010 that the world prevalence of diabetes among adults aged 20–79 was 6.5 %, affecting over 285 million people [1]. This number is predicted to rise to over 400 million adults in the year 2030 as average life expectancy increases and the obesity epidemic grows in developed nations. Diabetic retinopathy has important public health implications as it is the leading cause of blindness in working age adults. Since nearly all patients with type I diabetes and up to 60 % of patients with type II diabetes will develop diabetic retinopathy 20 years from initial diagnosis, it has been imperative to identify strategies to prevent and/or limit morbidity from diabetic retinopathy [2].

Diabetic macular edema (DME) is the most common cause of vision loss in patients with diabetes and affects nearly 75,000 new patients in the United States each year. The treatment of DME was investigated by the Early Treatment of Diabetic Retinopathy Study (ETDRS), which was a landmark randomized, controlled, multicenter clinical trial performed from 1979 to 1989 [3]. The ETDRS further defined "clinically significant" DME (CSDME) for the purpose of treatment guidelines as seeing at least one of the following on clinical examination:

- Retinal thickening within 500 μm of the center of the fovea
- Hard exudates within 500 μm of the center of the macula with adjacent retinal thickening
- Retinal thickening at least 1 disk area in size, any part of which is within 1 disk diameter of the center of the macula

R. Turner, MD
Department of Ophthalmology, Medical University of South Carolina, Storm Eye Institute, 167 Ashley Avenue, 8th Floor, Charleston, SC 29425, USA

L.V. Del Priore, MD, PhD (✉)
Department of Ophthalmology, Yale University School of Medicine, New Haven, CT, USA
e-mail: ldelpriore@yahoo.com

S. Schaal, H.J. Kaplan (eds.), *Cystoid Macular Edema*,
DOI 10.1007/978-3-319-39766-5_5

Of note, the diagnosis of CSDME has historically been determined by slit lamp biomicroscopy or stereographic photos and not with fluorescein angiography. Optical coherence tomography (OCT) has emerged as a valuable diagnostic tool that is more sensitive in detecting early DME by determining the thickness of the macular center or central subfield thickness [4].

Although CSDME may present without visual-acuity changes, up to 30 % of patients with CSDME will develop moderate visual loss, defined as a doubling of the visual angle. The ETDRS-established laser photocoagulation as the initial gold standard therapy for DME. Laser photocoagulation is effective in preventing further vision loss from DME, but is less successful in improving visual acuity. Since the ETDRS, a better understanding of the pathophysiology of DME has occurred allowing new treatment strategies to be developed. Anti-VEGF agents have emerged as the favored treatment of center-involving DME with roughly 90 % of retina specialists in 2013 in the United States reportedly using anti-VEGF agents as their initial therapy [5].

Pathophysiology of DME

The pathophysiology of DME is a complex process caused by multiple factors which results in the breakdown of the blood-retina barrier (BRB). The BRB consists of an inner biological unit formed by tight junctional complexes between the retinal vascular endothelial cells and a network of glial cells, astrocytes, and Müller cells, to maintain a low permeability environment; the outer BRB is formed by tight junctions between the retinal pigment epithelium (RPE). Breakdown of the BRB leads to leakage of fluid, retinal thickening, and exudates that cause retinal dysfunction and vision loss [6].

Chronic hyperglycemia is generally accepted as the major pathological factor contributing to diabetic retinopathy and DME. Elevated blood glucose levels lead to increased intracellular levels of glucose which may then react with proteins, lipids, and nucleic acids to subsequently form advanced glycation end-products (AGEs). The receptor for AGEs is expressed on endothelial cells and is called RAGE. The binding of AGE to RAGE leads to endothelial dysfunction and breakdown of the BRB via oxidative stress, the release of proinflammatory cytokines, and increased expression of vascular endothelial growth factor-A (VEGF-A) [7].

VEGF-A was identified in 1983 as a 34–42 kDa protein that is able to induce significant vascular leakage. When compared to histamine on a molar basis, VEGF-A is estimated to be 50,000 times more effective at inducing vascular permeability. Fetal liver kinase-1 (FLK-1) is a tyrosine kinase receptor that has been identified as the principle mediator of VEGF-A's effect on vascular permeability and angiogenesis. Elevated levels of VEGF-A in the vitreous and anterior chamber have been shown to correlate with the severity of DME, making it a key player in the pathogenesis of DME [8].

Additional vasoactive factors implicated in the pathogenesis of DME are protein kinase C (PKC) and angiotensin II (AII). PKC is a family of serine-threonine kinases which are upregulated in diabetic patients and has been shown to increase vascular permeability and decrease retinal blood flow by increasing the expression of endothelins. Endothelins interact with receptors on pericytes to cause intracellular calcium-mediated vasoconstriction of the retinal microvasculature. AII has been shown to directly stimulate the secretion of VEGF in endothelial cells. Therapies targeting PKC and AII have been shown to reduce the retinal vascular changes associated with diabetes in animal models [9].

There have been many more factors identified in the pathogenesis of DME. This has led to the evolution in the management of DME as targeted therapies have developed. Further understanding of the causes of BRB breakdown will undoubtedly lead to new treatments both locally and systemically for DME.

Medical Management of DME

There are several effective treatment modalities for DME. Laser photocoagulation and surgical intervention will be covered in a later chapter. Current medical therapies include systemic risk factor modification, topical eye drops, and intravitreal injection of steroids and anti-VEGF agents. These treatments are summarized in Table 1.

Systemic Control [10, 11]

The primary goals of systemic intervention are to prevent the development of diabetic retinopathy/DME and to reduce vision loss in patients with existing retinopathy/DME. The mainstays of systemic control are blood sugar and blood pressure control. More recently, therapies targeting the renin-angiotensin system (RAS) and lipid-lowering agents have been investigated. Improvement in systemic risk factors alone can significantly decrease the risk of vision loss from DME.

Glycemic Control

The most effective systemic intervention to prevent the progression of diabetic retinopathy is improved glycemic control seen by a lowering of glycosylated hemoglobin (HbA1c). This was established by the Diabetes Control and Complications Trial (DCCT) in type 1 diabetics and the UK Prospective Diabetes Study (UKPDS) in type 2 diabetics. Both studies showed intensive glycemic control reduced the incidence and progression of diabetic retinopathy.

Not surprisingly, intensive glycemic control is associated with an increased risk of hypoglycemic events. Additionally, the Action to Control Cardiovascular Risk in

Table 1 Summary of medical therapies for DME

Treatment	Advantages/disadvantages	Literature support
Systemic risk factor modification		
Glycemic control	Decreases morbidity from retinopathy, nephropathy, and neuropathy Increased risk of hypoglycemic events	Diabetes Control and Complications Trial (DCCT) UK Prospective Diabetes Study (UKPDS) Action to Control Cardiovascular Risk in Diabetes (ACCORD)
Blood pressure control	Decreased risk of heart attack	Wisconsin Epidemiological Study of Diabetic Retinopathy (WESDR)
Renin-Angiotensin System (RAS)	Decreased risk of retinopathy progression	Diabetic Retinopathy Candesartan Trials (DIRECT) European Controlled Trial of Lisinopril in Insulin-Dependent Diabetes (EUCLID)
Lipid-lowering agents	Decreased risk of retinopathy progression, DME, and cardiovascular disease	Fenofibrate Intervention and Event Lowering in Diabetes (FIELD) Action to Control Cardiovascular Risk in Diabetes (ACCORD)
Topical Therapy		
NSAID and steroid eye drops	Low risk of treatment Ease of delivery	Uncontrolled, retrospective studies
Intravitreal Injection		
Anti-VEGF agents	Greatest improvement in visual-acuity and anatomic outcomes Need for frequent visits and repeated treatments, risk of infection, unknown long-term systemic side effects	RESTORE study BOLT study VISTA-DME and VIVID-DME trials
Steroids	Improvement in visual-acuity and anatomic outcomes May help cases poorly responsive to anti-VEGF Risk of cataract and glaucoma progression	MEAD study BEVORDEX study Fluocinolone Acetonide for Diabetic Macular Edema (FAME) A and B studies

Diabetes (ACCORD) trial was stopped because an increase in all-cause mortality was identified in patients whose glucose was extremely tightly controlled with insulin and multiple oral agents. The validity of this association has been questioned, but nonetheless it is important to be cognizant of the potential risk.

Optimal metabolic control in both type 1 and type 2 diabetics may be very difficult to achieve. Various interventions to improve patient education such as nurse education and group therapy sessions have been shown to improve HbA1c levels. Since diabetes is a chronic condition, it is imperative that patients have a thorough understanding of their illness which facilitates better compliance with medical therapies.

The American Diabetes Association and the European Association for the Study of Diabetes provided a consensus statement in 2009 which provided guidance for a treatment algorithm for type 2 diabetes. The guidelines emphasized a goal HbA1c

<7.0 %, initial therapy with lifestyle modifications and metformin, rapid addition of additional oral agents if glycemic goals are not achieved or sustained, and early addition of insulin therapy in patients who do not meet goals with oral medications. Based on these guidelines and results of clinical studies, it is fundamental for ophthalmologists to review their patients' HbA1c and emphasize the importance of metabolic control at each visit.

Blood Pressure Control

Hypertension has been shown to be a major risk factor for DME in studies such as the Wisconsin Epidemiological Study of Diabetic Retinopathy (WESDR). The WESDR found that higher diastolic blood pressure increased the risk of progression of diabetic retinopathy over a 4-year period. Furthermore, the UKPDS demonstrated that improved control of systolic blood pressure reduced the need for laser treatment of diabetic retinopathy in patients with type 2 diabetes. Based on these and other studies, the American Diabetes Association recommends a target blood pressure of less than 130/80 mmHg for patients with diabetes.

Renin-Angiotensin System Inhibition

The renin-angiotensin system (RAS) in the eye is activated by chronic hyperglycemia which leads to overexpression of AII. As mentioned previously, AII induces the release of VEGF as well as increases vascular permeability and promotes vasoconstriction. Clinical trials such as the Renin-Angiotensin System Study (RASS) have evaluated medications that target this system and their effects on diabetic retinopathy. The RASS compared the effect of the angiotensin-converting enzyme inhibitor enalapril, the angiotensin receptor blocker losartan, and placebo on diabetic retinopathy progression over a 5-year period in normotensive patients. Both drugs significantly reduced the progression of diabetic retinopathy independently of glycemic levels and changes in blood pressure. Similar studies such as the Diabetic Retinopathy Candesartan Trials (DIRECT) and the European Controlled Trial of Lisinopril in Insulin-Dependent Diabetes (EUCLID) study have shown favorable effects on diabetic retinopathy progression.

Lipid-Lowering Agents

Lipid-lowering therapy is vitally important to decrease the risk of cardiovascular disease in patients with diabetes. Statins and fibrates have been shown to reduce hard exudates, microaneurysms, and the risk of vision loss in diabetic retinopathy.

The Fenofibrate Intervention and Event Lowering in Diabetes (FIELD) study showed a decrease in the rate of DME development and need for laser photocoagulation in type 2 diabetic patients. The protective effects of fenofibrate were independent of blood glucose, blood pressure, and baseline lipid levels. Furthermore, the ACCORD study showed that the addition of fenofibrate to statin therapy resulted in a reduction in diabetic retinopathy progression compared to taking a statin alone. These effects of fibrate medications appear to be independent of lipid concentration and have raised questions as to their mechanism of action.

Topical Therapy

Nonsteroidal Anti-inflammatory Drugs (NSAIDS)

The benefits of topical NSAIDs for treatment of DME are mainly reported anecdotally or in uncontrolled retrospective studies. For example, one case series of 6 eyes with DME treated with nepafenac 0.1 % for 6 months showed improvement in the average foveal thickness from 417 to 267 μm. Authors also reported that four eyes gained vision with a modest improvement in mean visual acuity from 0.78 to 0.67 logMAR [12]. Such results have prompted larger, controlled studies by the Diabetic Retinopathy Clinical Research Network (DRCRN) and National Eye Institute (NEI) which have not yet been published. Overall, most clinicians use topical NSAIDs with or without topical steroids to treat macular edema in diabetic patients associated with cataract surgery. If a response is not achieved after 1–3 months or side effects are experienced, intravitreal or surgical intervention is typically pursued [13].

Steroids

Topical steroids have been shown in small, uncontrolled studies to improve retinal thickening and visual acuity in patients with DME after surgical procedures and are typically given in combination with topical NSAIDs [14]. The treatment effect of topical steroids as monotherapy for DME has not been studied extensively and is not recommended.

Other Topical Agents

A growing interest in topical therapy for the treatment of DME and other retinal diseases has emerged. Topical therapy would be greatly advantageous compared to intravitreal injection or surgical intervention. In animal models, ranibizumab

(Lucentis, Genentech, Inc., San Francisco, CA) has been shown to reach the vitreous cavity and retina with topical application [15]. Other studies have evaluated coupling anti-VEGF drugs with various agents to improve intraocular penetration with topical administration. Even more exciting perhaps is the development of new drugs which target different pathological factors involved with DME. For example, the drug FOV-2304 (Fovea Pharmaceuticals SA) is delivered as a topical drop and targets the kallikrein-kinin system (KKS), which has been shown to induce vascular permeability in diabetic rats [16]. A phase II randomized, placebo-controlled trial evaluating the safety and efficacy of FOV-2304 was begun in 2011 with final results pending.

Intraocular Therapy

The treatment of DME drastically changed with the advent of intravitreal injections. Intravitreal steroids and anti-VEGF agents are superior to laser photocoagulation with regard to improving visual acuity. This has led to a paradigm shift in the treatment of DME.

Steroids

Several studies have shown the effectiveness of intravitreal injection of steroid with or without focal/grid laser. Cataract formation and intraocular pressure (IOP) rise are important adverse effects of steroid therapy that are frequently encountered with sustained release steroid injections that need to be considered.

The Diabetic Retinopathy Clinical Research Network (DRCRnet) has investigated the effects of intravitreal triamcinolone acetate on DME. The DRCRnet has shown that triamcinolone plus focal/grid laser is more effective than laser alone in pseudophakic eyes with DME. However, phakic eyes showed no improvement with the addition of triamcinolone compared to focal/grid laser alone and were much more likely to develop cataracts and an increase in IOP [17, 18].

Despite the lack of significant success with triamcinolone, other intravitreal steroids have shown to be effective in treating DME. The MEAD study was a 3-year, randomized, sham-controlled trial of Ozurdex (dexamethasone intravitreal implant; Allergan, Inc, Irvine, CA) in patients with center-involving DME. Ozurdex is a biodegradable implant delivered via a preloaded, single-use 22-gauge needle. In the study, roughly 20 % of patients experienced ≥15-letter improvement in BCVA from baseline with about 4 Ozurdex injections over the 3-year period, which achieved the predefined primary efficacy endpoint for the US Food and Drug Administration (FDA). However, it is important to consider that roughly 65 % of patients who received Ozurdex compared to 20 % of patients in the sham group developed cataracts.

The BEVORDEX study compared Ozurdex 0.7 mg with bevacizumab 1.25 mg (Avastin, Genentech, Inc., South San Francisco, CA) for center-involving DME. Both achieved similar rates of visual improvement with roughly 40 % of patients gaining 10 or more letters of best-corrected visual acuity (BCVA). Ozurdex achieved superior anatomic outcomes compared to bevacizumab with a mean improvement in central macular thickness of 187 μm compared with 122 μm. Also, Ozurdex-treated eyes required fewer injections with a mean of 2.7 injections of the implant compared to a mean of 8.6 injections in the bevacizumab group. Similar to the MEAD study, patients in the Ozurdex group developed cataract at a much higher rate compared with those treated with anti-VEGF agents, and roughly 1 % of patients treated with Ozurdex required glaucoma surgery due to uncontrolled increase in IOP. Combined, the BEVORDEX and MEAD studies helped gain Ozurdex FDA approval for the treatment of DME [19, 20].

In September 2014, the FDA approved another intravitreal steroid drug, Iluvien (fluocinolone acetonide, Alimera Science, Alpharetta, GA), for the treatment of DME. The FDA approval recommends that patients be treated with a course of topical steroids and show a lack of clinically significant rise in IOP prior to being treated with Iluvien. Iluvien is a non-erodible cylindrical tube with a central drug-polymer matrix that releases 0.19 mg of fluocinolone acetonide into the vitreous cavity via a 25-gauge intravitreal injection. It releases small doses of fluocinolone acetonide for at least 3 years. No systemic absorption has been documented [21].

The Fluocinolone Acetonide for Diabetic Macular Edema (FAME) A and B studies showed Iluvien significantly improved visual acuity with 28 % of treated patients compared to 19 % of control patients gaining 15 letters of BCVA at 3 years follow-up. Cataract formation occurred in over 80 % of patients treated with Iluvien compared to 50 % of control patients; however, visual-acuity gains remained improved after subsequent cataract surgery. Incisional IOP-lowering surgery was required in 4.8 % of Iluvien patients compared to 0.5 % in the sham group. Subgroup analysis has shown that Iluvien is more effective for patients with chronic DME, lasting greater than 3 years despite laser photocoagulation [22].

There are many factors to consider when deciding to use intravitreal steroids to treat DME. Cost is a significant consideration given that the product cost alone for these steroids is around $2,000 for Ozurdex and $8,000 for Iluvien in the USA. However, the duration of action of these drugs could decrease the burden of frequent office visits. Overall, it seems the intravitreal steroids are most useful in treating center-involving DME in pseudophakic patients with a low risk of developing glaucoma.

Anti-VEGF

VEGF is one of the most important players in the pathogenesis of DME. It is not surprising that intravitreal anti-VEGF agents have shown to be so successful in treating DME. The three main anti-VEGF agents used to treat DME include bevacizumab (Avastin, Genentech, Inc., San Francisco, CA, USA), ranibizumab, and eylea (Aflibercept, Regeneron Pharmaceuticals, Inc., Tarrytown, NY, USA). While the ETDRS-established laser photocoagulation could prevent further vision loss in DME, several studies evaluating anti-VEGF agents have shown superior improvement in visual acuity compared to laser. These effects are even greater for center-involving DME [23, 24].

Ranibizumab, a recombinant humanized antibody fragment that is active against all isoforms of VEGF-A, is the most studied anti-VEGF agent for the treatment of DME. The RESTORE study published in 2011 was a randomized, double-masked, multicenter controlled study which compared ranibizumab 0.5 mg monotherapy to combined therapy with laser and to laser alone. At 12 months, patients treated with ranibizumab alone gained an average of 6.1 letters of BCVA compared to 5.9 and 0.8 in the ranibizumab plus laser and laser-alone treatment groups, respectively [25]. The DRCRnet found similar results in a study with 2-year follow-up which again showed that patients treated with ranibizumab with or without prompt laser achieved about 5 letters of BCVA compared to laser alone [26].

The FDA approved ranibizumab for the treatment of DME in August 2012 after the results of the RIDE and RISE trials. These trials were identically designed, parallel, double-masked, 3-year placebo-controlled studies which evaluated the safety and efficacy of intravitreal ranibizumab with rescue laser if needed. At 24 months, 34 % of patients in the RIDE arm and 45 % in the RISE arm gained at least 15 letters of BCVA compared to 12 and 18 % in the control groups. These visual improvements were maintained through the 3-year study period. These studies established ranibizumab as a better approach to DME management [27].

Bevacizumab is a full-length recombinant humanized antibody active against all forms of VEGF-A. It is not FDA approved for the treatment of DME but has also been shown to be an effective therapy. In 2007, the DRCRnet published a phase II, prospective, randomized, multicenter clinical trial to determine bevacizumab's safety and possible benefits in DME. The study showed bevacizumab improved central subfoveal thickness and BCVA but only followed patients for 24 weeks [28]. The BOLT study published in 2012 provided a prospective randomized controlled trial with 2 years of outcome data comparing bevacizumab to macular laser therapy in patients with center-involving DME. The study found that patients treated with bevacizumab gained an average of 8.6 letters of BCVA compared to a loss of 0.5 letters in the laser group at 2 years. Additionally, 32 % of patients in the bevacizumab group gained 15 or more letters compared to just 4 % in the laser group [29]. Since bevacizumab is considerably cheaper than the other anti-VEGF agents, many clinicians prefer an initial trial with this agent before using either ranibizumab or aflibercept.

Aflibercept is a recombinant fusion protein consisting of the VEGF-binding portions from the extracellular domains of human VEGF receptors 1 and 2 that are fused to the Fc portion of the human IgG immunoglobulin. The FDA approved aflibercept for the treatment of DME in August 2014 based on the results from the phase III VISTA-DME and VIVID-DME trials. These similarly designed, double-masked, randomized studies compared aflibercept 2 mg given monthly, aflibercept

2 mg given every 2 months (after five initial monthly injections), or macular laser photocoagulation (at baseline and then as needed). After 1 year, the mean letters gained in BCVA for the monthly and every 2-month aflibercept groups were 12.5 and 10.7, compared to 0.2 letters in the laser group. Furthermore, 41 and 31 % of eyes treated with aflibercept gained ≥15 letters compared to 8 % treated with laser. Similar efficacy was noted with aflibercept injection at 4-week intervals compared to 8-week intervals after the standard 5 initial monthly injections [30].

Studies comparing the anti-VEGF agents head to head for DME are emerging. One study comparing ranibizumab to bevacizumab for DME showed similar improvements in BCVA, but ranibizumab required less injections (7.7) compared to the bevacizumab group (9.8) over the 12 months of the study [31]. In February 2015, the DRCRnet reported results from a multicenter, randomized controlled trial comparing the 3 anti-VEGF agents. This study evaluated the effectiveness of aflibercept, ranibizumab, and bevacizumab on visual acuity and central subfield thickness over a 12-month period in roughly 350 patients with center-involving DME. The DRCRnet found that all 3 drugs significantly improved visual acuity and central subfield thickness in patients presenting with mild vision loss, 20/32–20/40 vision. However, in patients presenting with visual acuity of 20/50 or worse, aflibercept displayed a clinically meaningful advantage over ranibizumab and bevacizumab. Specifically, an improvement in the visual-acuity letter score of at least 15 (3 Snellen lines) was observed in 67 % of aflibercept-treated eyes compared to 50 and 41 % of eyes treated with ranibizumab and bevacizumab, respectively [32]. The study did not compare the costs associated with treatment but did mention the Medicare allowable charges for a single intravitreous injection is $1,950 for aflibercept (at a dose of 2.0 mg), $50 for bevacizumab (under the assumption that 10 mg is used to repackage a 1.25-mg dose), and $1,200 for ranibizumab (at a dose of 0.3 mg), making cost a significant factor when choosing an anti-VEGF agent for an individual patient.

Summary

The medical management of DME has evolved since the first reports of the ETDRS showed a 50 % reduction in vision loss with focal/grid laser. A better understanding of the factors involved with the pathophysiology of DME has led to the development of more effective treatments. Expert panels and review articles are beginning to establish new treatment recommendations based on the growing body of evidence that anti-VEGF agents are superior to laser for the treatment of DME. It is generally recommended to treat center-involving DME with vision loss with an anti-VEGF agent with or without focal/grid laser since studies have consistently shown anti-VEGF agents can recover BCVA. Laser photocoagulation should be reserved for non-center-involving DME without significant vision loss. The role of intraocular steroids is less clear. Most clinicians reserve their use for poorly responsive cases in patients that are pseudophakic and have low risk of glaucomatous optic neuropathy [33, 34]. A simplified algorithm for the treatment of DME is presented in Fig. 1.

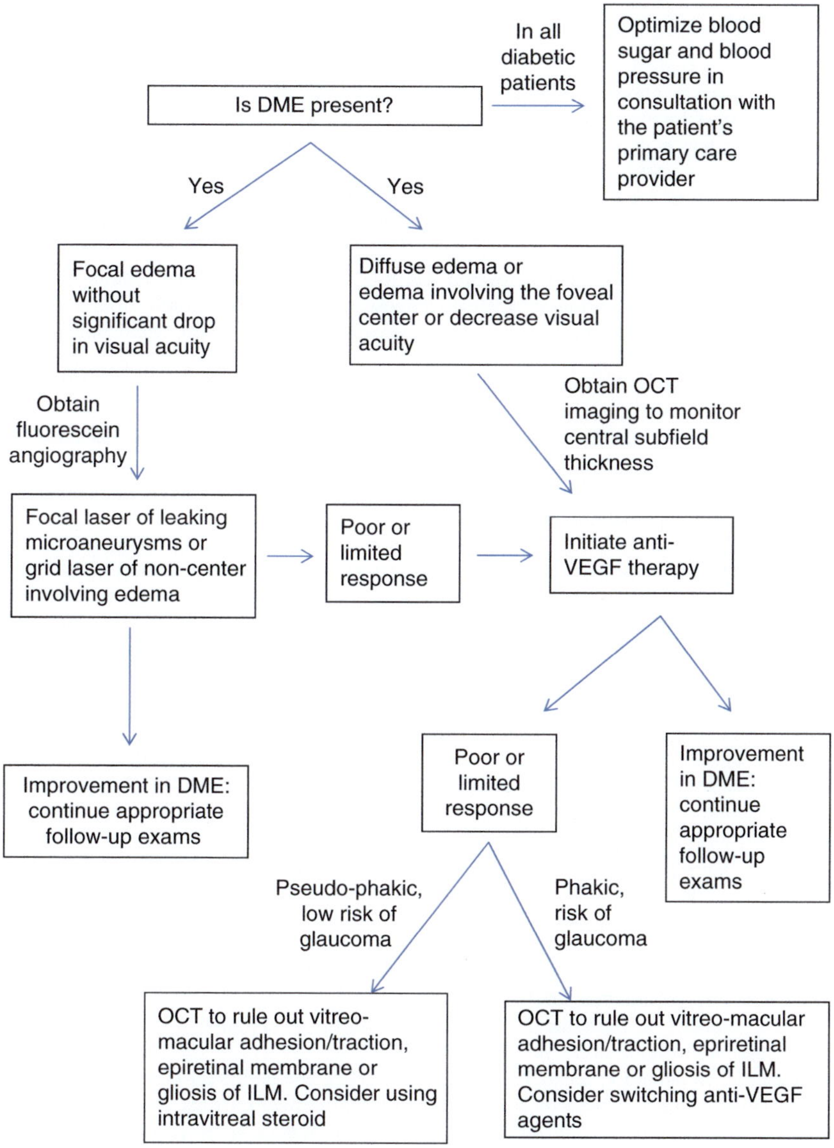

Fig. 1 A simplified algorithm for the treatment of DME

Ophthalmologists have several effective treatment options available for the management of DME. The strategy employed is based on several factors that are specific to each patient. Cost, number of treatments, and response to therapy are all significant variables involved with the decision-making process. Further studies will help clarify treatment protocols for DME.

References

1. Shaw J, Sicree R, Zimmet P. Global estimates of the prevalence of diabetes for 2010 and 2030. Diabetes Res Clin Pract. 2010;87(1):4–14.
2. Moss SE, Klein R, Klein BE. The 14-year incidence of visual loss in a diabetic population. Ophthalmology. 1998;105:998–1003.
3. Photocoagulation for diabetic macular edema. Early treatment diabetic retinopathy study report number 1. Early treatment diabetic retinopathy study research group. Arch Ophthalmol. 1985;103(12):1796–806.
4. Virgili G, Menchini F, Dimastrogiovanni AF, Rapizzi E, Menchini U, Bandello F, Chiodini RG. Optical coherence tomography versus stereoscopic fundus photography or biomicroscopy for diagnosing diabetic macular edema: a systematic review. Invest Ophthalmol Vis Sci. 2007;48(11):4963–73.
5. American Society of Retina Specialists Preference and Trends (PAT) Survey 2013 (http://www.asrs.org/asrs-community/pat-survey).
6. Zhang X, Zeng H, Bao S, Wang N, Gillies MC. Diabetic macular edema: new concepts in pathophysiology and treatment. Cell Biosci. 2014;4:27.
7. Bhagat N, Grigorian RA, Tutela A, Zarbin MA. Diabetic macular edema: pathogenesis and treatment. Surv Ophthalmol. 2009;54:1–32.
8. Roh MI, Kim HS, Song JH, et al. Effect of intravitreal bevacizumab injection on aqueous humor cytokine levels in clinically significant macular edema. Ophthalmology. 2009;116:80–6.
9. Funatsu H, Yamashita H, Nakamura S, et al. Vitreous levels of pigment epithelium-derived factor and vascular endothelial growth factor are related to diabetic macular edema. Ophthalmology. 2006;113:294–301.
10. Kiire C, Porta M, Chong V. Medical management for the prevention and treatment of diabetic macular edema. Surv Ophthalmol. 2013;58:459.
11. Abbate M, Cravedi P, Iliev I, Remuzzi G, Ruggenenti P. Prevention and treatment of diabetic retinopathy: evidence from clinical trials and perspectives. Curr Diabetes Rev. 2011;7:190–200.
12. Hariprasad SM, Akduman L, Clever JA, Ober M, Recchia FM, Mieler WF. Treatment of cystoid macular edema with the new-generation NSAID nepafenac 0.1%. Clin Ophthalmol. 2009;3(1):147–54.
13. Russo A, Costagliola C, Delcassi L, Parmeggiani F, Romano M, dell'Omo R, Semeraro F. Topical nonsteroidal anti-inflammatory drugs for macular edema. Mediators Inflamm. 2013;2013:476525. Epub 2013 Oct 21.
14. Nakano S, Yamamoto T, Kirii E, Abe S, Yamashita H. Steroid eye drop treatment (difluprednate ophthalmic emulsion) is effective in reducing refractory diabetic macular edema. Graefes Arch Clin Exp Ophthalmol. 2010;248(6):805–10.
15. Chen J, Ebmeier S, Sutherland W, Ghaz N. Potential penetration of topical ranibizumab (Lucentis) in the rabbit eye. Eye. 2011;25:1504–11.
16. Pruneau D, Bélichard P, Sahel J, Combal J. Targeting the kallikrein-kinin system as a new therapeutic approach to diabetic retinopathy. Curr Opin Investig Drugs. 2010;11(5):507–14.
17. Diabetic Retinopathy Clinical Research Network (DRCR.net). Three-year follow up of a randomized trial comparing focal/grid photocoagulation and intravitreal triamcinolone for diabetic macular edema. Arch Ophthalmol. 2009;127(3):245–51.
18. Diabetic Retinopathy Clinical Research Network, Elman MJ, Aiello LP, Beck RW, Bressler NM, Bressler SB, Edwards AR, Ferris 3rd FL, Friedman SM, Glassman AR, Miller KM, Scott IU, Stockdale CR, Sun JK. Randomized trial evaluating ranibizumab plus prompt or deferred laser or triamcinolone plus prompt laser for diabetic macular edema. Ophthalmology. 2010;117(6):1064–1077.e35.
19. Gillies MC, Lim LL, Campain A, Quin GJ, Salem W, Li J, Goodwin S, Aroney C, McAllister IL, Fraser-Bell S. A randomized clinical trial of intravitreal bevacizumab versus intravitreal dexamethasone for diabetic macular edema: the BEVORDEX study. Ophthalmology. 2014;121(12):2473–81.

20. Boyer DS, Yoon YH, Belfort Jr R, Bandello F, Maturi RK, Augustin AJ, et al. Ozurdex MEAD study group. Three-year, randomized, sham-controlled trial of dexamethasone intravitreal implant in patients with diabetic macular edema. Ophthalmology. 2014;121(10):1904–14.
21. Mariana C, Steven Y, Thomas AA. Sustained-release corticosteroid options. J Ophthalmol. 2014; 2014:Article ID 164692, 5 pages.
22. FAME Study Group. Sustained delivery fluocinolone acetonide vitreous inserts provide benefit for at least 3 years in patients with diabetic macular edema. Ophthalmology. 2012;119(10):2125–32.
23. Early photocoagulation for diabetic retinopathy. ETDRS report number 9. Early Treatment Diabetic Retinopathy Study Research Group. Ophthalmology. 1991;98(5 Suppl):766–85.
24. Virgili G, Parravano M, Menchini F, Evans JR. Anti-vascular endothelial growth factor for diabetic macular oedema. Cochrane Database Syst Rev. 2014;(10):CD007419.
25. Mitchell P, Bandello F, Schmidt-Erfurth U, et al. The RESTORE study: ranibizumab monotherapy or combined with laser versus laser monotherapy for diabetic macular edema. Ophthalmology. 2011;118:615–25.
26. Diabetic Retinopathy Clinical Research Network. Expanded 2-year follow-up of ranibizumab plus prompt or deferred laser or triamcinolone plus prompt laser for diabetic macular edema. Ophthalmology. 2011;118(4):609–14.
27. Nguyen QD, Brown DM, Marcus DM, et al. Ranibizumab for diabetic macular edema: results from 2 phase III randomized trials: RISE and RIDE. Ophthalmology. 2012;119:789–801.
28. Diabetic Retinopathy Clinical Research Network, Scott IU, Edwards AR, Beck RW, Bressler NM, Chan CK, Elman MJ, Friedman SM, Greven CM, Maturi RK, Pieramici DJ, Shami M, Singerman LJ, Stockdale CR. A phase II randomized clinical trial of intravitreal bevacizumab for diabetic macular edema. Ophthalmology. 2007;114(10):1860–7.
29. Rajendram R, Fraser-Bell S, Kaines A, Michaelides M, Hamilton R, Esposti S, et al. A 2-year prospective randomized controlled trial of intravitreal bevacizumab or laser therapy (BOLT) in the management of diabetic macular edema: 24-month data: report 3. Arch Ophthalmol. 2012;130(8):972–9.
30. Korobelnik JF, Do DV, Schmidt-Erfurth U, Boyer DS, Holz FG, Heier JS, et al. Intravitreal aflibercept for diabetic macular edema. Ophthalmology. 2014;121(11):2247–54.
31. Nepomuceno AB, Takaki E, Paes de Almeida FP, et al. A prospective randomized trial of intravitreal bevacizumab versus ranibizumab for the management of diabetic macular edema. Am J Ophthalmol. 2013;156:502–10.
32. The Diabetic Retinopathy Clinical Research Network. Aflibercept, bevacizumab, or ranibizumab for diabetic macular edema. N Engl J Med. 2015;372(13):1193–203.
33. Mitchell P, Wong TY, Diabetic Macular Edema Treatment Guideline Working Group. Management paradigms for diabetic macular edema. Am J Ophthalmol. 2014;157(3):505–13.e1-8.
34. Bandello F, Cunha-Vaz J, Chong NV, Lang GE, Massin P, Mitchell P, et al. New approaches for the treatment of diabetic macular oedema: recommendations by an expert panel. Eye (Lond). 2012;26(4):485–93.

Chapter 6
Management of Macular Edema in Vitreo-Maculopathies

Matin Khoshnevis and J. Sebag

Key Concepts

1. Anomalous PVD is the fundamental cause of vitreo-maculopathies with vitreo-macular traction and macular pucker, both associated with macular edema.
2. Vitreo-macular adhesion can be an important contributor to macular edema resulting from diabetic retinopathy, retinal vein occlusion, and exudative age-related macular degeneration.
3. Vitreous surgery, which has been the mainstay of therapy for macular edema due to vitreo-maculopathy, may be replaced or augmented by pharmacologic vitreolysis, which can also aid in the management of macular edema from comorbidities. In the future, pharmacologic vitreolysis may be used to induce prophylactic PVD to mitigate macular edema from both primary vitreo-maculopathies and comorbid conditions.

Introduction

Macular edema can be broadly defined as abnormal thickening of the macula due to the accumulation of fluid in the extracellular compartment of the neurosensory retina. When cysts form within the outer plexiform layer, the term "cystoid macular

M. Khoshnevis, MD
VMR Institute for Vitreous Macula Retina,
7677 Center Avenue, suite 400, Huntington Beach, CA 92647, USA

Temple University, Department of Ophthalmology, Philadelphia, PA, USA

J. Sebag, MD, FACS, FRCOphth, FARVO (✉)
VMR Institute for Vitreous Macula Retina,
7677 Center Avenue, suite 400, Huntington Beach, CA 92647, USA
e-mail: jsebag@VMRinstitute.com

S. Schaal, H.J. Kaplan (eds.), *Cystoid Macular Edema*,
DOI 10.1007/978-3-319-39766-5_6

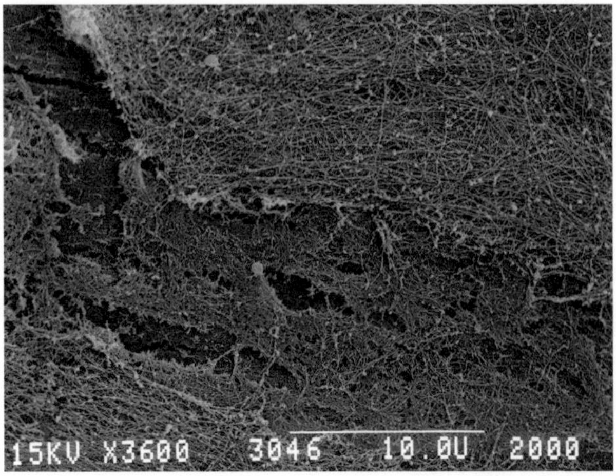

Fig. 1 Human posterior vitreous cortex. Scanning electron microscopy showing a dense network of collagen fibrils. Bar = 10 microns (Reprinted with permission from Sebag [5], p. 266)

edema" (CME) is applicable [1]. In this chapter, the term "CME" will be reserved for edema in the macula that has a petaloid pattern on fluorescein angiography without any identifiable cause, such as vitreo-macular adhesion/traction, diabetic retinopathy, retinal vein occlusions, exudative AMD, etc. Macular edema from identifiable causes will be referred to as "macular edema" (ME). The following discusses the role of vitreous in the pathogenesis of all forms of ME.

The hallmark of all vitreo-maculopathies is vitreo-macular adhesion (VMA); when it exerts traction on the macula causing structural alterations, it is called vitreo-macular traction (VMT) [2]. The prevalence of VMA is greater than commonly appreciated. Optical coherence tomography (OCT) has shown VMA not detected by biomicroscopy in 30 % of cases [3]. In pathologic studies of posterior vitreous detachment (PVD), remnants of the posterior vitreous cortex (Fig. 1) were found on the inner retina in 42 % of cases [4].

VMA and VMT influence the macula via different mechanisms. In the case of VMA, effects are molecular and physiologic, while untoward effects in VMT result from traction. Traction arising from anomalous posterior vitreous detachment (PVD) with persistent VMA between the posterior vitreous cortex and the inner limiting membrane (ILM) of the retina can be either tangential to the surface of the retina, axial, or both.

This chapter will briefly review vitreous biochemistry, structure, and physiology, as well as aging, PVD, and anomalous PVD causing VMT. The role of VMA as a comorbidity in exudative age-related macular degeneration and diabetic macular edema will be discussed. Lastly, the medical management of vitreo-maculopathies will be described, while surgical management will be covered elsewhere and only briefly addressed herein.

Vitreous Biochemistry and Structure

The main component of vitreous is water, which constitutes more than 98 % of the vitreous body. Roughly 15–20 % of this water is attached to glycosaminoglycans

(GAGs), primarily hyaluronan. The other major structural macromolecule of vitreous is collagen. Variations in the concentrations of hyaluronan and collagen in different species account for differences in the rheologic (gel/liquid) state of the vitreous body [5, 6].

The three main GAGs of vitreous are hyaluronan, chondroitin sulfate, and heparan sulfate:

- Hyaluronan (HA) is the major CAG of the human vitreous. HA synthesis begins after birth and plateaus in adulthood. As there is no extracellular degradation [7–10], the levels of HA tend to remain constant because HA molecules escape via the anterior segment of the eye [11]. It has previously been shown that HA acts like an ion-exchange resin in that an electrostatic interaction can occur between small charges of mobile ions in the tissue and the electrostatic envelope of this stationary polyelectrolyte [12]. This interaction explains the properties of HA in vitreous and its influences on ion transport and distribution, osmotic pressure, and electric potentials within the vitreous body.
- Chondroitin sulfate (CS) is an important component of the extracellular matrix throughout the body. In vitreous, CS may serve as a link between HA and collagen. Versican, a vitreous CS, has been shown to house the pathogenic mutation in Wagner's Vitreo-Retinal Dystrophy [13, 14].
- Heparan sulfate (HS) is a renewable proteoglycan that has been found in small amounts in human vitreous. Its function is speculated to be the maintenance of an adequate distance between vitreous collagen fibrils to achieve transparency [15].

Type II collagen comprises 75 % of all vitreous collagens [16]. Stickler syndrome is a mutation that occurs in exon 2 of COL2A1, resulting in liquefied vitreous [16, 17] and an increased risk of retinal detachment. Type IX collagen comprises 10–15 % of vitreous collagen and interacts with collagen II fibrils and other collagens. It has been hypothesized that changes in the quantity and the location of type IX collagen are the reasons for many of the important phenomena in age-related vitreous changes [18, 19]. Lastly, a hybrid collagen type V/XI makes up about 10 % of all vitreous collagen [20]. Types II and V/XI often combine to form a heterotypic fibril that helps keep the distance between vitreous collagen fibrils to minimize light scattering [20].

Vitreous body structure consists primarily of interpenetrating networks of HA molecules and collagen fibrils. Collagen fibrils provide a rigid structure that is "filled" by the hydrophilic HA creating a solid gel in youth (Fig. 2). If collagen is removed from the vitreous body, HA forms a viscous solution, while removal of HA causes the gel to shrink [12]. Type II collagen is very rich in proteoglycans and has a strong collagen-proteoglycan interaction. It has also been shown that proteoglycans have a stabilizing effect upon collagen [21]. Swann et al. [22] postulated that HA-collagen interaction in the human vitreous might involve a third molecule that represents a "link" composed of either a glycoprotein or proteoglycans. This is consistent with previous studies that have shown HA to interact with link proteins [23], as well as an HA-binding glycoprotein, known as hyaluronectin [24]. Such organization to keep the vitreous collagen fibrils a critical distance apart minimizes light scattering [24] achieving transparency.

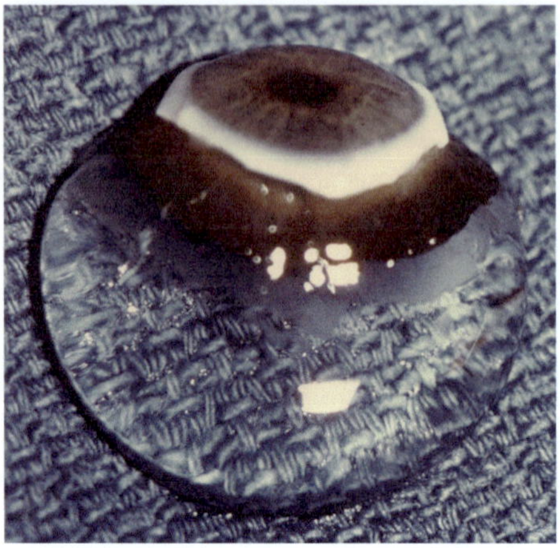

Fig. 2 Vitreous body of an eye obtained at autopsy from a 9-month-old child. The sclera choroid and retina were dissected off the vitreous body, which remains attached to the anterior segment. A band of gray tissue can be seen posterior to the ora serrata. This is the neural retina that was firmly adherent to the vitreous base and could not be dissected. Due to the young age of the donor, the vitreous body is almost entirely gel. Thus, it is solid and maintains its shape, although situated on a surgical towel exposed to room air (Reprinted with permission from Sebag [5], cover photo)

The vitreo-retinal interface is composed of the inner limiting membrane of the retina, the outer layer of the vitreous body, known as the posterior vitreous cortex (Fig. 1), and an intervening extracellular matrix containing laminin, fibronectin, and other constituents [25]. Opticin is a structural protein found at the vitreo-retinal interface, where it is speculated to play an important role in vitreo-retinal adhesion and the prevention of neovascularization [26, 27].

Aging and PVD

The vitreous body undergoes dramatic changes with age (Fig. 3) likely related to changes in collagen/proteoglycans composition and organization. In nondiabetic patients, the average half-life of vitreous collagen is estimated to be 15 years, similar to the skin [28]. In aging and especially in diabetes, vitreous pentosidine [25] and AGEs increase significantly [29, 30]. HA and CS, which are both attached to core proteins to form proteoglycans [20], are believed to play important roles in the structural changes with aging [30]. CS primarily interacts with type IX collagen and may be important in collagen aggregation [19, 31], while HS seems to play a role at the vitreo-retinal interface [20].

After age 40 there is a significant decrease in gel volume and a concurrent increase in liquid vitreous, which mainly accumulates centrally [32, 33]. These changes within the vitreous body lead to pockets of liquid vitreous known as "lacunae." Oksala [34] used ultrasonography to detect echoes from the gel/liquid interfaces in the aging vitreous body. Recent studies with swept source

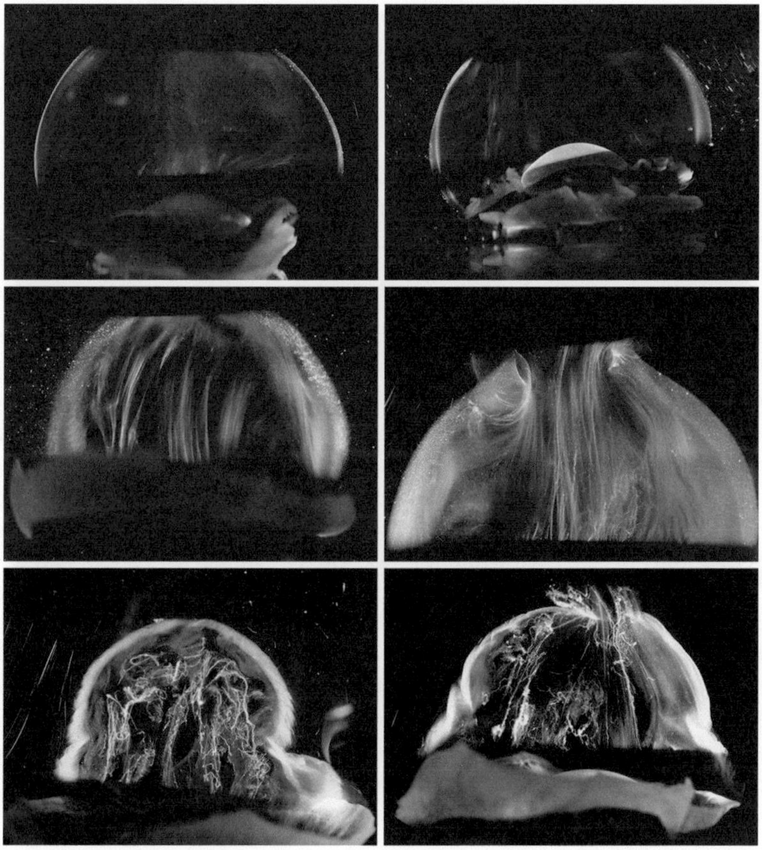

Fig. 3 Aging changes in human vitreous structure. Dark-field slit microscopy of fresh unfixed whole human vitreous body with the sclera, choroid, and retina dissected off the vitreous body, which remains attached to the anterior segment. A slit lamp beam illuminates from the side, creating a horizontal optical section with an illumination– observation angle of 90°, maximizing the Tyndall effect. The anterior segment is below and the posterior pole is above in all specimens. *Top Panel*: the vitreous bodies of an 11-year-old girl (*left*) and a 14-year-old boy (*right*) demonstrate a homogeneous structure with no significant light scattering within the vitreous body, only at the periphery where the vitreous cortex is comprised of a dense matrix of collagen fibrils. The posterior aspect of the lens is visible at the bottom of each image. *Middle Panel*: vitreous structure in a 56-year-old (*left*) and a 59-year-old (*right*) subject features macroscopic fi bers in the central vitreous body with an antero-posterior orientation. These form when hyaluronan molecules no longer separate collagen fibrils, allowing cross-linking and aggregation of collagen fibrils into visible fibers. *Bottom Panel*: in old age the fibers of the central vitreous become significantly thickened and tortuous, as demonstrated in the two eyes of an 88-year-old woman. Adjacent to these large fibers are areas of liquid vitreous, at times forming pockets, called lacunae. (Reprinted from Sebag et al. [224]).

OCT imaging [35] have challenged the previous belief that the posterior lacuna is solely a manifestation of age-related liquefaction [35, 36]. Rather, this seems to represent an anatomic structure, most likely the bursa premacularis of Worst, since it is found in youth [37]. Nonetheless, with aging there is increasing liquefaction with additional lacuna formation, leading to destabilization of the vitreous body and ultimately collapse due to the currents and countercurrents of liquid vitreous occurring during head/eye movement. Posterior vitreous detachment (PVD) occurs when there is sufficient liquefaction to promote collapse of the vitreous body accompanied by sufficient weakening of vitreo-retinal adhesion to allow anterior separation of the posterior vitreous cortex away from the ILM of the retina. With adequate weakening of vitreo-retinal adhesion, PVD occurs without pathologic consequences [5, 38–40].

The most common cause of PVD is aging; however, myopia, diabetes, and several other conditions (Marfan syndrome, Ehlers-Danlos syndrome, Stickler syndrome [41]) are also predisposing factors. It has been shown that surgical removal of the crystalline lens results in a higher incidence of complete PVD [42]. Another study demonstrated the importance of posterior capsule integrity [43]. In a recent prospective study of 575 eyes without PVD prior to cataract surgery, 5 %, 8 %, 11 %, 18 %, and 30 % developed PVD at 3, 6, 12, 24, and 36 months postoperatively, respectively [44]. This is perhaps due to a reduction in the concentration of hyaluronan [45] resulting from increased diffusion into the anterior chamber, amplified by absence of an intact posterior capsule [45, 46]. As a result of HA loss, vitreous viscoelasticity decreases lowering shock-absorbing ability [47], resulting in increased force transmission to the remaining vitreo-retinal attachments during ocular saccades and head movement. Persistent vitreo-retinal adhesion during PVD can have serious untoward consequences.

Anomalous PVD

When gel liquefaction exceeds the degree of weakening in vitreo-retinal adherence, traction is exerted at the vitreo-retinal interface with a variety of potential ill effects, collectively known as anomalous PVD (APVD). Full-thickness APVD occurs when the entire (full-thickness) posterior vitreous cortex stays attached to the retina, such as in vitreo-macular traction syndrome or retinal tears/detachment. Partial-thickness APVD occurs when there is a split in the posterior vitreous cortex, called vitreoschisis (VS; Fig. 4). Figure 5 outlines the various possible consequences of APVD that vary depending upon the area(s) of greatest vitreous liquefaction and where the posterior vitreous cortex is most firmly adherent to the retina. While peripheral and optic disk APVD are important, this chapter will only consider vitreo-maculopathies. These will be discussed as either "primary," where APVD is the cause, or "comorbid," where vitreo-macular adhesion contributes to the underlying maculopathy, typically either exudative AMD or ME due to diabetes or retinal vein occlusions.

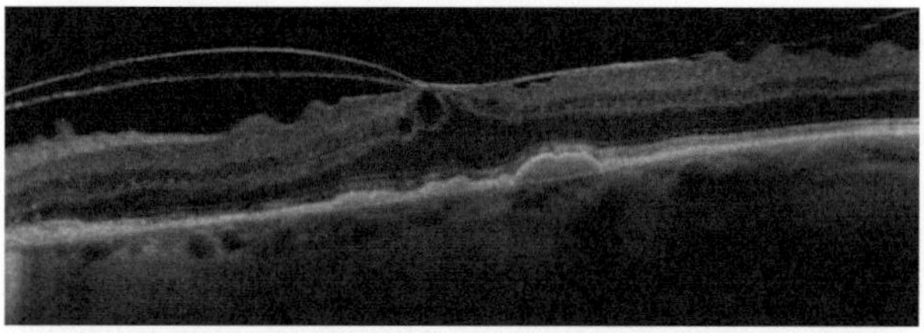

Fig. 4 Vitreoschisis. In vivo SD-OCT imaging of the human vitreo-retinal interface demonstrates a split in the posterior vitreous cortex, called vitreoschisis (Image courtesy of Jay Duker, MD)

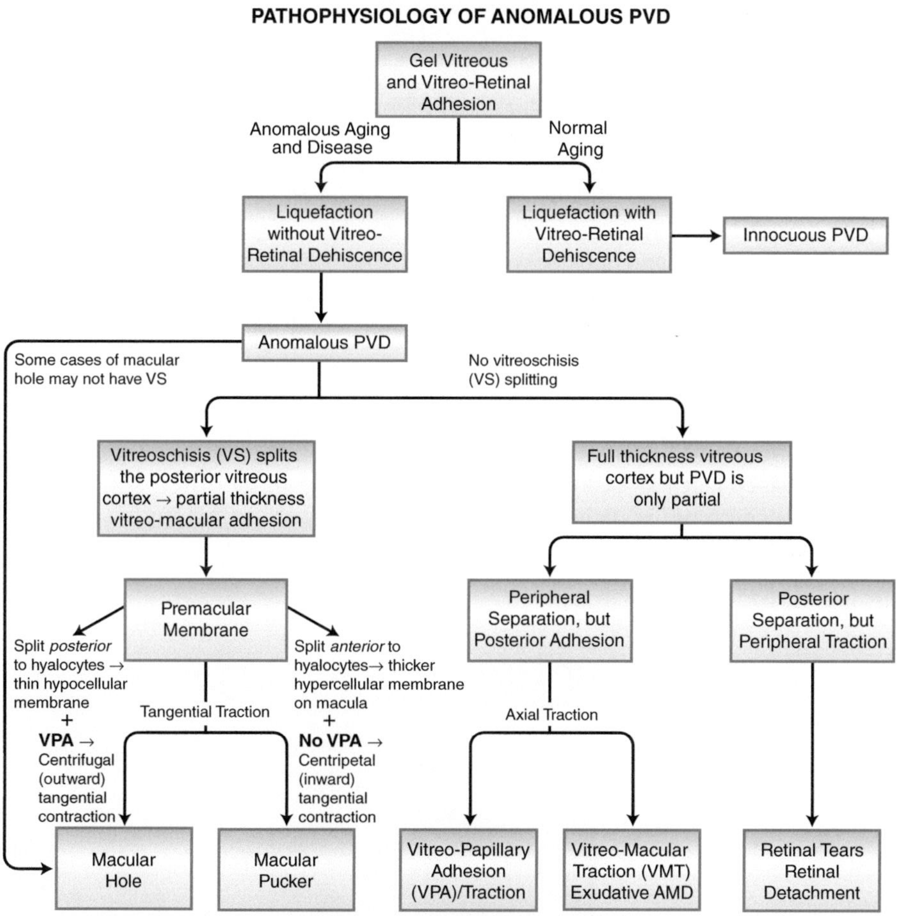

Fig. 5 Mechanisms and clinical manifestations of anomalous PVD. The mechanisms and various clinical consequences of anomalous PVD are shown. The different manifestations depend upon the area(s) of greatest vitreous gel liquefaction and where the posterior vitreous cortex is most firmly adherent to the retina

Primary Vitreo-Maculopathies (APVD Is the Primary Cause)

Vitreo-Macular Traction (VMT)

VMT is defined as vitreo-macular adhesion with structural changes in the underlying macula [2]. At the International Vitreomacular Traction Study (IVTS) group conference in 2012, a new classification system of vitreo-macular traction was developed, based solely upon anatomic changes as found with OCT imaging. To diagnose VMT, the following changes should be observed: (1) evidence of perifoveal vitreous cortex detachment from the retinal surface, (2) macular attachment of the posterior vitreous cortex within a 3-mm radius of the fovea, and (3) distortion of the foveal surface, intraretinal structural changes, elevation of the fovea above the RPE, or a combination of these anatomical changes [2]. VMT is classified by the size of vitreous attachment: focal, if less than 1500 μm, or broad, if greater than 1500 μm.

In the classic form of VMT, the posterior vitreous cortex is separated from the retina in the peripheral fundus but remains attached posteriorly, resulting in antero-posterior traction on a broad, often dumbbell-shaped region encompassing the macular area and optic nerve [49–52] (Fig. 6). The zone of vitreo-macular attachment can be small as seen in Fig. 6 or measure several disk areas in size [51, 52]. Associated findings include a premacular membrane and varying degrees of macular edema with fluorescein leakage. If VMT is severe, traction macular detachment can result, as seen in Fig. 6. Symptoms tend to progress with time, but a full-thickness macular hole rarely develops [53]. Vitreo-retinal surgery to relieve VMT is often associated with anatomic and visual improvement [50, 51, 54–57]. It has been suggested that traction on the fovea arising from APVD is a contributing pathogenic factor in some cases of CME following cataract surgery [58].

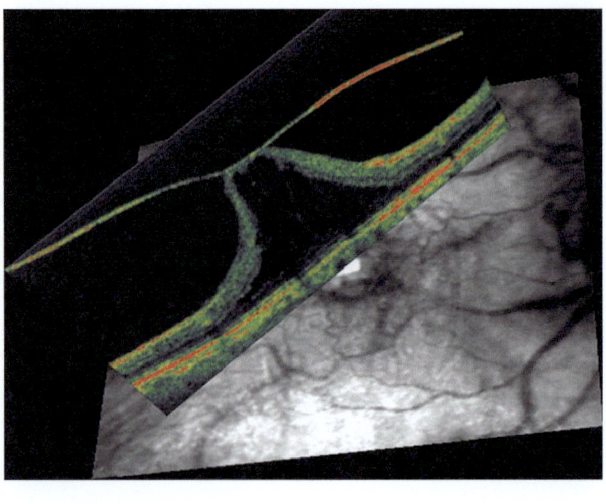

Fig. 6 Anomalous PVD with vitreo-macular traction. Persistent vitreo-macular adhesion results in axial vitreo-macular traction with elevation of the central macula

Macular Holes (MH)

A full-thickness macular hole (FTMH) is defined as a foveal lesion with interruption of all retinal layers from the ILM to the RPE, usually diagnosed by OCT imaging. The exact pathophysiologic mechanism is unknown; however, many theories have been proposed, such as vitreous traction, trauma, foveal degeneration, high myopia, and involutional thinning with PVD. The IVTS differentiated FTMHs based on size (small $\leq$250 µm, medium >250 to <400 µm, large $\geq$400 µm), vitreous status (with or without VMA), and associated conditions (primary vs. secondary) [41]. This classification has been shown to be useful as it predicts the anatomic and functional success after treatment with pharmacologic vitreolysis or surgical intervention [2].

There is typically no macular edema in MH because the cysts surrounding the hole are tractional rather than exudative [59–62]. The tangential traction theory [63] suggests that shrinkage of the perifoveal vitreous cortex induces an FTMH in four stages [64]. The possible mechanisms that can cause tangential vitreous traction are: fluid vitreous movement and countercurrents, cellular remodeling of the cortical vitreous, and contraction of a cellular membrane on the tapered cortical vitreous after vitreoschisis [65–67]. Indeed, vitreoschisis has been found in half of the eyes with MH [67]. In addition, vitreo-papillary adhesion (VPA) may play a crucial role in the development of MH, since VPA is present in 88.2 % of MH eyes [68]. VPA is also more prevalent in eyes with intraretinal cystoid spaces in both lamellar macular holes and macular pucker [68, 69]. Thus, it has been suggested that VPA influences the vector of tangential forces on the macula causing outward (centrifugal) traction opening a central dehiscence in an FTMH, foveal splitting in lamellar MH, and the formation of intraretinal cysts. In contrast, macular puckers have a very low incidence of VPA, and the vector of tangential forces is believed to be inward (centripetal).

Macular Pucker (MP)

When anomalous PVD is associated with vitreoschisis, a vitreous membrane remains on the macular surface. The term epiretinal membrane (ERM) is often used in literature to refer to this membrane. However, this term is inaccurate for two reasons: The term "epi-" indicates a location next to or beside a structure, in this case, the retina. Thus, the term "epiretinal" could refer to a subretinal location, which is clearly not the case. In addition, all of the related conditions are maculopathies, not retinopathies. Therefore, the accurate term is "premacular membrane" (PMM), which will be used throughout this chapter. In addition, the term "idiopathic" ERM is no longer appropriate, as we know that the cause of this condition is vitreous.

Following APVD with vitreoschisis, premacular membranes (PMM) can contract and cause metamorphopsia and visual impairment. Light microscopic studies of these membranes have shown the presence of astrocytes and RPE cells. However, there are likely other cells that have a similar morphological appearance, namely, hyalocytes. Zhao et al. examined ILM from 79 patients with macular pucker or VMT and found that hyalocytes are one of the major cell types [70]. These cells can elicit the migration of monocytes from the circulation further increasing the population of

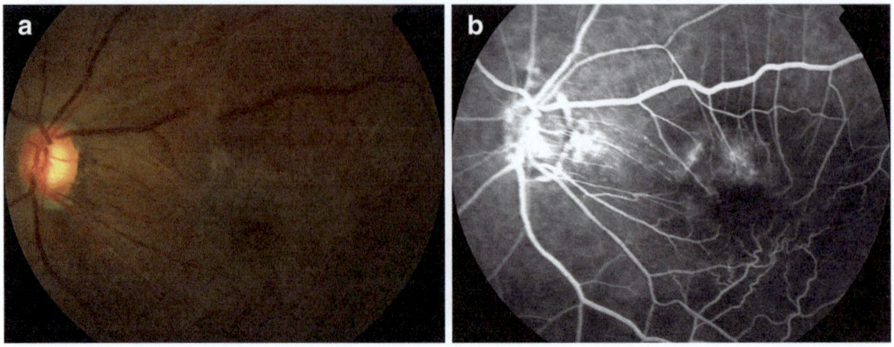

Fig. 7 Macular pucker. (**a**) Color fundus photograph of the left eye in a 65-year-old man showing macular pucker. (**b**) Premacular membrane (PMM) contraction in macular pucker has resulted in the disruption of the blood-retinal barrier with leakage and macular edema as demonstrated on fluorescein angiography

mononuclear phagocytes in these membranes. Sebag hypothesized that MP results when VS splits the posterior vitreous cortex anterior to the hyalocytes, leaving a thick and cellular membrane attached to the macula. A recent study found that half of all eyes with MP have more than one site of retinal contraction leading to a higher incidence of intraretinal cysts and significantly more macular thickening [71]. It is not clear whether these cysts are the result of traction as in the case of MH, or exudation and macular edema, which is found in about 40 % of eyes with MP [72].

Premacular membranes (PMM) are associated with macular dysfunction most likely due to an impairment of the neural retinal layers, particularly disruption of the inner and outer segments of photoreceptors [73, 74]. With time, PMM contraction in MP can result in disruption of the blood-retinal barrier in the underlying retina with exudation, identifiable on fluorescein angiography (Fig. 7). The extracellular accumulation of fluid can lead to cystoid changes, particularly in chronic MP. Thus, in addition to the distortions induced by the PMM in MP, ME causes blurred vision subjectively and decreased visual acuity objectively [75].

Vitreous surgery is the definitive cure for MP, with reduction/elimination of distortions [76], resolution of ME, and restoration of normal macular thickness and function. Visual acuity improves in 87 % of cases with restoration of normal macular thickness in 94 % of patients [77, 78]. MP does not presently appear to be treatable by pharmacologic vitreolysis, as the presence of a PMM is a relative contraindication to this form of therapy for vitreo-maculopathies (see below).

Comorbid Vitreo-Maculopathies (Vitreous Contributes)

Vitreous in Exudative AMD

It has been shown that full-thickness vitreo-macular adhesion (VMA) and traction (VMT) play a role in exudative age-related macular degeneration (AMD).

Anomalous PVD with persistent VMA is believed to promote or at least predispose to choroidal neovascularization, while a total PVD appears to be somewhat protective against wet AMD [79–82]. Clinical studies [79] found a twofold higher prevalence of PVD (diagnosed by ultrasound) in eyes with dry AMD compared to exudative AMD and a fivefold higher prevalence of VMA (diagnosed by OCT) in wet AMD compared to eyes with dry AMD. This was subsequently confirmed in two separate paired eye studies [79, 83] and was recently confirmed by a meta-analysis of 1,025 qualified articles, which found that wet AMD has double the prevalence of VMA and is less likely to have PVD [84]. Thus, although the exact mechanism is yet to be discovered, anomalous PVD seems to be a risk factor for exudative AMD [85–87]. A recent study [88] looked at 30 eyes of 25 patients with VMA surrounded by shallow detachment of the posterior vitreous cortex. The area of adhesion corresponded to a site of retinal angiomatous proliferation (RAP) in 88.2 %. In 73.3 % there was evidence of visible vitreo-retinal traction lines directed toward the choroidal neovascular membrane. Additionally, vitreo-papillary adhesion could be detected on the temporal margin of the optic disk in 83.3 %, about as often as in macular holes [68, 69], and the posterior vitreous cortex seemed to be split in the area of vitreo-papillary attachment, constituting vitreoschisis.

Vitreous in Diabetic Macular Edema (DME)

The biochemistry [30] and structure [89] of vitreous is altered by diabetes resulting in diabetic vitreopathy [48], which plays a role in the pathobiology of proliferative diabetic vitreo-retinopathy. Ultrasonography [90] and histopathology [91] have demonstrated vitreoschisis in proliferative diabetic retinopathy as well as in DME [92], which is the most common cause of vision loss in diabetic patients. In DME, cytokines and chemokines such as VEGF, fibroblast growth factor-2, and protein kinase C induce proliferation of hyalocytes and astrocytes in the posterior vitreous cortex [93]. These cells may strengthen adhesion of the posterior vitreous cortex to the ILM and perpetuate VMA, promoting VMT and contributing to DME [93]. Clinical studies have shown that the surgical removal of the posterior vitreous in DME patients contributes to less ischemia and decreased vasopermeability [94–96]. These findings may not only be due to relief of VMT by vitrectomy but also the removal of various molecules that promote DME, since vitreous appears to be a repository for various molecules that promote DME [97, 98]. Recent studies have shown that diabetic patients have more pro-inflammatory molecules in the vitreous body compared to nondiabetics [99]. In particular, IL-1B, caspase 1, and chemokines are increased significantly in vitreous, suggesting that chronic low-grade inflammation may be a factor in the pathogenesis of DME [99]. TNFα, which is also found in vitreous of patients with DME, is known to increase retinal endothelial permeability [100]. Other key molecules thought to promote DME by breakdown of the blood-retinal barrier are endothelial adhesion molecules, such as ICAM1, VCAM1, platelet-endothelial cell adhesion molecule 1 (PECAM-1), and P-selectin [101, 102].

Vitreous in Macular Edema due to Retinal Vein Occlusion (RVO)

Globally, an estimated 13.9 million people are affected by branch retinal vein occlusion (BRVO) and 2.5 million by central retinal vein occlusion (CRVO) [103], affecting males and females equally with a mean age of 65 years for CRVO. Five percent of RVO occurs in people over 80 years of age [104, 105]. The primary risk factor for RVO is atherosclerosis [105, 106], although arterial hypertension, cardiovascular disease, hyperlipidemia, diabetes mellitus, hypercoagulation, thrombophilia, and inflammatory disease have also been associated with RVO.

Retinal vein thrombosis causes elevation of intravascular pressure in vessels distal to the occlusion. The increased transmural hydrostatic pressure gradient in retinal capillaries results in transudation of fluid into the extracellular space. Associated hypoxia releases cytokines such as VEGF that break down the blood-retinal barrier, causing further leakage in both central and branch RVOs [107–110]. Although the exact etiology of RVO is not understood, vitreous seems to play a role [111]. Vitreopapillary adhesion has been documented in patients with ischemic central retinal vein occlusion (CRVO), resulting in a secondary serous neurosensory detachment that usually involves the macula [112]. Thick peripapillary tissue may be due to the growth of fibrous tissue in the area of VPA following hemorrhagic CRVO.

Although the current mainstay in treating ME due to RVO is intravitreal anti-VEGF injection [113], vitrectomy has been shown to be relatively beneficial for non-ischemic CRVO [114–116] and BRVO [116–119]. In addition, pharmacologic vitreolysis with autologous plasmin enzyme in eyes with BRVO has resulted in PVD and significant reduction of ME and improvement of VA in 88 % of eyes [119]. These observations suggest a role for the cortical vitreous and PVD status in BRVO. Future studies should explore whether pharmacologic vitreolysis could provide a useful adjunct to other forms of therapy for ME due to RVO.

Therapy

Surgical

The surgical management of vitreo-maculopathies is covered elsewhere in this book. However, two aspects that deserve emphasis here are chromodissection and reoperations.

Chromodissection

Chromodissection is a term that refers to the use of dyes to stain the ILM so as to facilitate membrane peeling [120]. This technique is especially useful in macular hole surgery [121], achieving a primary anatomic closure rate of 94 % using indocyanine green (ICG) chromodissection and 89 % with trypan blue [122].

ILM removal by chromodissection remains a controversial topic in macular pucker (MP) surgery. The rationale for ILM removal relates to the high incidence of vitreoschisis in MP and the risk of leaving a layer behind if ILM removal is not performed. Further, removal of ILM may reduce the incidence of MP recurrence due to removal of a scaffold that would enable cells to re-proliferate.

Reoperations of Macular Holes (MH) and Macular Pucker (MP)

Failure of MH surgery results from the incomplete peeling of the posterior vitreous cortex, the presence of subclinical premacular membrane (PMM) causing a residual traction at the hole, or inadequate gliosis [123, 124]. After initial successful closure, there can also be reopening of an MH, sometimes even years later [122, 123, 125–128]. The presence and progression of PMM formation has been correlated with MH recurrence, the mechanism thought to be that the PMM exerts tangential traction causing foveal dehiscence [123, 124].

Macular edema (ME) is associated with a sevenfold increase in the reopening of MH [129], with inflammatory fibrinolysis considered to be the causative process [122, 128]. Post-vitrectomy cataracts occur in 76 % of cases after 2 years [130–134], and cataract surgery after MH surgery has been associated with the reopening of the hole within 6 months of cataract extraction [122, 125, 128]. The proposed hypothesis for this event is the development of ME and/or PMM formation after cataract surgery due to breakdown of the blood-retinal barrier introducing postoperative inflammatory mediators. In order to avoid these complications, some surgeons have elected to combine MH surgery with phacoemulsification [130–132]. Lastly, YAG capsulotomy of posterior capsular opacification has been implicated in MH reformation [133], with the mechanism thought to be a perifoveal vitreous contraction related to the laser pulse, although it is not clear how this could occur.

Reoperation for recurrent/persistent MH and MP is successful if the cause is incomplete removal of the PMM. In this instance, ILM peeling with chromodissection can be performed with a number of stains such as ICG, trypan blue, triamcinolone acetonide, and Brilliant Blue G [67, 135–138]. In cases where adequate PMM and ILM peeling have been performed in the central macula, it has been suggested that more extensive ILM removal toward the vascular arcades may be an option [139]. However, reoperations can at times be associated with profound loss of vision [140]. Patients usually describe the sudden onset of a scotoma that occurs soon after surgery. There is significant loss of visual acuity, an afferent pupillary defect (APD), and altitudinal visual field loss. This presentation has been identified as resulting from vitrectomy with membrane peeling that has injured the retinal nerve fiber layer, resulting in an inner retinal optic neuropathy (IRON) [141]. Unlike AION, the visual field loss in IRON is not altitudinal, and no disk edema is present [141]. Studies [141] have determined that the risk of IRON is markedly diminished if reoperations are undertaken at least 6 months after the initial surgery. This is presumably due to the protection of the inner retina provided by resynthesis of the ILM, a process that takes many months [142].

Medical Management

Macular Edema (ME) in Retinal Vein Occlusion (RVO)

The current mainstay of treating ME from RVO is VEGF inhibition with ranibizumab, bevacizumab, or aflibercept. Frequent injections are usually needed to show benefit [143, 144], and rebound edema is sometimes worse than pretreatment edema [145]. In addition, the possible neurotoxic effect of chronic pan-VEGF suppression in an ischemic retina has raised concerns [146]. Other therapies have been advocated such as laser-induced chorio-retinal anastomosis, retinal intravascular tPA infusion, and surgery by radial optic neurotomy or arteriovenous sheathotomy [147]. Considering the aforementioned putative role of vitreous in RVO, there may be value in performing only vitrectomy with surgical induction of PVD or pharmacologic vitreolysis to induce PVD as an adjunct to the medical management of ME from RVO.

Diabetic Macular Edema (DME)

DME is the leading cause of vision loss in patients with both types 1 and 2 diabetes. Corticosteroids have been used to suppress inflammatory cell proliferation and migration and block the upregulation and/or activity of many pro-inflammatory cytokines involved in leukocyte stasis and breakdown of the blood-retinal barrier [148], but there are complications that follow repeated steroid injections. VEGF inhibition is an FDA-approved pharmacologic approach for the management of DME. Studies using pegaptanib [149], ranibizumab [150, 151], and bevacizumab [152] have demonstrated favorable clinical responses. It has recently been shown that aflibercept is superior to ranibizumab, which is in turn superior to bevacizumab in the treatment of DME [153].

Vitreous seems to play an important role in DME, both via VMA (see above) and VMT [154, 155]. There is also evidence that even subclinical perifoveal vitreous detachment may play a role in DME [156]. Thus, it would be reasonable to consider that the induction of PVD by pharmacologic vitreolysis could provide a useful adjunct to the medical therapy of DME.

Macular Edema in Age-Related Macular Degeneration (AMD)

Leakage from choroidal neovascularization (CNV) in neovascular age-related macular degeneration (AMD) results in intraretinal, as well as subretinal, fluid accumulation [157–159]. Studies have found that in exudative AMD, decreased visual acuity correlates with increased macular thickness [159, 160]. Anti-VEGF treatment with intravitreous ranibizumab has resulted in significant reduction of central retinal thickness (which includes both intraretinal and subretinal fluid components) as early as 1 day after the first injection [160]. Clinical trials have shown a significant reduction in central retinal thickness and improvement in visual acuity with anti-VEGF therapy [160]. It is important to note that reduction of macular edema overlying the CNV is not always accompanied by visual gain, most likely due to the atrophy of photoreceptors, loss of RPE, fibrotic scarring, and other irreversible alterations.

The importance of vitreous in the pathophysiology of exudative AMD was described above. Vitreous also appears to play a role in the therapy of exudative AMD [161]. In eyes with VMA, the attached posterior vitreous cortex might create a barrier effect interfering with the influx of nutrients and oxygen to, as well as the efflux of pro-angiogenic cytokines from, the macula [84]. A study in 110 eyes with wet AMD but no VMA found that there was significant improvement in VA after treatment with anti-VEGF injections ($P<0.05$) [162], while eyes with VMA did not have a significant improvement. This was confirmed by another study [163] of 255 treatment-naïve subjects, also finding that eyes with PVD improved with fewer injections. Thus, inducing PVD may not only eliminate any contribution of vitreous to the pathophysiology of exudative AMD but may be a way to enhance the pharmacotherapy of AMD as well. This was recently achieved via pharmacologic vitreolysis using ocriplasmin in 100 patients with exudative AMD and VMA. Those patients who achieved VMA resolution required fewer anti-VEGF injections [164]. These findings were recently confirmed by a study of p.r.n. dosing with ranibizumab in 34 treatment-naïve eyes with VMT, compared to 29 treatment-naïve eyes without VMT, as well as to other variable dosing studies (CATT, HARBOR, PrONTO, SUSTAIN). The findings showed that after 1 year of treatment, eyes with VMT had no significant improvement in visual acuity or central macular thickness, while eyes without VMT had significant improvements in both, and the degree of improvement was comparable to those of previous large studies [165].

Given the apparent role of vitreous in both the pathophysiology [166] and therapy [84] of exudative AMD, there may be benefit in eliminating the contribution of vitreous through adjunctive therapy to separate vitreous from the macula. While this can be effectively achieved with vitrectomy, a less invasive approach is preferable, such as with pharmacologic vitreolysis.

Pharmacologic Vitreolysis

Vitrectomy surgery is the mainstay of therapy to eliminate the role of vitreous in various retinal diseases, but it is considerably invasive, expensive, and can lead to complications [141, 167, 168]. Thus, alternative methods for the induction of PVD have been investigated, in particular, pharmacologic vitreolysis [169]. To this end, various agents have been tested over the past 20 years. According to their mechanism of action, these agents can be categorized as "enzymatic" or "nonenzymatic." Enzymatic agents include tissue plasminogen activator (tPA) [170], plasmin [171], microplasmin [172], nattokinase [173], chondroitinase [174], dispase [175], and hyaluronidase [176]. Nonenzymatic agents include urea/Vitreosolve and arginine-glycine-aspartate peptides [177].

Table 1 Pharmacologic vitreolysis classification based on biologic action

Liquefactants (agents that liquefy the gel vitreous)
Nonspecific:
tPA, plasmin, ocriplasmin, nattokinase, Vitreosolve[a]
Substrate specific:
Hyaluronidase
Interfactants (agents that weaken/lyse vitreo-retinal adhesion)
Nonspecific:
tPA, plasmin, ocriplasmin, nattokinase, Vitreosolve[a]
Substrate specific:
Dispase, chondroitinase, RGD-peptides[a]

Note: tPA, plasmin, ocriplasmin, nattokinase, and Vitreosolve are believed to be liquefactants and interfactants
tPA tissue plasminogen activator
[a]Nonenzymatic agents

Recently, Sebag [177] proposed a classification system in which pharmacologic vitreolysis agents are categorized based on their biologic effect: those that induce vitreous liquefaction (liquefactants) and those that induce dehiscence at the vitreo-retinal interface (interfactants). Table 1 classifies agents based on these biologic activities. Of note is that there have been seven agents tested to date. Five projects have failed or been disbanded, one agent is currently under continuing investigation, and only one agent has been approved for clinical pharmacologic vitreolysis.

Tissue Plasminogen Activator (tPA)

tPA is a serine protease that converts plasminogen into plasmin, the main enzyme responsible for blot clot lysis [178]. A randomized study [179] compared an intra-vitreal injection of 25 μg tPA to balanced salt solution (BSS) in ten patients before vitrectomy for proliferative diabetic vitreo-retinopathy. The use of tPA purportedly resulted in disintegration of the vitreo-retinal interface by PVD, thus facilitating vitrectomy without severe side effects [179]. In early studies the use of intravitreal tPA injection to treat subretinal hemorrhage encountered complications such as vitreous hemorrhage related to the fibrinolytic activity of tPA, which has been a concern [180, 181]. This is not frequent, however, and intraocular tPA is used routinely to lyse and displace submacular hemorrhage [182].

Plasmin

This nonspecific protease plays an active role in biologic processes such as fibrinolysis, neovascularization, and the activation of enzymes such as matrix metalloproteinases [183, 184]. Plasmin acts directly on fibronectin and laminin, which are in part responsible for adhesion between the posterior vitreous cortex and the ILM [171, 185]. Plasmin has been used to induce PVD in several animal models [171, 183, 185–189]. Intravitreal plasmin injection before or during vitrectomy has been studied in case series for DME with an adherent thick posterior vitreous cortex [190], macular holes [191, 192], proliferative diabetic retinopathy [193], diabetic tractional retinal detachment [194], VMT syndromes [195], and retinopathy of prematurity [196, 197]. Studies evaluating the use of plasmin during macular hole surgery suggest that plasmin facilitates membrane peeling [191, 192, 198, 199], especially in pediatric macular holes [197]. Other studies evaluated the use of plasmin during vitrectomy in six patients with bilateral proliferative diabetic retinopathy [193]. Surgical time was reduced (68 vs 89 min, $p=0.04$) and the incidence of retinal tears (0 vs. 3 eyes) was lower in the plasmin group than untreated fellow eyes, although there were no significant differences in vision outcomes [193]. Tsukhara et al. [196] successfully employed plasmin in six eyes with stage five ROP, four with a closed-funnel retinal detachment.

The intraoperative use of plasmin in eyes with DME associated with posterior vitreous cortex contraction found no significant difference in final retinal thickness, but plasmin-treated eyes had significantly better visual acuity than controls [190]. Another study evaluated the use of intravitreal plasmin as an adjunct to vitrectomy for 16 patients with refractory (to laser) DME [200]. One month post injection, central macular thickness was reduced and visual acuity was significantly increased in the plasmin-treated eyes [200]. The investigators concluded that pharmacologic vitreolysis effectively reduces central macular thickness and improves visual acuity in DME patients refractory to conventional laser treatment. However, because plasmin is derived preoperatively from the patient's blood by affinity chromatography, followed by a complicated process of sterilization and refrigeration before use [201], this technique is time consuming, cumbersome, and difficult. Further, plasmin is not commercially available for clinical use, and the enzyme activity is dependent on several variables. Thus, plasmin has not gained widespread use [202].

Ocriplasmin

The development of recombinant ocriplasmin has solved many of the problems with plasmin. Ocriplasmin contains only the enzymatic portion of the plasmin molecule [203] and is thus smaller (28 vs. 80 KD) [204]. Research with experimental models demonstrated that in both feline and human cadaver eyes there is dose- and time-dependent cleavage between the posterior vitreous cortex and the ILM without adverse effects on retinal structure [205]. Gandorfer et al. found that doses of 125 μg (the current clinical dose) or more caused a complete PVD with bare ILM in human eyes as demonstrated by electron microscopy. These findings were confirmed by DeSmet et al. [206] in porcine eyes. Their findings were corroborated by Sakuma et al. [172] in rabbit eyes using doses of ocriplasmin from 12.5 to 250 μg; although doses of 125 μg of ocriplasmin or greater induced a complete PVD, lower doses induced a partial PVD. Recently, Chen et al. [203] used immunofluorescent histochemistry in rat eyes to determine that ocriplasmin causes degradation of fibronectin and laminin not only at the vitreo-retinal interface but also at the photoreceptor layer in the outer retina, a potentially untoward effect.

Clinically, ocriplasmin has been found to induce PVD and vitreous liquefaction without evidence of retinal toxicity [172]. In addition to salubrious mechanical effects, there may be physiologic benefits to ocriplasmin pharmacologic vitreolysis. Sebag et al. [207] reported that pharmacologic vitreolysis with ocriplasmin increases vitreous diffusion coefficients as determined by dynamic light scattering. Another study [208] showed that PVD induction by ocriplasmin increases oxygen levels in the vitreous body, perhaps assisting in the management of ischemic retinopathies with exudative maculopathy like DME and ME from RVOs (see above).

Pharmacologic vitreolysis [177, 209, 210] with ocriplasmin is now approved to treat symptomatic VMA in the USA and VMT in Europe, specifically macular holes based upon the results of phase III studies [211]. A recent review article by Khoshnevis and Sebag [212] summarized the rationale and the therapeutic potential of ocriplasmin in treating vitreo-retinal disorders. Based on post-approval analyses of the phase III trials in Europe and the USA, the following criteria have been identified as favorable clinical characteristics: (1) female gender, (2) age less than 65 years old, (3) phakic lens status, (4) VMA < 1500 μm in extent, (5) FTMH ≤ 400 μm (best results < 250 μm) in diameter, and (6) the absence of a premacular membrane with macular pucker [211]. Thus, ocriplasmin represents a viable alternative approach to surgery in selected cases.

Nattokinase

Nattokinase is a strong fibrinolytic agent that is derived from natto, a popular soybean cheese in Japan [169, 173]. Nattokinase is a serine protease produced by *Bacillus subtilis* (natto). It can be administered orally and is available in foods prepared from soybeans. One study [173] injected nattokinase into rabbit eyes and found that this induced complete PVD with a smooth ILM surface.

Chondroitinase

Chondroitinase is an enzyme complex that cleaves chondroitin-sulfate-containing glycosaminoglycan (GAG) side chains of proteoglycan "core" molecules [213]. Since GAGs play an important role at the vitreo-retinal interface, chondroitinase has the potential to be a potent interfactant. Studies testing chondroitinase in human, primate, and pig eyes showed that adhesion between the collagen/hyaluronan matrix of the posterior vitreous cortex and the retina, optic disk, and lens was markedly reduced [214, 215]. Phase I/II FDA testing showed some evidence of efficacy; however, its development has not been further pursued for several reasons, including cost [213, 216].

Vitreolysin™ (Purified Dispase)

Purified dispase (Vitreolysin™) is a protease produced by *Paenibacillus polymyxa* that has been developed for the pharmacologic induction of PVD [217]. By degrading type IV collagen and fibronectin at the vitreo-retinal interface, this agent cleaves posterior vitreous cortex attachment to the ILM. The low affinity of dispase for type II collagen allows this agent to induce PVD without disrupting the macromolecular structure of the vitreous body. One study [218] injected dispase into human and porcine cadaver eyes and after 15 min of incubation showed partial or total PVD in the majority of the eyes. Microscopic examinations of retinal cell viability were equivalent in dispase-treated and control eyes [218]. The investigators concluded that dispase might be useful in removing cortical vitreous at surgery. Another study found that purified dispase was useful in PVD induction [219]. While initially some studies reported harmful effects from dispase such as retinal hemorrhages, cataract, or lens subluxation [175, 220, 221], subsequent studies found that purified dispase (Vitreolysin™) does not induce toxicity [217]. Human studies investigating the efficacy and safety of pharmacologic vitreolysis with purified dispase are still pending.

Hyaluronidase

Vitrase®, a highly purified bovine hyaluronidase [176, 222], acts on the glycosidic bonds of hyaluronan (HA) and other mucopolysaccharides, causing liquefaction of the vitreous gel [185]. Because HA does not play a role in maintaining vitreo-retinal adhesion, Vitrase has no effect upon the vitreo-retinal interface. Thus, rather than release vitreo-retinal adhesion, Vitrase could induce anomalous PVD (see above). Consequently, phase III clinical trials to assess the efficacy of Vitrase in accelerating the clearance of vitreous hemorrhage did not provide sufficient evidence to demonstrate clinical efficacy, and the FDA did not approve this drug for pharmacologic vitreolysis. The underlying reason for the failure of Vitrase is the fact that HA is not important in maintaining vitreo-retinal adhesion, and thus, hyauronidase is not an interfactant but only a liquefactant (Table 1) and does not weaken vitreo-retinal adhesion [185, 223]. In diabetic patients with proliferative diabetic vitreo-retinopathy, this will lead to persistent traction upon the neovascular complexes that have grown into the posterior vitreous cortex and lead to recurrent vitreous hemorrhage and vision loss. Because Vitrase has a high likelihood of inducing anomalous PVD, it should not be used to clear vitreous hemorrhage except perhaps in the setting of existing PVD.

References

1. Tso MOM. Pathology of cystoid macular edema. Ophthalmology. 1982;89:902–15.
2. Duker JS, Kaiser PK, Binder S, de Smet MD, Gaudric A, Reichel E, Sadda SR, Sebag J, Spaide RF, Stalmans P. The International Vitreomacular Traction Study Group classification of vitreomacular adhesion, traction, and macular hole. Ophthalmology. 2013;17:2611–9.
3. Carpineto P, Di Antonio L, Aharrh-Gnama A, Ciciarelli V, Mastropasqua L. Diagnosing and treating vitreomacular adhesion. Eur Ophthalmic Rev. 2011;5(1):69–73.
4. Kishi S, Demaria C, Shimizu K. Vitreous cortex remnants at the fovea after spontaneous vitreous detachment. Int Ophthalmol. 1986;9:253–60.

5. Sebag J. The vitreous: structure, function, and pathobiology. New York: Springer; 1989.
6. Jacobson B. Degradation of glycosaminoglycans by extracts of calf vitreous hyalocytes. Exp Eye Res. 1984;39(3):373–85.
7. Breen M, Bizzell JW, Weinstein HG. A galactosamine containing proteoglycan in human vitreous. Exp Eye Res. 1977;24(4):409–12.
8. Allen WS, Otterbein EC, Wardi AH. Isolation and characterization of the sulfated glycosaminoglycans of the vitreous body. Biochim Biophys Acta. 1977;498(1):167–75.
9. Kamei A, Totani A. Isolation and characterization of minor glycosaminoglycans in the rabbit vitreous body. Biochme Biophys Res Commun. 1982;109(3):881–7.
10. Hultsch E, Freeman MI, Balazs EA. Transport and regeneration of hyaluronic acid in extracellular ocular compartments. Annual meeting of the Association for Research in Vision and Ophthalmology (ARVO). Invest Ophthalmol. 1974;11:97.
11. Borzacchiell A, Netti PA, Ambrosio L, Nicolais L. Hyaluronic acid derivatives mimic the rheological properties of vitreous body. In: Abatangelo G, Weigel PH, editors. New frontiers in medical sciences: redefining hyaluronan: proceedings of the symposium held in Padua. 17–19 June 1999. Amsterdam: Elsevier; 2000. p. 195–202.
12. Comper WD, Laurent TC. Physiological function of connective tissue polysaccharides. Physiol Rev. 1978;58(1):255–315.
13. Reardon A, Heinegard D, McLeod D, Seehan JK, Bishop PN. The large chondroitin sulphate proteoglycan versican in mammalian vitreous. Matrix Biol. 1988;17(5):325–33.
14. Kloeckener-Gruissem B, Bartholdi D, Abdou MT, Zimmermann DR, Berger W. Identification of the genetic defect in the original Wagner syndrome family. Mol Vis. 2006;12:350–5.
15. Goes RM, Nader HB, Porcionatto MA, Haddad A, Laicine EM. Chondroitin sulfate proteoglycans are structural renewable constituents of the rabbit vitreous body. Curr Eye Res. 2005;30(5):405–13.
16. Bishop P, Crossman M, McLeod D, Ayad S. Extraction and characterization of the tissue forms of collagen types II and IX from bovine vitreous. Biochem J. 1994;299(Pt 2):497.
17. Richards AJ, Martin S, Yates JRW, Scott JD, Baguley DM, Pope FM, et al. COL2A1 exon 2 mutations: relevance to the Stickler and Wagner syndromes. Br J Ophthalmol. 2000;84(4):364–71.
18. Bishop P, McLeod D, Ayad S. Extraction and characterization of the intact form of bovine vitreous type IX collagen. Biochem Biophys Res Commun. 1992;185(1):392–7.
19. Bos K, Holmes D, Meadows R, Kadler K, McLeod D, Bishop P. Collagen fibril organization in mammalian vitreous by freeze etch/rotary shadowing electron microscopy. Micron. 2001;32(3):3016.
20. Bishop PN, McLeod D, Reardon A. Effects of hyaluronan lyase, hyaluronidase, and chondroitin ABC lyase on mammalian vitreous gel. Invest Ophthalmol Vis Sci. 1999;40(10):2173–8.
21. Jackson DS. Chondroitin sulphuric acid s a factor in the stability of tendon. Biochem J. 1953;54(4):638–41.
22. Swann DA, Constable IJ, Caulfield JB. Vitreous structure. IV. Chemical composition of the insoluble residual protein fraction from the rabbit vitreous. Invest Ophthalmol. 1975;14(8): 613–6.
23. Scott JE. Supramolecular organization of extracellular matrix glycosaminoglycans, in vitro and in the tissues. FASEB J. 1992;6(9):2639–45.
24. Scott JE. The chemical morphology of the vitreous. Eye (Lond). 1992;6(Pt6):553–5.
25. Halfter W, Sebag J, Cunningham EC. Vitreo-retinal interface and inner limiting membrane. In: Sebag J, editor. Vitreous – in health & disease. New York: Springer; 2014. p. 165–91.
26. Russell SR. What we know (and do not know) about vitreoretinal adhesion. Retina. 2012;32: S181–6.
27. Hindson VJ, Gallagher JT, Halfter W, Bishop PN. Opticin binds to heparan and chondroitin sulfate proteoglycans. Invest Ophthalmol Vis Sci. 2005;46(12):4417–23.
28. Le Goff M, Bishop P. Adult vitreous structure and postnatal changes. Eye. 2008;22(10): 1214–22.
29. Van Deemter M, Ponsioen T, Bank R, Snabel J, Van der Worp R, Hooymans J, et al. Pentosidine accumulates in the aging vitreous body: a gender defect. Exp Eye Res. 2009;88(6):1043–50.

30. Sebag J, Buckingham B, Charles MA, Reiser K. Biochemical abnormalities in vitreous of humans with proliferative diabetic retinopathy. Arch Ophthalmol. 1992;110:1472–9.
31. Sebag J. Vitreous – from biochemistry to clinical relevance. In: Tasman W, Jaeger E, editors. Duane's foundation of clinical ophthalmology. Philadelphia: Lippincott Williams & Wilkins; 1998. p. 1–34.
32. Schmut O, Mallinger R, Paschke E. Studies on a distinct fraction of bovine vitreous body collagen. Graefes Arch Clin Exp Ophthalmol. 1984;221(6):286–9.
33. Scott JE, Chen Y, Brass A. Secondary and tertiary structures involving chondroitin and chondroitin sulphates in solution, investigated by rotary shadowing/electron microscopy and computer simulation. Eur J Biochem. 1992;209(2):675–80.
34. Oksala A. Ultrasonic and biomicroscopic observations on the vitreous space in patients with idiopathic detachment of the retina. Albrecht Von Graefes Arch Klin Exp Ophthalmol. 1980;214(3):205–12.
35. Itakura H, Kishi S, Li D, Akiyama H. Observation of posterior precortical vitreous pocket using swept-source optical coherence tomography. Invest Ophthalmol Vis Sci. 2013;54(5): 3102–7.
36. Shimada H, Hirose T, Yamamoto A, Nakashizuka H, Httori T, Yuzawa M. Depiction of the vitreous pocket by optical coherence tomography. Int Ophthalmol. 2011;31(1):51–3.
37. Kakeshashi A, Kado M, Akiba J, Kirokawa H. Biomicroscopic findings of premacular posterior vitreous. Nihon Ganka Gakkai Zasshi. 1995;99(3):323–8.
38. Balazs EA, Denlinger JL. Aging changes in the vitreous. In: Sekuler R, Kline D, Dismukes K, editors. Aging and human visual function. New York: Liss; 1982. p. 45–7.
39. Eisner G. Posterior vitreous detachment. Klin Monbl Augenheilkd. 1989;194(5):389–92.
40. Foos RY, Wheeler NC. Vitreoretinal juncture. Synchysis senilis and posterior vitreous detachment. Ophthalmology. 1982;89(12):1502–12.
41. Snead MP, Yates JR. Clinical and molecular genetics of Stickler syndrome. J Med Genet. 1999;36(5):353–9.
42. Heller MD, Straatsma BR, Foos RY. Detachment of the posterior vitreous in phakic and aphakic eyes. Mod Probl Ophthalmol. 1972;10:23–36.
43. McDonnell PJ, Patel A, Green WR. Comparison of intrascapular and extrascapular cataract surgery. Histopathologic study of eyes obtained postmortem. Ophthalmology. 1985;92(9):1208–25.
44. Hikichi T. Time course of development of posterior vitreous detachment after phacoemulsification surgery. Ophthalmology. 2012;119(10):2102–7.
45. Osterlin S. Macromolecular composition of the vitreous in the aphakic owl monkey eye. Exp Eye Res. 1978;26(1):77–84.
46. Osterlin S. Changes in the molecular morphology of the vitreous after intraocular surgery. Acta Ophthalmol. 1970;48(4):829.
47. Kawano SI, Honda Y, Negi A. Effects of biological stimuli on the viscosity of the vitreous. Acta Ophthalmol. 1982;60(6):977–91.
48. Sebag J. Diabetic vitreopathy. Ophthalmology. 1996;103(2):205–6.
49. Jaffe NS. Vitreous traction at the posterior pole of the fundus due to alterations in the vitreous posterior. Trans Am Acad Ophthalmol Otolaryngol. 1967;71:642–52. 2.
50. Smiddy WE, Michels RG, Glaser BM, deBustros S. Vitrectomy for macular traction caused by incomplete vitreous separation. Arch Ophthalmol. 1988;106:624–8.
51. McDonald HR, Johnson RN, Schatz H. Surgical results in the vitreomacular traction syndrome. Ophthalmology. 1994;101:1397–403.
52. Smiddy WE. Vitreomacular traction syndrome. In: Yanoff M, Duker JS, editors. Ophthalmology. 2nd ed. St. Louis: CV Mosby; 2004. p. 951–5.
53. Margherio RR, Trese MT, Margherio AR, Cartright K. Surgical management of vitreomacular traction syndromes. Ophthalmology. 1989;96:1437–45.
54. Melberg NS, Williams DF, Balles MW, et al. Vitrectomy for vitreomacular traction syndrome with macular detachment. Retina. 1995;15:192–7.
55. Massin P, Erginay A, Haouchine B, et al. Results of surgery of vitreomacular traction syndromes. J Fr Ophthalmol. 1997;20:539–47.

56. Pournaras CJ, Kapetanios AD, Donati G. Vitrectomy for traction macular edema. Doc Ophthalmol. 1999;97:439–47.
57. Koerner F, Garweg J. Vitrectomy for macular pucker and vitreomacular traction syndrome. Doc Ophthalmol. 1999;97:449–58.
58. Tolentino FI, Schepens CL. Edema of posterior pole after cataract extraction. Arch Ophthalmol. 1965;74:781–6.
59. Spaide RF, Wong D, Fisher Y, Goldbaum M. Correlation of vitreous attachment and foveal deformation in early macular hole states. Am J Ophthalmol. 2002;133:226–9.
60. Gaudric A, Haouchine B, Massin P, Paques M, Blain P, Erginay A. Macular hole formation. New data provided by optical coherence tomography. Arch Ophthalmol. 1999;117:744–51. [PubMed].
61. Haouchine B, Massin P, Gaudric A. Foveal pseudocyst as the first step in macular hole formation: a prospective study by optical coherence tomography. Ophthalmology. 2001;108(1): 15–22.
62. Takahashi A, Yoshida A, Nagaoka T, Takamiya A, Sato E, Kagokawa H, et al. Idiopathic full-thickness macular holes and the vitreomacular interface: a high-resolution spectral-domain optical coherence tomography study. Am J Ophthalmol. 2012;154:881–92.
63. Haritoglou C, Reiniger IW, Schaumberger M, Gass CA, Priglinger SG, Kampik A. Fiver-year follow up of macular hole surgery with peeling of the internal limiting membrane: update of a prospective study. Retina. 2006;26(6):618–22.
64. Johnson RN, Gass JD. Idiopathic macular holes. Observations, stages of formation, and implications for surgical intervention. Ophthalmology. 1988;95(7):917–24.
65. Sebag J. Anomalous posterior vitreous detachment: a unifying concept in vitreo-retinal disease. Graefes Arch Clin Exp Ophthalmol. 2004;242(8):690–8.
66. Gartner J. Electron-microscopic study on the fibrillar network and fibrocyte-collagen interactions in the vitreous cortex at the ora serrata of human eyes with special regard to the role of disintegrating cells. Exp Eye Res. 1986;42(1):21–33.
67. Sebag J. Vitreous: the resplendent enigma. Br J Ophthalmol. 2009;93(8):989–91. Available at: http://www.ncbi.nlm.nih.gov/pubmed/19633281.
68. Sebag J, Wang MY, Nguyen D, Sadun AA. Vitreopapillary adhesion in macular diseases. Trans Am Ophthalmol Soc. 2009;107:35–44.
69. Wang MY, Nguyen D, Hindoyan N, Sadun AA, Sebag J. Vitreo-papillary adhesion in macular hole and macular pucker. Retina. 2009;29:644–50.
70. Zhao F, Gandorfer A, Haritoglou C, Scheler R, Schaumberger MM, Kampik A, et al. Epiretinal cell proliferation in macular pucker and vitreomacular traction syndrome: analysis of flat mounted internal limiting membrane specimens. Retina. 2013;33(1):77–88.
71. Gupta P, Saddun AA, Sebag J. Multifocal retinal contraction in macular pucker analyzed by combined optical coherence tomography/scanning laser ophthalmoscopy. Retina. 2008;28(3): 447–52.
72. Fatum S, Trevino A, Ophir A. Non-diabetic diffuse macular edema associated with extrafoveal vitreous traction. Isr Med Assoc J. 2009;11(5):286–90.
73. Tanikawa A, Horiguchi M, Kondo M, et al. Abnormal focal macular electroretinograms in eyes with idiopathic epimacular membrane. Am J Ophthalmol. 1999;127:559–64.
74. Inoue M, Morita S, Watanabe Y, Kaneko T, Yamane S, Kobayashi S, Arakawa A, Kadonosono K. Preoperative inner segment/outer segment junction in spectral-domain optical coherence tomography as a prognostic factor in epiretinal membrane surgery. Retina. 2011;31(7):1366–72. doi:10.1097/IAE.0b013e318203c156.
75. Hillenkamp J, Saikia P, Gora F, et al. Macular function and morphology after peeling of idiopathic epiretinal membrane with and without the assistance of indocyanine green. Br J Ophthalmol. 2005;89(4):437–43.
76. Nguyen J, Yee KMP, Sadun AA, Sebag J: Quantifying visual dysfunction and the response to surgery in macular pucker. Ophthalmology. E-pub ahead of print April 27, 2016 pii: S0161-6420(16)00382-1. doi: 10.1016/j.ophtha.2016.03.022.

77. de Bustros S, Rice TA, Michels RG, Thompson JT, Marcus S, Glaser BM. Vitrectomy for macular pucker after treatment of retinal tears or retinal detachment. Arch Ophthalmol. 1988;106:758–60.
78. Lee PY, Cheng KC, Wu WC. Anatomic and functional outcome after surgical removal of idiopathic macular epiretinal membrane.Kaohsiung. J Med Sci. 2011;27:268–75.
79. Robison CD, Krebs I, Binder S, Barbazetto IA, Kotsolis AI, Yannuzzi LA, Sadun AA, Sebag J. Vitreomacular adhesion in active and end-stage age-related macular degeneration. Am J Ophthalmol. 2009;148:79–82.
80. Krebs I, Glittenberg C, Binder S, Weber-Krause B, Eckardt C. Incidence of PVD in the elderly. Ophthalmologe. 1997;94:619–23.
81. Binder S, Krebs I, Hilgers RD, et al. Outcome of transplantation of autologous retinal pigment epithelium in age-related macular degeneration: a prospective trial. Invest Ophthalmol Vis Sci. 2004;45:4151–60.
82. Krebs I, Brannath W, Glittenberg C, Zeiler F, Sebag J, Binder S. Posterior vitreo-macular adhesion: a potential risk factor for exudative age-related macular degeneration? Am J Ophthalmol. 2007;144(5):741–6.
83. Lee SJ, Lee CS, Koh HJ. Posterior vitreo-macular adhesion and risk of exudative age-related macular degeneration: paired eye study. Am J Ophthalmol. 2009;147:621–6.
84. Jackson TL, Nicod E, Angelis A, Grimaccia F, Prevost AT, Simpson AR, Kanavos P. Vitreous attachment in age-related macular degeneration, diabetic macular edema, and retinal vein occlusion: a systematic review and metanalysis. Retina. 2013;33(6):1099–108. doi:10.1097/IAE.0b013e31828991d6.
85. Mayr-Sponer U, Waldstein SM, Kundi M, Ritter M, Golbaz I, Heiling U, et al. Influence of the vitreomacular interface on outcomes of Ranibizumab therapy in neovascular age-related macular degeneration. Ophthalmology. 2013;120(12):2620–9.
86. Uney GO, Unlu N, Acar MA, Hazirolan D, Altiparmak UE, Yalniz-Akkaya Z, et al. Role of posterior vitreous detachment on outcome of anti-vascular endothelial growth factor treatment in age-related macular degeneration. Retina. 2014;34:32–7.
87. Sebag J, Glittenberg C, Krebs I, et al. Vitreomacular adhesion in active and end-stage age-related macular degeneration author reply. Am J Ophthalmol. 2010;149:172e3.
88. Krebs I, Glittenberg C, Zeiler F, Binder S. Spectral domain optical coherence tomography for higher precision in the evaluation of vitreoretinal adhesions in exudative age-related macular degeneration. Br J Ophthalmol. 2011;95:1415–8.
89. Sebag J. Abnormalities of human vitreous structure in diabetes. Graefes Arch Clin Exp Ophthalmol. 1993;231(5):257–60.
90. Chu TG, Lopez PF, Cano MR, Freeman WR, Lean JS, Liggett PE, et al. Posterior vitreoschisis. An echographic finding in proliferative diabetic retinopathy. Ophthalmology. 1996;103(2):315–22.
91. Schwatz SD, Alexander R, Hiscott P, Gregor ZJ. Recognition of vitreoschisis in proliferative diabetic retinopathy. A useful landmark in vitrectomy for diabetic traction retinal detachment. Ophthalmology. 1996;103(2):323–8.
92. Sebag J. Vitreoschisis in diabetic macular edema. Invest Ophthalmol Vis Sci. 2011;52(11):8455–6. Author reply 6–7.
93. Bhagat N, Grigorian RA, Tutela A, Zarbin MA. Diabetic macular edema: pathogenesis and treatment. Surv Opthalmol. 2009;54:1–32.
94. Nguyen QD, Shah SM, Van Anden E, et al. Supplemental oxygen improved diabetic macular edema: a pilot study. Invest Ophthalmol Vis Sci. 2004;45:617–24.
95. Flaxel CJ, Edwards AR, Aiello LP, et al. Factors associated with visual acuity outcomes after vitrectomy for diabetic macular edema: diabetic retinopathy clinical research network. Retina. 2010;30:1488–95.
96. Haller JA, Qin H, Apte RS, et al; Diabetic Retinopathy Clinical Research Network Writing Committee. Vitrectomy outcomes in eyes with diabetic macular edema and vitreomacular traction. Ophthalmology. 2010;117(6):1087–93.

97. Deissler H, Deissler H, Lang S, Lang GE. VEGF-induced effects on proliferation, migration and tight junctions are restored by ranibizumab (Lucentis) in microvascular retinal endothelial cells. Br J Ophthalmol. 2008;92:839–43.
98. Lang GE. Vitreous in retino-vascular diseases and diabetic macular edema. In: Sebag J, editor. Vitreous – in health & disease. New York: Springer; 2014. p. 407–19.
99. Zhang W, Liu H, Al-Shabraway M, Caldwell RW, Caldwell RB. Inflammation and diabetic retinal microvascular complications. J Cardiovasc Dis Res. 2011;2:96–103.
100. Simo-Servat O, Hernandez C, Simo R. Usefulness of the vitreous fluid analysis in the translational research of diabetic retinopathy. Mediators Inflamm. 2012;2012:872978.
101. Olson JA, Whitelaw CM, McHardy KC, Pearson DW, Forrester JV. Soluble leucocyte adhesion molecules in diabetic retinopathy stimulate retinal capillary endothelial cell migration. Diabetologia. 1997;40:1166–71.
102. Klein BE, Knudtson MD, Tsai MY, Klein R. The relation of markers of inflammation and endothelial dysfunction to the prevalence and progression of diabetic retinopathy: Wisconsin epidemiologic study of diabetic retinopathy. Arch Ophthalmol. 2009;127:1175–82.
103. Laouri M, Chen E, Looman M, Gallagher M. The burden of disease of retinal vein occlusion: review of the literature. Eye. 2011;25:981–8.
104. Rogers S, McIntosh M, Cheung N, Lim L, Wang JJ, Mitchel P, Kowalski JW, Nguyen H, Wong TY. The international eye disease consortium: the prevalence of retinal vein occlusion: pooled data from population studies from the United States, Europe, Asia, and Australia. Ophthalmology. 2010;117:313–9.
105. Jaulim A, Ahmed B, Khanam T, Chatziralli IP. Branch retinal vein occlusion: epidemiology, pathogenesis, risk factors, clinical features, diagnosis and complications. An update of the literature. Retina. 2013;33:901–10.
106. Stern MS, Talwar N, Comer GM, Stein JD. A longitudinal analysis of risk factors associated with central vein occlusion. Ophthalmology. 2013;120:362–70.
107. Sidd R, Fine S, Owens S, Patz A. Idiopathic preretinal gliosis. Am J Opthalmol. 1982;94(1):44.
108. Cunha-Vaz JG. The blood–retinal barriers. Doc Ophthalmol. 1976;41(287–327):12.
109. Vinores SA, Amin A, Derevjanik NL, Green WR, Campochiaro PA. Immunohistochemical localization of blood-retinal barrier breakdown sites associated with post-surgical macular edema. Histochem J. 1994;26(655–665):13.
110. Vinores SA, Youssri AI, Luna JD, Chen YS, Bhargave S, Vinores MA, Schoenfeld CL, Peng B, Chan CC, LaRochelle W, Green WR, Campochiaro PA. Upregulation of vascular endothelial growth factor in ischemic and non-ischemic human and experimental retinal disease. Histol Histopathol. 1997;12(99–109):14.
111. Hikichi T, Konno S, Trempe CL. Role of the vitreous in central retinal vein occlusion. Retina. 1995;15(1):29–33.
112. Rumelt S, Karatas M, Pikkel J, Majlin M, Ophir A. Optic disc traction syndrome with central retinal vein occlusion. Arch Opthalmol. 2003;121:1093–7.
113. Lazić R, Boras I, Vlasić M, Gabrić N, Tomić Z. Anti-VEGF in treatment of central retinal vein occlusion. Coll Antropol. 2010;34 Suppl 2:69–72.
114. Noma H, Funatsu H, Mimura T, Shimada K. Visual acuity and foveal thickness after vitrectomy for macular edema. Ophthalmologica. 2010;224(367–373):24.
115. Park DH, Kim IT. Long-term effects of vitrectomy and internal limiting membrane peeling for macular edema secondary to central retinal vein occlusion and hemiretinal vein occlusion. Retina. 2010;30(117–124):25.
116. Raszewska-Steglinska M, Gozdek P, Cisiecki S, Michalewska Z, Michalewski J, Nawrocki J. Pars plana vitrectomy with ILM peeling for macular edema secondary to retinal vein occlusion. Eur J Ophthalmol. 2009;19(1055–1062):26.
117. Shah GK, Sharma S, Fineman MS, Federman J, Brown MM, Brown GC. Arteriovenous adventitial sheathotomy for the treatment of macular edema associated with branch retinal vein occlusion. Am J Ophthalmol. 2000;129(104–106):27.
118. Tsujikawa A, Fujihara M, Iwawaki T, Yamamoto K, Kurimoto Y. Triamcinolone acetonide with vitrectomy for treatment of macular edema associated with branch retinal vein occlusion. Retina. 2005;25(861–867):28.

119. Sakuma T, Mizota A, Inoue J, Tanaka M. Intravitreal injection of autologous plasmin enzyme for macular edema associated with branch retinal vein occlusion. Am J Ophthalmol. 2010;150(6):876–82.
120. Haritoglou C, Gandorfer A, Kampik A. Chromodissection in vitreo-retinal surgery. In: Sebag J, editor. Vitreous – in health & disease. New York: Springer; 2014. p. 601–11.
121. Hartioglou C, Sebag J. Indications and considerations for chromodissection. Retinal Phys. 2014;11(5):34–9.
122. Haritoglou C, Gass CA, Schaumberger M, Gandorfer A, Ulbig MW, Kampik A. Long-term follow-up after macular hole surgery with internal limiting membrane peeling. Am J Ophtalmol. 2002;134(5):661–6. Available at: http://www.ncbi.nlm.nih.gov/pubmed/12429240. Accessed 15 Jan 2014.
123. Paques M, Massin P, Santiago PY, Spielmann AC, Le Gargasson JF, Gaudric A. Late reopening of successfully treated macular holes. Br J Ophthalmol. 1997;81(8):658–62. Available at http://www.pubmedcentral.nih.gov/articlerender.fcgi?artid=1722272&tool=pmcentrez&rendertype=abstract.
124. Yosida M, Kishi S. Pathogeneis of macular hole recurrence and its prevention by internal limiting membrane peeling. Retina (Philadelphia, Pa). 2007;27(2):169–73. Available at http://www.ncbi.nlm.nih.gov/pubmed/17290198. Accessed 20 Apr 2012.
125. Brooks HL. Macular hole surgery with and without internal limiting membrane peeling. Ophthalmology. 2000;107(10):1939–48; discussion 1948–9. Available at http://www.ncbi.nlm.nih.gov/pubmed11013203.
126. Christmas NJ, Smiddy WE, Flynn HW. Reopening of macular holes after initially successful repair. Ophthalmol. 1998;105(10)1835–8. Available at http://www.ncbi.nlm.nih.gov/pubmed/9787352.
127. Scott IU, Moraczweski AL, Smiddy WE, Flynn HW, Feuer WJ. Long-term anatomic and visual acuity outcomes after initial anatomic success with macular hole surgery. Am J Ophthalmol. 2003;135(5):633–40. Available at: http://www.ncib.nlm.nih.gov/pubmed12719070. Accessed 15 Jan 2014.
128. Paques M, Massin P, Blain P, Duquesnoy AS, Gaudric A. Long-term incidence of reopening of macular holes. Ophthalmol. 2000;107(4):760–5; discussion 766. Available at: http://www.ncbi.nlm.nih.gov/pubmed/10768340.
129. Bhatnagar P, Kaiser PK, Smith SD, Meisler DM, Lewis H, Sears JE. Reopening of previously closed macular holes after cataract extraction. Am J Ophthalmol. 2007;144(2):252–9. Available at: http://www.ncbi.nlm.nih.gov/pubmed/17543876. Accessed 13 Apr 2012.
130. Gottlieb CC, Martin JA. Phacovitrectomy with internal limiting membrane peeling for idiopathic macular hole. Can J Ophthalmol. 2002;37(5):227–82; discussion 282. Available at: http://www.ncbi.nlm.nih.gov/pubmed/12322859. Accessed 15 Jan 2014.
131. Theocharis IP, Alexandridou A, Gili NJ, Tomic Z. Combined phacoemulsification and pars plana vitrectomy for macular hole treatment. Acta Opthalmol Scand. 2005;83(2):172–5. Available at: http://www.ncbi.nlm.nih.gov/pubmed/15799728. Accessed 15 Jan 2014.
132. Kotecha AV, Sinclair SH, Gupta AK, Tipperman R. Pars plana vitrectomy for macular holes combined with cataract extraction and lens implantation. Ophthalmic Surg Lasers. 2000;31(5):387–93. Available at: http://www.ncbi.nlm.nih.gov/pubmed/11011707. Accessed 15 Jan 2014.
133. Garcia-Arumi J, Palau MM, Espax AB, Martinez-Castillo V, Garrido HB, Corcostegui B. Reopening of 2 macular holes after neodymium:YAG capsulotomy. J Cataract Refract Surg. 2006;32(2):363–6. Available at: http://www.ncbi.nlm.nih.gov/pubmed/16565020. Accessed 15 Jan 2014.
134. Kwok AK, Li WW, Pang CP, et al. Indocyanine green staining and removal of internal limiting membrane in macular hole surgery: histology and outcome. Am J Ophthalmol. 2001;132(2):178–83. Available at: http://www.ncbi.nlm.nih.gov/pubmed/11476676. Accessed 21 Apr 2012.
135. Kampik A, Kenyon KR, Michels RG, Green WR, de la Cruz ZC. Epiretinal and vitreous membranes. Comparative study of 56 cases. Arch Ophthalmol. 1981;99(8):1445–54.
136. Gibran SK, Flemming B, Stappler T, et al. Peel and peel again. Br J Ophthalmol. 2008;92(3):373–7. Available at: http://www.ncbi.nlm.nih.gov/pubmed/18055573. Accessed 20 Apr 2012.

137. Ducournau Y, Ducournau D. Aspects anatomopathologiques des membranes epiretiniennes idiopathiques et secondaires. Dans "La Chirigie de la Macula." Bulletin des Societes d'Ophtalmologie de France, Rapport Annuel. 1996:87–119.
138. Kwow AK, Lai TY, Yuen KS. Epiretinal membrane surgery with or without internal limiting membrane peeling. Clin Experiment Ophthalmol. 2005;33(4):379–85. Available at: http://www.ncbi.nlm.nigh.gov/pubmed/16033350. Accessed 15 Jan 2014.
139. Park DW, Dugel PU, Garda J, et al. Macular pucker removal with and without internal limiting membrane peeling: pilot study. Ophthalmol. 2003;110(1):62–4. Available at: http://www.ncbi.nlm.nih.gov/pubmed/18536602. Accessed 21 Apr 2012.
140. Pan BX, Yee KM, Ross-cisneros FN, Sadun AA, Sebag J. Macular hole and macular pucker surgery with special emphasis on reoperation. In: Sebag J, editor. Vitreous – in health & disease. New York: Springer; 2014. p. 613–28.
141. Pan BX, Yee KM, Ross- Cisneros FN, Sadun AA, Sebag J. Inner retinal optic neuropathy: vitreomacular surgery–associated disruption of the inner retina. J Invest Ophthalmol Vis Sci. 2014;55:6756–64. doi:10.1167/iovs.14-15235.
142. Katira RC, Zamani M, Beristein DM, Garfinkel RA. Incidence and characteristics of macular pucker formation after primary retinal detachment repair by pars plana vitrectomy alone. Retina. 2008;28:744–8.
143. Mitry D, Bunce C, Charteris D. Anti-vascular endothelial growth factor for macular oedema secondary to branch retinal vein occlusion. Cochrane Database Syst Rev. 2013;(1):CD009510. doi:10.1002/14651858.CD009510.pub2.
144. Braithwaite T, Nanji AA, Lindsley K, Greenberg PB. Anti-vascular endothelial growth factor for macular oedema secondary to central retinal vein occlusion. Cochrane Database Syst Rev. 2014;(5):CD007325. doi:10.1002/14651858.CD007325.pub3.
145. Matsumoto Y, Freund KB, Peiretti E, Cooney MJ, Ferrara DC, Yannuzzi LA. Rebound macular edema following bevacizumab (Avastin) therapy for retinal venous occlusive disease. Retina. 2007;27:426–31.
146. Nishijima K, Ng YS, Zhong L, et al. Vascular endothelial growth factor-A is a survival factor for retinal neurons and a critical neuroprotectant during the adaptive response to ischemic injury. Am J Pathol. 2007;171:53–67.
147. Garcia-Arumi J, Binder S, Leila M, Victori M. Vitreous surgery of arterial and venous retinovascular diseases. In: Sebag J, editor. Vitreous – in health & disease. New York: Springer; 2014. p. 647–61.
148. Tamura H, Miyamoto K, Kiryu J, et al. Intravitreal injection of corticosteroid attenuates leukostasis and vascular leakage in experimental diabetic retina. Invest Ophthalmol Vis Sci. 2005;46:1440–4.
149. Cunningham Jr ET, Adamis AP, Altaweel M, et al. A phase II randomized double-masked trial of pegaptanib, an antivascular endothelial growth factor aptamer, for diabetic macular edema. Ophthalmology. 2005;112:1747–57.
150. Chun DW, Heier JS, Topping TM, Duker JS, Bankert JM. A pilot study of multiple intravitreal injections of ranibizumab in patients with center-involving clinically significant diabetic macular edema. Ophthalmology. 2006;113:1706–12.
151. Nguyen QD, Tatlipinar S, Shah SM, et al. Vascular endothelial growth factor is a critical stimulus for diabetic macular edema. Am J Ophthalmol. 2006;142:961–9.
152. Diabetic Retinopathy Clinical Research Network. A phase II randomized clinical trial of intravitreal bevacizumab for diabetic macular edema. Ophthalmology. 2007;114:1860–7.
153. Wells JA, Glassman AR, Ayala AR, et al. Diabetic Retinopathy Clinical Research Network. Aflibercept, bevacizumab, or ranibizumab for diabetic macular edema. N Engl J Med. 2015;372(13):1193–203. doi: 10.1056/NEJMoa1414264. Epub 2015 Feb 18.
154. Lewis H, Abrams GW, Blumenkranz MS, Campo RV. Vitrectomy for diabetic macular traction and edema associated with posterior hyaloidal traction. Ophthalmology. 1992;99:753–9.
155. Massin P, Duguid G, Erginay A, Haouchine B, Gaudric A. Optical coherence tomography for evaluating diabetic macular edema before and after vitrectomy. Am J Ophthalmol. 2003;135:169–77.

156. Gaucher D, Tadayoni R, Erginay A, Haouchine B, Gaudric A, Massin P. Optical coherence tomography assessment of the vitreoretinal relationship in diabetic macular edema. Am J Ophthalmol. 2005;139:807–13.
157. Hee MR, Baumal CR, Puliafito CA. Optical coherence tomography of age-related macular degeneration and choroidal neovascularization. Ophthalmology. 1996;103:1260–70.
158. Ting TD, Oh M, Cox TA, Meyer C, Toth CA. Decreased visual acuity associated with cystoid macular edema in neovascular age-related macular degeneration. Arch Ophthalmol. 2002;120: 731–7.
159. Fung AE, Lalwani GA, Rosenfeld PJ, et al. An optical coherence tomography-guided, variable dosing regimen with intravitreal ranibizumab (Lucentis) for neovascular age-related macular degeneration. Am J Ophthalmol. 2007;143:566–83.
160. Krebs I, Stolba U, Glittenberg C, Seyeddain O, Benesch T, Binder S. Prognosis of untreated occult choroidal neovascularization. Graefes Arch Clin Exp Ophthalmol. 2007;245:376–84.
161. Sebag J. Vitreous in AMD therapy – the medium is the message. (Guest Editorial) Retina. 2015;35(9):1715–8.
162. Lee SJ, Koh HJ. Effects of vitreo-macular adhesion on anti-vascular endothelial growth factor treatment for exudative age-related macular degeneration. Ophthalmology. 2011;118(1): 101–10. doi:10.1016/j.ophtha.2010.04.015.
163. Waldstein SM, Ritter M, Simader C, Mayr-Sponer U, Kundi M, Schmidt-Erfurth U. Impact of vitreo-macular adhesion on ranibizumab mono- and combination therapy for neovascular age-related macular degeneration. Am J Ophthalmol. 2014;158(2):328–336.e1. doi:10.1016/j.ajo.2014.04.028.
164. Novack RL, Staurenghi G, Girach A, Narendran N, Tolentino M. Safety of intravitreal ocriplasmin for focal vitreo-macular adhesion in patients with exudative age-related macular degeneration. Ophthalmology. 2015;122(4):796–802. doi:10.1016/j.ophtha.2014.10.006.
165. Krishnan R, Arora R, De Salvo G, Stinghe A, Goverdhan S. Vitreo-macular traction affects anti-vascular endothelial growth factor treatment outcomes for exudative age-related macular degeneration. Retina. 2015;35(9):1750–6.
166. Krebs I, Glittenberg C, Binder S. Vitreous in age-related macular degeneration. In: Sebag J, editor. Vitreous – in health & disease. New York: Springer; 2014. p. 329–46.
167. Russell SR, Hageman GS. Optic disc, foveal, and extrafoveal damage due to surgical separation of the vitreous. Arch Ophthalmol. 2001;119:1653–8.
168. Recchia FM, Scott IU, Brown GC, Brown MM, Ho AC, Ip MS. Small-gauge pars plana vitrectomy: a report by the American Academy of Ophthalmology. Ophthalmology. 2010;117(9):1851–7. doi:10.1016/j.ophtha.2010.06.014.
169. Sebag J. Pharmacologic vitreolysis. In: Sebag J, editor. Vitreous – in health & disease. New York: Springer; 2014. p. 799–816.
170. Hesse L, Nebeling B, Schroeder B, Heller G, Kroll P. Induction of posterior vitreous detachment in rabbits by intravitreal injection of tissue plasminogen activator following cryopexy. Exp Eye Res. 2000;70:31–9.
171. Uemura A, Nakamura M, Kachi S, Nishizawa Y, Asami T, Miyake Y, et al. Effect of plasmin on laminin and fibronectin during plasmin-assisted vitrectomy. Arch Ophthalmol. 2005;123: 209–13.
172. Sakuma T, Tanaka M, Mizota A, Inoue J, Pakola S. Safety of *in vivo* pharmacologic vitreolysis with recombinant microplasmin in rabbit eyes. Invest Ophthalmol Vis Sci. 2005;46(9): 3295–9.
173. Takano A, Hirata A, Ogasawara K, Sagara N, Inomata Y, Kawaji T, et al. Posterior vitreous detachment induced by nattokinase (subtilisin NAT): a novel enzyme for pharmacologic vitreolysis. Invest Ophthalmol Vis Sci. 2006;47:2075–9.
174. Hageman GS, Russell SR. Chondroitinase-mediated disinsertion of the primate vitreous body. Invest Ophthalmol Vis Sci. 1994;35:1260.
175. Wang F, Wang Z, Sun X, Wang F, Xu X, Zhang X. Safety and efficacy of dispase and plasmin in pharmacologic vitreolysis. Invest Ophthalmol Vis Sci. 2004;45:3286–90.

176. Kuppermann BD, Thomas EL, de Smet MD, Grillone LR, Vitrase for Vitreous Hemorrhage Study Groups. Pooled efficacy results from two multinational randomized controlled clinical trials of a single intravitreous injection of highly purified bovine hyaluronidase (Vitrase) for the management of vitreous hemorrhage. Am J Ophthalmol. 2005;140:573–84.
177. Sebag J. Pharmacologic vitreolysis-premise and promise of the first decade. Retina. 2009;29:871–4.
178. Kroll P, Hesse L. Pharmacologic vitreolysis with tissue plasminogen activator. In: Sebag J, editor. Vitreous – in health & disease. New York: Springer; 2014. p. 825–31.
179. Hesse L, Chofflet J, Kroll P. Tissue plasminogen activator as a biochemical adjuvant in vitrectomy for proliferative diabetic vitreo-retinopathy. Ger J Ophthalmol. 1995;4:323–7.
180. Chung J, Park YH, Lee YC. The effect of Nd:YAG laser membranotomy and intravitreal tissue plasminogen activator with gas on massive diabetic premacular hemorrhage. Ophthalmic Surg Lasers Imaging. 2008;39:114–20.
181. Hillenkamp J, Surguch V, Framme C, Gabel VP, Sachs HG. Management of submacular hemorrhage with intravitreal versus subretinal injection of recombinant tissue plasminogen activator. Graefes Arch Clin Exp Ophthalmol. 2010;248:5–11.
182. Binder S, Chong LP. Age-related macular degeneration surgery. In: Sebag J, editor. Vitreous – in health & disease. New York: Springer; 2015. p. 553–70.
183. Takano A, Hirata A, Inomata Y, Kawaji T, Nakagawa K, Nagata S, et al. Intravitreal plasmin injection activates endogenous matrix metalloproteinase-2 in rabbit and human vitreous. Am J Ophthalmol. 2005;140:654–60.
184. Verstraeten Thierry C. Pharmacologic vitreolysis with plasmin: basic science experiments. In: Sebag J, editor. Vitreous – in health & disease. New York: Springer; 2014. p. 831–7.
185. Wang ZL, Zhang X, Xu X, Sun XD, Wang F. PVD following plasmin but not hyaluronidase: implications for combination pharmacologic vitreolysis therapy. Retina. 2005;25:38–43.
186. Verstraeten TC, Chapman C, Hartzer M, Winkler BS, Trese MT, Williams GA. Pharmacologic induction of posterior vitreous detachment in the rabbit. Arch Ophthalmol. 1993;111:849–54.
187. Kim NJ, Yu HG, Yu YS, Chung H. Long-term effect of plasmin on the vitreolysis in rabbit eyes. Korean J Ophthalmol. 2004;18:35–40.
188. Hikichi T, Yanagiya N, Kado M, Akiba J, Yoshida A. Posterior vitreous detachment induced by injection of plasmin and sulfur hexafluoride in the rabbit vitreous. Retina. 1999;19:55–8.
189. Gandorfer A, Kampik A. Enzyme-assisted vitrectomy in enucleated pig eyes. Curr Eye Res. 2005;30:821–2.
190. Azzolini C, D'Angelo A, Maestranzi G, Codenotti M, Della Valle P, Prati M, et al. Intrasurgical plasmin enzyme in diabetic macular edema. Am J Ophthalmol. 2004;138:560–6.
191. Margherio AR, Margherio RR, Hartzer M, Trese MT, Williams GA, Ferrone PJ. Plasmin enzyme-assisted vitrectomy in traumatic pediatric macular holes. Ophthalmology. 1998;105:1617–20.
192. Trese MT, Williams GA, Hartzer MK. A new approach to stage 3 macular holes. Ophthalmology. 2000;107:1607–11.
193. Hirata A, Takano A, Inomata Y, Yonemura N, Sagara N, Tanihara H. Plasmin-assisted vitrectomy for management of proliferative membrane in proliferative diabetic retinopathy: a pilot study. Retina. 2007;27:1074–8.
194. Williams JG, Trese MT, Williams GA, Hartzer MK. Autologous plasmin enzyme in the surgical management of diabetic retinopathy. Ophthalmology. 2001;108:1902–5.
195. Díaz-Llopis M, Udaondo P, Cervera E, García-Delpech S, Salom D, Quijada A, et al. Enzymatic vitrectomy by intravitreal autologous plasmin injection as initial treatment for macular epiretinal membranes and vitreomacular traction syndrome. Arch Soc Esp Oftalmol. 2009;84:91–100.
196. Tsukahara Y, Honda S, Imai H, Kondo N, Fujii S, Yokoyama N, et al. Autologous plasmin-assisted vitrectomy for stage 5 retinopathy of prematurity: a preliminary trial. Am J Ophthalmol. 2007;144:139–41.

197. Wu WC, Drenser KA, Lai M, Capone A, Trese MT. Plasmin enzyme-assisted vitrectomy for primary and reoperated eyes with stage 5 retinopathy of prematurity. Retina. 2008;28(3 Suppl):S75–80.
198. Wu WC, Drenser KA, Trese MT, Williams GA, Capone A. Pediatric traumatic macular hole: results of autologous plasmin enzyme-assisted vitrectomy. Am J Ophthalmol. 2007;144: 668–72.
199. Sakuma T, Tanaka M, Inoue M, Mizota A, Souri M, Ichinose A. Efficacy of autologous plasmin for idiopathic macular hole surgery. Eur J Ophthalmol. 2005;15:787–94.
200. Diaz-Llopis M, Udaondo P, Arevalo F, Salom D, Garcia-Delpech S, Quijada A, et al. Intravitreal plasmin without associated vitrectomy as a treatment for refractory diabetic macular edema. J Ocul Pharmacol Ther. 2009;25:379–84.
201. Trese MT. Enzymatic-assisted vitrectomy. Eye. 2002;16:365–8.
202. Gandorfer A. Enzymatic vitreous disruption. Eye (Lond). 2008;22:1273–7.
203. Chen W, Huang X, Ma XW, Mo W, Wang WJ, Song HY. Enzymatic vitreolysis with recombinant microplasminogen and tissue plasminogen activator. Eye (Lond). 2008;22:300–7.
204. De Smet Marc D, Bart J. Pharmacologic vitreolyssi with ocriplasmin. In: Sebag J, editor. Vitreous – in health & disease. New York: Springer; 2014. p. 845–53.
205. Gandorfer A, Rohleder M, Sethi C, et al. Posterior vitreous detachment induced by microplasmin. Invest Ophthalmol Vis Sci. 2004;45(2):641–7.
206. De Smet MD, Valmaggia C, Zarranz-Ventura J, Willekens B. Microplasmin: *ex vivo* characterization of its activity in porcine vitreous. Invest Ophthalmol Vis Sci. 2009;50(2):814–9.
207. Sebag J, Ansari RR, Suh KI. Pharmacologic vitreolysis with microplasmin increases vitreous diffusion coefficients. Graefes Arch Clin Exp Ophthalmol. 2007;245(4):576–80.
208. Quiram PA, Leverenz VR, Baker RM, Dang L, Giblin FJ, Trese MT. Microplasmin-induced posterior vitreous detachment affects vitreous oxygen levels. Retina. 2007;27:1090–6.
209. Sebag J. Pharmacologic vitreolysis (Guest Editorial). Retina. 1998;18:1–3.
210. Sebag J. Is pharmacologic vitreolysis brewing? (Guest Editorial). Retina. 2002;22:1–3.
211. Stalmans P, Benz MS, Gandorfer A, et al. Enzymatic vitreolysis with ocriplasmin for vitreomacular traction and macular holes. N Engl J Med. 2012;367:606–15.
212. Khoshnevis M, Sebag J. Pharmacologic vitreolysis with ocriplasmin: rationale for use and therapeutic potential in vitreo-retinal disorders. BioDrugs. 2015;29(2):103–12. doi:10.1007/s40259-015-0120-y.
213. Russell Stephen R, Hageman Gregory S. Chondroitinase as a vitreous interfactant: vitreous disinertion in the human. In: Sebag J, editor. Vitreous – in health & disease. New York: Springer; 2014. p. 881–95.
214. Jivrajka RV, KIM JK, Fink W, Saddun AA, Sebag J. Quantitative analysis of central visual field defects in macular edema using three-dimensional computer-automated threshold Amsler grid testing. Graefes Arch Clin Exp Opthalmol. 2009;247:165–70.
215. Kang SW, Hyung S-M, Choi MY, Lee J. Induction of vitreolysis and vitreous detachment with hyaluronidase and perfluoropropane gas. Korean J Ophthalmol. 1995;9:69–78.
216. Russel SR. What we know (and don't know) about the vitreoretinal interface. Retina. 2012;32(Suppl):S181–6.
217. Tezel Tongalp H, Del Priore Lucian V, Kaplan Henry J. Pharmacologic vitreolysis with purified dispase (VitreolysinTM). In: Sebag J, editor. Vitreous – in health & disease. New York: Springer; 2014. p. 869–81.
218. Tezel TH, Del Priore LV, Kaplan HJ. Posterior vitreous detachment with dispase. Retina. 1998;18:7–15.
219. Oliveira LB, Tatebayashi M, Mahmoud TH, Blackmon SM, Wong F, McCuen 2nd BW. Dispase facilitates posterior vitreous detachment during vitrectomy in young pigs. Retina. 2001;21:324–31.
220. Jorge R, Oyamaguchi EK, Cardillo JA, Gobbi A, Laicine EM, Haddad A. Intravitreal injection of dispase causes retinal hemorrhages in rabbit and human eyes. Curr Eye Res. 2003;26: 107–12.

221. Zhu D, Chen H, Xu X. Effects of intravitreal dispase on vitreoretinal interface in rabbits. Curr Eye Res. 2006;31:935–46.
222. De Smet Marc D, Lisa G. Hyaluronidase as a vitreous liquefactant. In: Sebag J, editor. Vitreous – in health & disease. New York: Springer; 2014. p. 863–9.
223. Hikichi T, Kado M, Yoshida A. Intravitreal injection of hyaluronidase cannot induce posterior vitreous detachment in the rabbit. Retina. 2000;20(2):195–8.
224. Sebag J, Niemeyer M, Koss, M. Anomalous PVD and Vitreoschisis. In: Sebag J, editor. Vitreous – in health & disease. New York: Springer; 2014. p. 245.

Chapter 7
Medical Management of CME Associated with Retinal Vascular Occlusions

Wolf Buehl and Ursula M. Schmidt-Erfurth

Introduction

The term "retinal vascular occlusion" covers two different disease entities: retinal artery occlusion (RAO) and retinal vein occlusion (RVO). Depending on the site of the occlusion, both disease types may be subdivided into two primary categories, namely, occlusion of the central retinal vessel (central retinal artery occlusion (CRAO) and central retinal vein occlusion (CRVO)) and occlusion of a peripheral (branch) retinal vessel (branch retinal artery occlusion (BRAO) and branch retinal vein occlusion (BRVO)) [1].

While retinal artery occlusion typically leads to sudden and irreversible vision loss, retinal vein occlusion has a better prognosis and often shows a delayed onset of clinical symptoms, mainly caused by the subsequent macular edema [2]. As cystoid macular edema (CME) rarely occurs in cases of retinal artery occlusion [3], this chapter will focus on medical treatment of macular edema associated with central or branch retinal vein occlusion (CRVO, BRVO).

BRVO occurs more commonly than CRVO. CRVO may be divided into ischemic or nonischemic, whereby the nonischemic type usually has a better prognosis than the ischemic. The visual acuity in untreated BRVO generally improves over time, whereas it typically decreases over time in untreated CRVO eyes. About 5–15 % of eyes with BRVO develop macular edema over 1 year, and the majority of patients with CRVO have signs of macular edema at presentation. The natural history and clinical course of vision and ocular complications differ between BRVO and CRVO [4]. Although development of macular edema is common in BRVO eyes (around 10 % in 1 year), about 18–40 % of cases with macular edema at baseline resolve over time, and visual acuity may improve over time without intervention, with

W. Buehl, MD • U.M. Schmidt-Erfurth, MD (✉)
Department of Ophthalmology, Medical University of Vienna,
Waehringer Guertel 18-20, Vienna A-1090, Austria
e-mail: ursula.schmidt-erfurth@meduniwien.ac.at

S. Schaal, H.J. Kaplan (eds.), *Cystoid Macular Edema*,
DOI 10.1007/978-3-319-39766-5_7

between 37 and 74 % of eyes showing a two-line improvement. In CRVO cases, visual acuity at diagnosis is usually poor (<20/40) and decreases further over time. Compared with nonischemic CRVO, ischemic CRVO is associated with lower mean visual acuity both at diagnosis and during the follow-up periods. Macular edema is frequently present at the time of CRVO diagnosis, which resolves in 30 % of non-ischemic CRVO eyes and in up to 73 % of ischemic CRVO eyes in 15 months [4].

Treatment Options

During the past decades, diverse treatment methods have been developed for retinal vein occlusion. Most therapies focus on eliminating the complications and vision-disturbing effects of RVO which are mainly caused by macular edema.

Acute Therapy

Although this chapter focuses on medical treatment of macular edema associated with RVO, it should be mentioned that because of the complex pathogenesis, treatment, and prophylaxis of RVO, treatment is an interdisciplinary task. All patients with acute RVO should be referred to an internal medicine specialist, and any underlying disease should be diagnosed and treated, if necessary. Rheological therapy has been considered to be first-line treatment in acute RVO. Several specialists accept isovolemic hemodilution as a first-line treatment within the first 8 weeks after RVO, as it increases retinal perfusion and may prevent capillary closure and further retinal ischemia. The therapy is usually well tolerated; side effects include headache, dyspnea, deep vein thrombosis, and hypotension [5]. Nevertheless, patients have to be carefully selected and should not have any severe cardiorespiratory or renal disease. Early treatment seems to be important in order to reduce the risk of ischemic complications.

Other rheological substances that have been tested for treatment of BRVO include troxerutin and pentoxifylline. The first is thought to improve microcirculation in capillaries and venules by inhibiting erythrocyte and platelet aggregation improving erythrocyte deformability [6]. Pentoxifylline leads to vessel dilation and improves retinal blood flow [7]. Both substances have been used in the treatment of peripheral (extremities) vein occlusions. However, the efficacy of these drugs in patients with BRVO has not sufficiently been proven in prospective studies [2].

Treatment of Macular Edema

Based on the results of the branch retinal vein occlusion study (BVOS), laser photocoagulation had been the standard of care for treatment of macular edema associated with BRVO for several decades [8]. However, in many cases visual acuity does not increase significantly after laser photocoagulation, and its use is not recommended in the first 3 months after the onset of BRVO. In contrast to BRVO, the central vein occlusion study (CVOS) showed no benefit for grid laser photocoagulation over no treatment in patients with macular edema secondary to CRVO at any follow-up point [9]. Therefore, the standard of care for CRVO was observation until the recent development of medical treatment options.

During the past decade, a number of new treatments for RVO-associated complications have been investigated and proven to be effective. In 2009, a dexamethasone intravitreal implant (Ozurdex, Allergan, Inc., Irvine, CA, USA) was granted approval for the treatment of macular edema following BRVO or CRVO in the Unites States and the European Union based on two multicenter, double-blind, randomized studies (GENEVA). Following dexamethasone, in 2010 ranibizumab (Lucentis, Genentech, Inc., South San Francisco, CA, USA; Novartis Pharma AG, Basel, Switzerland) was approved in the United States for the same indication on the basis of two multicenter, randomized, double-masked clinical trials (BRAVO and CRUISE). Recently, aflibercept (Eylea, Regeneron Pharmaceuticals, Inc., Tarrytown, NY, USA; Bayer HealthCare Pharmaceuticals, Berlin, Germany) has been granted approval for the treatment of CRVO (2012) and BRVO (2014) on the basis of three multicenter, randomized, double-masked clinical trials (COPERNICUS, GALILEO, and VIBRANT).

Corticosteroid Therapy

Corticosteroids lead to reduced permeability of the affected vessels and have an anti-inflammatory and angiostatic effect, thereby reducing macular edema and the associated chronic damage to photoreceptors [10].

Several studies have shown a positive effect of intravitreal injections of triamcinolone acetonide (IVTA) [2]. In vitro, corticosteroids also inhibit vascular endothelial growth factor (VEGF) expression and may thus prevent neovascularization and reduce the VEGF-mediated increase in retinal capillary permeability. However, triamcinolone acetonide has not been approved for the treatment of any ocular disease and must therefore be used on an off-label basis only. Besides, the positive effect of IVTA is usually temporary, and several re-treatments are necessary in most cases to avoid reoccurrence of the macular edema and associated loss in visual acuity. This in turn raises the risk for side effects of the treatment, mainly increased intraocular pressure, cataract formation, and endophthalmitis [11–13]. Early treatment seems to be important, because chronic macular edema often does not respond well to the treatment with intravitreal steroids, or steroid treatment does not lead to an increase in visual acuity. Unfortunately, most of the available clinical studies were not randomized or did not distinguish between different types (ischemic/non-ischemic) of BRVO or CRVO [2].

The standard care vs. corticosteroid for retinal vein occlusion (SCORE) study was a multicenter, randomized phase III trial designed to assess the efficacy and safety of standard care versus IVTA for the treatment of macular edema associated with CRVO and BRVO. The SCORE BRVO study compared IVTA (1 and 4 mg) to standard of care (prompt or deferred grid laser photocoagulation, depending on the presence of dense macular hemorrhage) in patients with macular edema secondary to BRVO [14]. The study showed no advantage for IVTA over laser treatment. Rates of intraocular pressure (IOP) rise and cataract progression were similar in the standard of care and 1 mg IVTA groups and higher in the 4 mg IVTA group. In contrast to the SCORE BRVO study, the SCORE CRVO study comparing IVTA (1 and 4 mg) to observation in patients with macular edema secondary to CRVO showed superiority for IVTA treatment in these patients [15]. IVTA-treated patients lost fewer letters than the observation group, and a higher proportion of patients in the IVTA groups gained 15 letters from baseline to 1 year. Again, rates of IOP changes and cataract progression were similar in the observation and 1 mg IVTA groups and higher in the 4 mg IVTA group [16].

For a longer-lasting therapeutic effect, the implantation of a sustained-release, intravitreal dexamethasone delivery system (DEX implant; OZURDEX®, Allergan, Inc., Irvine, CA) has also been shown to be effective in the treatment of BRVO [17]. It was the first FDA-approved drug therapy for the treatment of macular edema following retinal vein occlusion. The side effects, mainly IOP rise, are similar to repeated IVTA treatment. The phase III GENEVA studies were two identical, multicenter, masked, randomized, 6-month, sham-controlled clinical trials (each of which included patients with BRVO and patients with CRVO) comparing the DEX implant (0.35 or 0.7 mg) with sham treatment, followed by an open-label 6-month extension phase in which patients could receive a second DEX implant (0.7 mg) based on best-corrected visual acuity (BCVA) and retinal thickness [18, 19]. The studies showed a significantly higher mean VA improvement in the DEX groups than in the sham group up to 3 months after each injection. Rates of elevated IOP were overall higher in the DEX groups than in the sham group. Rates of cataracts were not significantly different between the DEX and sham groups at 6 months. However, at 12 months, patients who received two 0.7 mg DEX implants had a higher rate of cataract progression compared with sham [16].

Positive effects on visual acuity have also been shown for retrobulbar injections of triamcinolone; however, these were lower than after intravitreal application of corticosteroids, and there is no approved drug for retrobulbar application [2]. Besides, systemic application of steroids has been reported to reduce macular edema and improve visual acuity, but because of the possible side effects, it should only be considered for younger patients with concurrent optic disc edema or with an inflammatory component, especially in patients with systemic vasculitic disorder. However, currently there are only reports on the effectiveness of systemic steroid therapy in patients with CRVO, but no data regarding its usefulness in the treatment of BRVO [2].

Anti-VEGF Therapy

Retinal vein occlusion leads to increased expression of vascular endothelial growth factors (VEGF) into the vitreous body, causing vascular hyperpermeability with subsequent breakdown of the blood retina barrier and thus macular edema. VEGF overexpression may also cause neovascularization, another important complication of RVO. All currently available VEGF inhibitors (bevacizumab, pegaptanib, ranibizumab, aflibercept) have been applied successfully in the treatment of RVO, and two of them (ranibizumab, aflibercept) have gained approval based on several large randomized controlled trials. In contrast, there are only few randomized controlled studies on the (off-label) use of bevacizumab in RVO.

Bevacizumab (Avastin®)

Bevacizumab (Avastin®; Genentech Inc., San Francisco, CA, USA, and Roche Pharmaceuticals, Basel, Switzerland) is a recombinant humanized monoclonal antibody that blocks angiogenesis by inhibiting vascular endothelial growth factor A (VEGF-A). Bevacizumab was approved by the US Food and Drug Administration (FDA) for certain metastatic cancers. Although it has no approval for the treatment of any eye disorder, it has successfully been used in the treatment of several ocular diseases, including RVO [2].

In 2012, Epstein and colleagues evaluated intravitreal bevacizumab in CRVO [20]. Patients received either intravitreal bevacizumab 1.25 mg or sham injection every 6 weeks over a period of 6 months. After this, an open-label extension followed during which all patients received bevacizumab 1.25 mg every 6 weeks. Each group comprised 30 patients, who showed symptoms of CRVO. CRVO patients treated with bevacizumab every 6 weeks from baseline gained +16.1 letters, compared to +4.6 letters in those treated with sham injections followed by bevacizumab ($p<0.05$). The percentage of BCVA gain of more than 15 letters was 60 % (bevacizumab) vs. 33.3 % (sham/bevacizumab), respectively ($p<0.05$). The authors reported no case of endophthalmitis, or retinal tear/detachment in both groups. In the sham group, 16.7 % developed neovascularization of the iris (NVI), compared to none in the bevacizumab group. By month 12, no new development of NVI was found in both groups. Furthermore, in all previous NVI cases, neovascularization regressed completely after treatment changed from sham to bevacizumab 1.25 mg. There were no serious non-ocular adverse effects. However, one patient from the sham/bevacizumab group suffered from a transient ischemic attack and dropped out of the study [21].

Russo et al. compared intravitreal bevacizumab 1.25 mg based on an as-needed (pro-re-nata, PRN) treatment scheme versus grid laser photocoagulation in 30 patients with BRVO over 12 months [22]. Inclusion criterion was duration of macular edema of at least 3 months. They found a change in BCVA of +15.5 letters in bevacizumab-treated patients and +10 letters in grid laser photocoagulation ($p<0.05$) after a mean number of 1.7 intravitreal bevacizumab injections and 1.5 grid applications. No adverse events occurred during the study [21].

Pegaptanib Sodium (Macugen®)

Pegaptanib sodium (Macugen®; EyetechPharmaceuticals and Pfizer Inc., New York, NY, USA) is a VEGF aptamer (a single strand of nucleic acid) that specifically binds to the 165 isoform of VEGF. It gained FDA approval for the treatment of neovascular

AMD in 2004. There are only few (mostly non-randomized) clinical trials assessing the efficacy of pegaptanib sodium for the treatment of macular edema associated with CRVO or BRVO [23]. However, pegaptanib sodium has not been approved for treating RVO and plays a minor role since approval of ranibizumab and aflibercept and because of the availability of bevacizumab at lower costs. Moreover, all of the other agents show a higher affinity to VEGF-A than pegaptanib sodium [24].

Ranibizumab (Lucentis®)

Ranibizumab (Lucentis®; Genentech Inc., San Francisco, CA, USA, and Novartis Pharma AG, Basel, Switzerland) is a humanized, affinity-matured VEGF antibody fragment that binds to and neutralizes all isoforms of VEGF. The BRAVO (branch retinal vein occlusion) and CRUISE (central retinal vein occlusion) studies were large randomized phase III trials for the approval of ranibizumab for the treatment of macular edema secondary to RVO [25, 26]. Patients with macular edema secondary to BRVO or CRVO were randomized 1:1:1 to receive 6-monthly intravitreal injections of ranibizumab 0.3 mg, ranibizumab 0.5 mg, or sham, followed by a 6-month PRN phase, during which all patients could receive ranibizumab treatment. In the BRAVO study, patients could receive rescue laser treatment once during the treatment period and once during the observation period if prespecified criteria were met. In both studies, ranibizumab treatment was associated with significant improvements in BCVA, which were sustained over 12 months of treatment. In the BRAVO study, the mean increase in BCVA from baseline at month 6 was +18.3 letters in the ranibizumab 0.5 mg group compared with +7.3 letters in the sham group ($p<0.0001$). At month 12, mean BCVA improvements were +18.3 letters for ranibizumab 0.5 mg versus +12.1 letters with delayed treatment ($p<0.01$) [27]. In the CRUISE study, the mean increase in BCVA at 6 months was +14.9 letters in the ranibizumab 0.5 mg group compared with +0.8 letters in the sham group ($p<0.0001$). At month 12, mean BCVA improvements were +13.9 letters with ranibizumab 0.5 mg and +7.3 letters with delayed treatment ($p<0.001$) [27].

In both studies, ranibizumab-treated eyes showed a significantly greater mean reduction in central foveal thickness (CFT). At month 6 of the BRAVO study, the mean CFT reduction was −345.2 μm with ranibizumab 0.5 mg and −157.7 μm with sham ($p<0.0001$). This reduction was sustained to month 12 with ranibizumab 0.5 mg (−347.4 μm) compared with a reduction of −273.7 μm in the delayed treatment group ($p<0.05$). Similarly, at month 6 of the CRUISE study, mean reductions in CFT of −452.3 μm and −167.7 μm were observed with ranibizumab 0.5 mg and sham, respectively ($p<0.0001$). At month 12, the mean CFT reduction was −462.1 μm with ranibizumab 0.5 mg compared with −427.2 μm with delayed treatment [27].

Ranibizumab was generally well tolerated. In the BRAVO study, 6.2 % of patients in the ranibizumab 0.5 mg group, 2.6 % after delayed treatment, and 3.1 % in the first 6 months of the sham group developed a cataract. There was one incidence of endophthalmitis in the ranibizumab 0.5 mg group. Six serious adverse events (SAE) potentially related to VEGF inhibition were reported with ranibizumab 0.5 mg (hemorrhagic stroke, acute myocardial infarction, unstable angina, hypertension, non-ocular hemorrhage and intestinal perforation). In the delayed treatment group, there was one SAE (hemorrhagic stroke) up to month 6 and two SAEs (acute myocardial infarction and hypertension) during months 6–12. In the CRUISE study, 7.0 % of patients treated with ranibizumab 0.5 mg, 1.8 % in the delayed treatment group, and no patient in the sham group developed a cataract. There were no cases of endophthalmitis in any treatment group. However, there were four SAEs possibly related to VEGF inhibition in the 0.5 mg group (ischemic stroke, transient ischemic attack, myocardial infarction, and angina pectoris). In the delayed treatment group, there were two SAEs (myocardial infarction and hypertension) [27].

Patients completing the BRAVO and CRUISE trials were eligible for the open-label HORIZON cohort 2 study [28]. One-year results (corresponding to 2 years of treatment) showed that PRN ranibizumab dosing was adequate to maintain visual acuity gains in patients with BRVO. Improvements of 17.5 letters and 15.6 letters from BRAVO baseline were observed for patients initially randomized to ranibizumab 0.5 mg and sham, respectively. Although some loss of efficacy was observed in patients with CRVO, there was an overall improvement of 12.0 letters and 7.6 letters, respectively, from the CRUISE baseline for patients initially randomized to ranibizumab 0.5 mg and sham. The negative effect of delayed treatment was reduced in BRVO patients over the 12-month period, possibly because of the availability of rescue laser photocoagulation from month 3 in the BRAVO study. During the entire 24-month study period, increased intraocular pressure was reported for two patients with BRVO and one patient with CRVO. There were no cases of traumatic cataract. Two patients with CRVO experienced endophthalmitis [27].

The ongoing 2-year CRYSTAL and BRIGHTER studies evaluate the efficacy and safety of ranibizumab for macular edema secondary to CRVO and BRVO based on an individualized stability criteria-driven PRN scheme after a loading phase of three consecutive monthly injections, as per the EU label of ranibizumab for RVO. The 6-month (for BRVO) and 12-month (for CRVO) primary endpoints demonstrated a mean BCVA gain of 14.4 letters for BRVO and of 12.3 letters for CRVO (Mones J, ARVO 2014). No new safety signs were reported.

Aflibercept (Eylea®)

Aflibercept (Eylea®; Regeneron Pharmaceuticals Inc., Tarrytown, New York, and Bayer Healthcare, Berlin, Germany) is a fully human, recombinant fusion protein that targets VEGF-A, VEGF-B, and placental growth factor. Aflibercept binds all isoforms of VEGF-A with a higher affinity than that of ranibizumab. Aflibercept has been investigated in patients with CRVO in the controlled, phase III COPERNICUS and GALILEO trials [29, 30]. In the COPERNICUS study, 189 patients with CRVO were included and received intravitreal aflibercept 2 mg (aflibercept group) compared to sham treatment (sham/aflibercept group) monthly at a randomization ratio of 2:1 during the first 6 months followed by PRN treatment of intravitreal aflibercept 2 mg in all patients. Primary endpoint was the proportion of patients with an improvement of BCVA ≥15 letters. CRVO patients in the aflibercept 2 mg group gained +16.2 letters at month 12, compared to +3.8 letters in the sham/aflibercept group ($p<0.001$). The percentage of patients with a gain of more than 15 letters was 55.3 % (aflibercept) and 30.1 % (sham/aflibercept), respectively ($p<0.001$). After 5.8 aflibercept injections until month 6, visual acuity was stabilized with an additional 2.7 injections during PRN. In the control group, patients with a mean of 5.3 sham injections in the beginning received a mean of 3.9 injections of aflibercept 2 mg until month 12. The most common adverse events for both groups were conjunctival hemorrhage, eye pain, reduced visual acuity, and increased intraocular pressure. The incidence of systemic adverse events did not differ significantly between groups [21].

In the GALILEO study, a total of 177 treatment-naive patients with macular edema secondary to CRVO were randomized in a 3:2 ratio to receive either 2-mg intravitreal aflibercept or sham injections every 4 weeks for 20 weeks. From week 24 to 48, the aflibercept group received aflibercept as needed (PRN), and the sham group continued receiving sham injections. The primary efficacy endpoint was the proportion of patients who gained 15 letters or more in BCVA. At week 52, the mean percentage of patients gaining 15 letters or more was 60.2 % in the aflibercept group and 32.4 % in the sham group ($p<0.001$). Aflibercept patients, compared with sham patients, had a significantly higher mean improvement in BCVA (+16.9 letters vs. +3.8 letters, respectively) and reduction in central retinal thickness (−423.5 μm vs. −219.3 μm, respectively) at week 52 ($p<0.0001$ for both). Aflibercept patients received a mean of 2.5 injections during PRN dosing. The most common ocular adverse events in the aflibercept group were related to the injection procedure or the underlying disease and included macular edema (33.7 %), increased intraocular pressure (17.3 %), and eye pain (14.4 %) [21].

The VIBRANT study was a double-masked, active-controlled, randomized, phase III trial to compare the efficacy and safety of intravitreal aflibercept injection with macular grid laser photocoagulation for the treatment of macular edema after BRVO [31]. Treatment-naïve eyes with macular edema after BRVO were included in the study if the occlusion occurred within 12 months, and BCVA was between ≤73 and ≥24 early treatment diabetic retinopathy study (ETDRS) letters (20/40-20/320 Snellen equivalent). Eyes (1 eye per patient) received either intravitreal aflibercept 2 mg every 4 weeks from baseline to week 20 or grid laser at baseline with a single-grid laser rescue treatment, if needed, from weeks 12 to 20. The proportion of eyes that gained ≥15 ETDRS letters from baseline at week 24 was 52.7 % in the aflibercept group compared with 26.7 % in the laser group ($p=0.0003$). The mean improvement from baseline BCVA at week 24 was 17.0 ETDRS letters in the aflibercept group and 6.9 ETDRS letters in the laser group ($p<0.0001$). The mean reduction in central retinal thickness (CRT) from baseline at week 24 was 280.5 μm in the aflibercept group and 128.0 μm in the laser group ($p<0.0001$). Traumatic cataract in an intravitreal aflibercept patient was the only ocular SAE that occurred. There were no cases of intraocular inflammation or endophthalmitis. The incidence of non-ocular SAEs was 8.8 % in the aflibercept group and 9.8 % in the laser group. One event of nonfatal stroke (1.1 %) and 1 death (1.1 %) due to pneumonia occurred during the 24 weeks of the study, both in patients in the laser group. Monthly intravitreal aflibercept injections provided significantly greater visual benefit and reduction in CRT at 24 weeks than grid laser photocoagulation in eyes with macular edema after BRVO [31].

Treatment Recommendations

Similar to the treatment of AMD, the introduction of anti-VEGF therapy has revolutionized the treatment of macular edema related to retinal vascular occlusion. Ranibizumab and aflibercept are indicated for the treatment of visual impairment due to macular edema secondary to BRVO or CRVO. Both have been shown to be highly effective in the treatment of RVO. Bevacizumab seems to have a comparable effect in the treatment of RVO; however, it has not been approved for the treatment of any ocular disease. Pegaptanib sodium was also shown to be effective, but has also not been approved for the treatment of macular edema secondary to RVO. Because of the favorable risk-benefit ratio of intravitreal anti-VEGF therapy, also compared to corticosteroid therapy, it should be considered as first-line therapy for the treatment of macular edema in RVO.

The correlation between the duration of macular edema and poorer visual outcomes in patients with RVO suggests that prompt initiation of treatment is beneficial. Although spontaneous resolution of macular edema is seen in some patients, it is difficult to predict the prognosis for patients with BRVO in the acute phase of the disease. Patients with untreated, symptomatic BRVO presenting with poor VA (baseline VA ranging from 20/40 to 20/200) may experience some VA improvement over time; however, vision rarely improves beyond 20/40 [27]. In the BRAVO and CRUISE studies, significant improvements in BCVA were observed as early as 7 days after the first ranibizumab injection [25, 26]. Delaying ranibizumab treatment by 3 months (retinal vein occlusion) or 6 months (BRAVO and CRUISE) resulted in slower overall anatomical improvements and lower improvements in BCVA at month 12. Reduced VA is a generally accepted indicator of visual impairment and the measure employed to indicate when ranibizumab treatment should commence. Although 20/40 has often been used as a threshold for VA impairment in clinical trials, many ophthalmologists would consider this too low [27]. There are different approaches to initiating treatment, ranging from immediate treatment to treatment after 1–3 months of observation so as not to treat transient decrease of vision associated with some forms of RVO. Although intravitreal therapy is not without risk, its risks may be negligible compared with delayed recovery and potential permanent damage from delaying treatment. Early treatment is recommended for patients with CRVO. In cases of BRVO in which VA is marginally affected, the benefit of observation versus early treatment should be thoroughly discussed with the patient. In general, early treatment is recommended to optimize long-term VA benefits [27]. The physician's own judgment may better determine which extent of VA loss or visual function loss is significant to the individual patient to commence treatment. There is no level of VA for which treatment is contraindicated as a rule; even patients

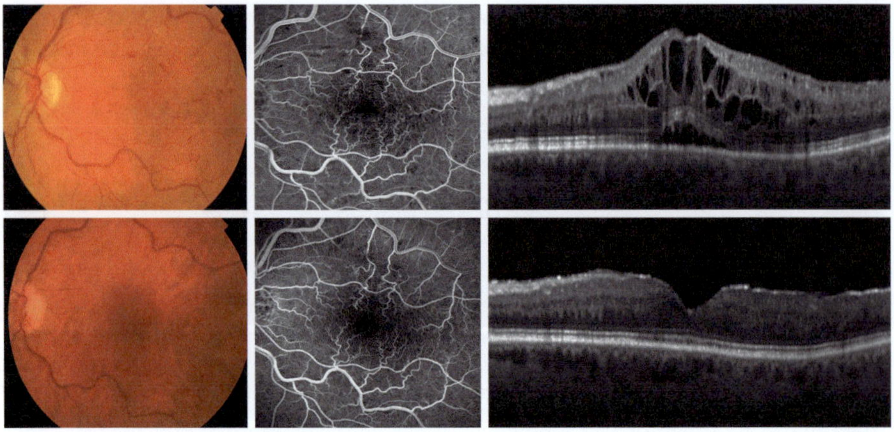

Fig. 1 *Left to right*: Fundus photographs, fluorescein angiography (FA) images, and optical coherence tomography (OCT) images of a patient with central retinal vein occlusion (CRVO) at baseline (*top*) and 2 years later after repeated intravitreal ranibizumab therapy (*bottom*)

with normal VA could present with significant impairment of contrast sensitivity or visual field. Therefore, although VA may be the leading indicator for treatment with ranibizumab in patients with RVO, other functional parameters may be useful on a patient-by-patient basis to finally determine the need for treatment [27].

Ranibizumab and aflibercept are recommended in the United States to be given as monthly intravitreal injections. However, it has been shown that in routine clinical practice, both therapies are not used as recommended by the manufacturers [32]. In accordance with the approved labels in the EU, ranibizumab or aflibercept treatment should be initiated with monthly injections and continued until the patient's VA is stable for three consecutive monthly assessments performed while on treatment. Evidence for this individualized stability-driven treatment regimen has been provided by the CRYSTAL and BRIGHTER studies (see Figs. 1, 2, and 3).

OCT permits detailed assessment and quantification of the degree and type of edema and is essential to determine whether visual impairment in patients with RVO is caused by macular edema. If patients do not experience any improvement in BCVA for the initial 3-monthly assessments while on treatment, continued treatment is not recommended. The attainment of stable VA for three consecutive months while on treatment (at least three injections when treatment is initiated and a minimum of two injections if treatment is restarted) is considered sufficient for a temporary interruption of treatment. Patients should continue to undergo monthly monitoring of VA. Monthly treatment is reinitiated when a loss of VA resulting from macular edema secondary to RVO is observed. No threshold for VA loss to trigger retreatment has been defined. OCT should be performed to determine the extent of macular edema; if VA has not changed but OCT clearly shows worsening, treatment may be considered on an individual basis [27].

When treating newly diagnosed RVO, physicians should be aware of common risk factors, to follow good clinical practice and refer patients to the appropriate specialist if necessary. Physicians should be aware of signs of rubeosis during

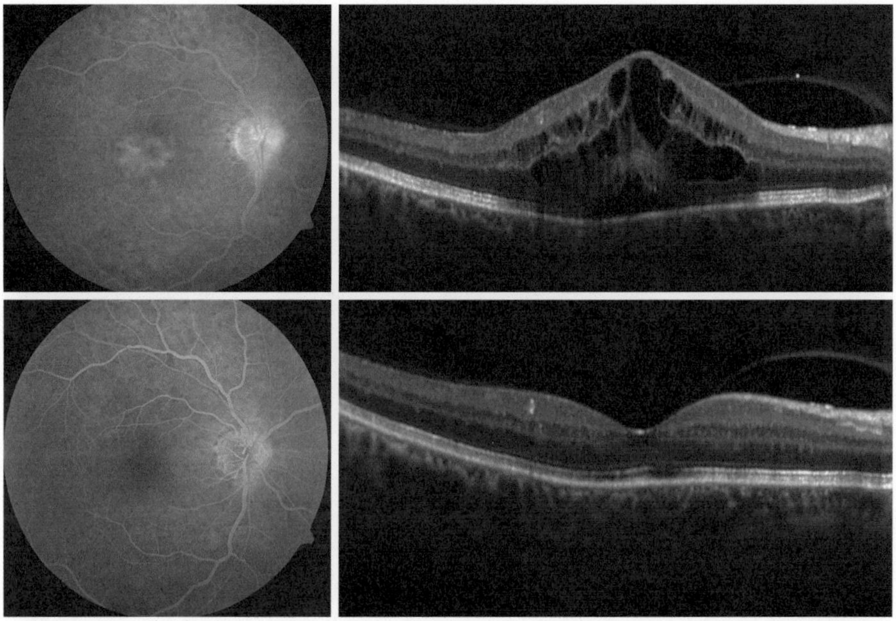

Fig. 2 *Left to right*: FA images and OCT images of a patient with recurrent macular edema after central retinal vein occlusion (CRVO) before (*top*) and 3 months later after 3 × intravitreal ranibizumab therapy (*bottom*)

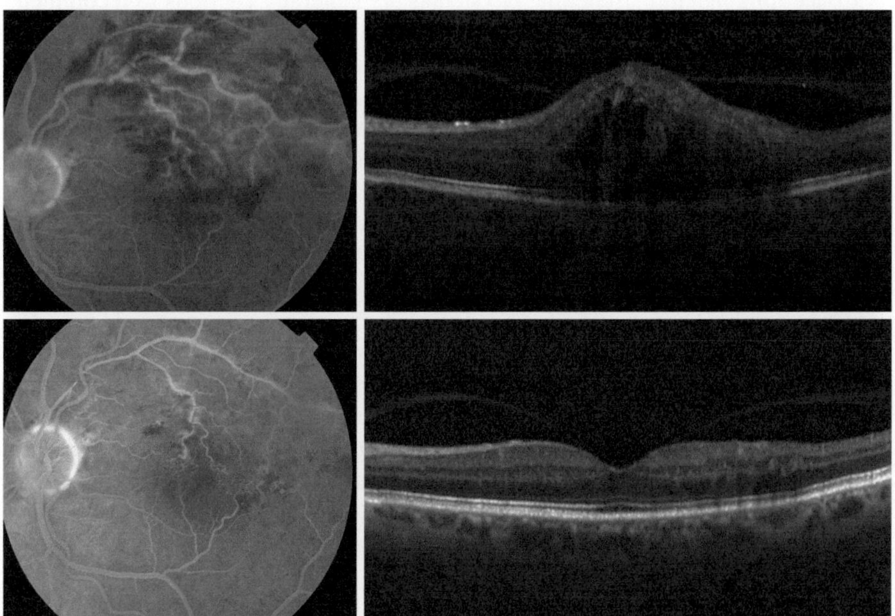

Fig. 3 *Left to right*: FA images and OCT images of a patient with branch retinal vein occlusion (BRVO) at baseline (*top*) and 3 months later after 3 × intravitreal ranibizumab therapy (*bottom*)

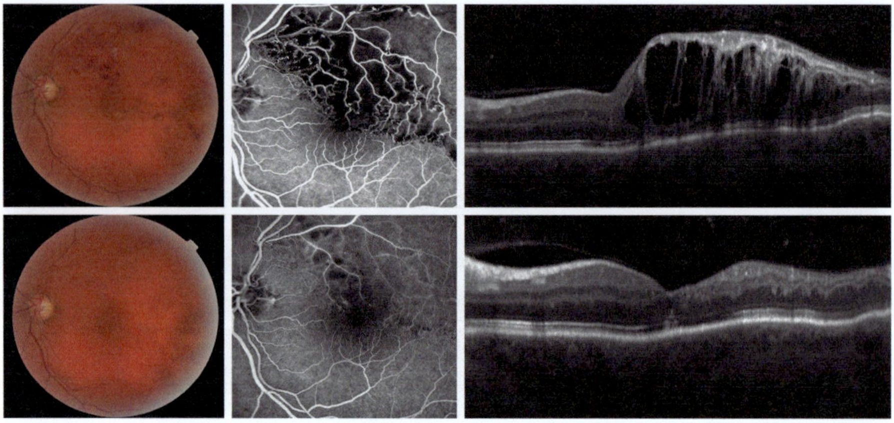

Fig. 4 *Left to right*: Fundus photographs, FA images, and OCT images of a patient with ischemic branch retinal vein occlusion (BRVO) at baseline (*top*) and 3 months later after 3×intravitreal ranibizumab therapy (*bottom*)

follow-up of all RVO cases, particularly CRVO. The role of anti-VEGF therapy in the prevention and management of rubeosis is still unclear and requires further study. In the BRAVO and CRUISE studies, no patients from the BRAVO and only two patients from the CRUISE study met the generally accepted definition for ischemic RVO (≥10 disc areas of capillary non-perfusion) [25, 26].

Concerning *macular* ischemia, physicians are generally cautious to recommend anti-VEGF therapy for patients presenting with ischemic visual loss because of the limited availability of phase III trial data in this patient population. At present, physicians should use their own judgment in patients with macular ischemia affecting the fovea as to whether any functional improvement might be achieved with anti-VEGF treatment. However, the primary endpoint data of the CRYSTAL and BRIGHTER studies provided evidence for similar functional efficacy of ranibizumab regardless of the status of macular ischemia at baseline (Ref. Mones J, ARVO 2015) (see Fig. 4). Fluorescein angiography may be performed during follow-up of these patients to evaluate any progression of ischemia, but is not considered essential [27].

The extent of *peripheral* ischemia in RVO may be the driving force in recurrent edema after intravitreal injections by affecting the levels of intravitreal VEGF and, in turn, modulating the severity of macular edema and its response to therapy. Surprisingly, patients with a greater extent of retinal non-perfusion on presentation were more likely to experience a greater improvement in macular edema and visual acuity in a study by Singer et al. [33]. The authors also showed that the level of non-perfusion changes dynamically in response to intravitreal anti-VEGF or dexamethasone treatment and correlates with the severity of edema and visual acuity loss.

There is still a lack of prospective, randomized head-to-head trials comparing the efficacy of ranibizumab and aflibercept and the sustained-release dexamethasone (DEX) implant in patients with RVO. A systematic literature review published by

Pielen et al. compared anti-VEGF agents (ranibizumab, bevacizumab, aflibercept) versus steroids (triamcinolone and Ozurdex) for macular edema in RVO [21]. All anti-VEGF agents showed a better visual acuity gain compared to steroids at month 12. The downside was that anti-VEGF therapy requires more frequent injections (around eight injections per year, compared to two injections in the steroid group). However, IOP increase and cataract progression are significantly higher in the patients treated with steroids compared to patients treated with anti-VEGF agents. These are substantial drawbacks for using steroids to treat macular edema in RVO. On the other hand, many affected patients may already be pseudophakic, and in these, the use of intraocular steroids may be reasonable [34]. Steroids may also have a place in the treatment pathway of patients who have failed on anti-VEGF therapy. Besides, the DEX implant may also be of value in vitrectomized eyes, where anti-VEGFs have shown significantly reduced half-life compared to non-vitrectomized eyes in previous reports [35], although some authors argue there is no difference [36].

Head-to-head trials comparing different anti-VEGF drugs are available for other conditions: Two similarly designed trials compared ranibizumab and aflibercept for the treatment of exudative age-related macular degeneration (VIEW 1 and 2) [37]. Similar efficacy and safety was found in both drugs. Aflibercept, compared with ranibizumab and bevacizumab, targets a wider range of cytokines and may have a stronger binding affinity [38]. Results suggested that aflibercept would require injections only every 8 weeks, which is fewer than ranibizumab, although ranibizumab was not tested every 8 weeks in VIEW. This was reflected in the FDA Dermatologic and Ophthalmic Drugs Advisory Committee recommendation that aflibercept should be given every 2 months following three initial monthly doses in neovascular age-related macular degeneration. Aflibercept also appeared to last longer in the eye than ranibizumab [39]. Age-related macular degeneration is a more aggressive condition than RVO, and so it is unlikely that more frequent dosing would be needed in RVO. Therefore, aflibercept may be preferred because it would reduce pressure on outpatient clinics [34]. Furthermore, there is some evidence from patients with age-related macular degeneration that aflibercept may be effective in patients who have not responded to ranibizumab [40, 41]. This may be due to the higher affinity and wider number of cytokines that are targeted. There is no reason to suspect that these effects are any different for the macular edema caused by RVO. However, there is as yet no evidence as to whether ranibizumab would be effective after aflibercept has failed [34].

There is little evidence that combining grid macular laser photocoagulation with anti-VEGF treatment provides additional clinical benefit for patients with visual impairment resulting from macular edema secondary to BRVO or CRVO [27, 42]. The randomized BRIGHTER study demonstrated similar functional efficacy for ranibizumab monotherapy versus ranibizumab combined with grid laser at the 6 months primary endpoint. Grid laser may lead to a reduced need for anti-VEGF injections; however, no prospective data are available as of yet. On the other hand, it has not been proven that anti-VEGF therapy may also treat peripheral ischemia. At present, anti-VEGF therapy should therefore be considered as supplemental therapy rather than replacement therapy in such cases. Some physicians recommend focal or pan-retinal laser photocoagulation in combination with anti-VEGF therapy for the treatment of ischemic retinal areas (for peripheral ischemia, most ophthalmologists consider a degree of ischemia of five disc diameters in BRVO and ten disc diameters in CRVO as significant). The rationale for this approach is to decrease the amount of VEGF by reducing the ischemic trigger. Although this approach seems logical, recent studies showed no benefit of laser treatment or combined treatment over anti-VEGF therapy in chronic RVO cases [42]. Furthermore, laser therapy should not be performed before initiation of intravitreal therapy because this may worsen macular edema [27].

Summary

Several studies have shown that intravitreal therapy with anti-VEGF medication or corticosteroids is currently the most effective medical treatment option for macular edema associated with retinal vascular occlusion (RVO). However, criteria for the retreatment of macular edema in RVO have yet to be defined, and there are currently no established protocols for long-term management of these patients. Most specialists currently favor an as-needed (PRN) or treat-and-extend treatment regimen after the initial, monthly anti-VEGF loading dose. Studies have yet to compare the long-term effectiveness and safety of repeated intravitreal anti-VEGF and/or corticosteroid injection regimens for treatment of RVO. In the extension studies of the large phase III trials for approval of ranibizumab and aflibercept, response to treatment varied considerably among patients with RVO. It appears that after the first year with monthly injections, one anti-VEGF injection every 3 months may be adequate to treat many patients with BRVO, but most patients with CRVO seem to require more frequent monitoring and treatment. The currently accepted (PRN) treatment regimen for anti-VEGF therapy in RVO aims at treating patients when they can benefit the most while minimizing the number of unnecessary intravitreal injections and hence the risk of side effects.

Similar to the treatment of exudative age-related macular degeneration, the use of aflibercept may allow for longer treatment intervals compared to ranibizumab or bevacizumab. Especially in chronic cases and nonresponders to anti-VEGF treatment, the continuous release of medication by the sustained-release dexamethasone (DEX) implant facilitates a stable level of drug within the eye, precluding the need for multiple repeated injections of other medications. Although its use is associated with significantly more side effects (especially cataract progression and IOP increase), as-needed treatment with the DEX implant typically results in only 2 or 3 injections per year, which is much less than that required with anti-VEGF therapy, therefore reducing other risks of repeated intravitreal injections. Hence, sustained-release corticosteroid therapy may be a valuable alternative treatment for patients with chronic macular edema after retinal vascular occlusion.

Further prospective trials are needed to compare long-term efficacy and adverse effects of both anti-VEGF and corticosteroid therapy. There is also a lack of evidence for the use of combination therapies for the treatment of RVO. Even supplemental laser coagulation has to be questioned since prospective randomized studies showed no advantage of combined anti-VEGF and laser therapy over anti-VEGF mono therapy in chronic cases. Head-to-head comparisons of the currently approved therapies are still ongoing and hopefully will aid in choosing the best medical option for treatment of macular edema secondary to retinal vascular occlusion.

References

1. Graham EM. The investigation of patients with retinal vascular occlusion. Eye (Lond). 1990;4(Pt 3):464–8. Review.
2. Buehl W, Sacu S, Schmidt-Erfurth U. Retinal vein occlusions. Dev Ophthalmol. 2010;46:54–72.
3. Ng WY, Wong DW, Yeo IY, Han DC. Cystoid macular edema in acute presentation of central retinal artery occlusion. Case Rep Ophthalmol Med. 2012;2012:530128. doi:10.1155/2012/530128. Epub 2012 Apr 4.
4. Laouri M, Chen E, Looman M, Gallagher M. The burden of disease of retinal vein occlusion: review of the literature. Eye (Lond). 2011;25(8):981–8. Review.
5. Rehak J, Rehak M. Branch retinal vein occlusion: pathogenesis, visual prognosis, and treatment modalities. Curr Eye Res. 2008;33(2):111–31.
6. Glacet-Bernard A, Coscas G, Chabanel A, et al. A randomized, double-masked study on the treatment of retinal vein occlusion with troxerutin. Am J Ophthalmol. 1994;118:421–9.
7. De Sanctis MT, Cesarone MR, Belcaro G, et al. Treatment of retinal vein thrombosis with pentoxifylline: a controlled, randomized trial. Angiology. 2002;53 Suppl 1:S35–8.
8. The Branch Vein Occlusion Study Group. The Branch Vein Occlusion Study Group: Argon laser photocoagulation for macular edema in branch vein occlusion. Am J Ophthalmol. 1984;98(3):271–82.
9. A randomized clinical trial of early panretinal photocoagulation for ischemic central vein occlusion. The Central Vein Occlusion Study Group N report. Ophthalmology. 1995;102(10): 1434–44.
10. McAllister IL, Vijayasekaran S, Chen SD, Yu DY. Effect of triamcinolone acetonide on vascular endothelial growth factor and occludin levels in branch retinal vein occlusion. Am J Ophthalmol. 2009;147(5):838–46.
11. Jonas JB, Degenring RF, Kreissig I, Akkoyun I, Kamppeter BA. Intraocular pressure elevation after intravitreal triamcinolone acetonide injection. Ophthalmology. 2005;112:593–8.
12. Jonas JB, Degenring RF, Kreissig I, Akkoyun I. Safety of intravitreal high-dose reinjections of triamcinolone acetonide. Am J Ophthalmol. 2004;138:1054–5.
13. Scott IU, Flynn Jr HW. Reducing the risk of endophthalmitis following intravitreal injections. Retina. 2007;27:10–2.
14. Scott IU, Ip MS, VanVeldhuisen PC, Oden NL, Blodi BA, Fisher M, Chan CK, Gonzalez VH, Singerman LJ, Tolentino M, SCORE Study Research Group. A randomized trial comparing the efficacy and safety of intravitreal triamcinolone with standard care to treat vision loss associated with macular Edema secondary to branch retinal vein occlusion: the Standard Care vs Corticosteroid for Retinal Vein Occlusion (SCORE) study report 6. Arch Ophthalmol. 2009;127(9):1115–28.
15. Ip MS, Scott IU, VanVeldhuisen PC, Oden NL, Blodi BA, Fisher M, Singerman LJ, Tolentino M, Chan CK, Gonzalez VH, SCORE Study Research Group. A randomized trial comparing the efficacy and safety of intravitreal triamcinolone with observation to treat vision loss associated with macular edema secondary to central retinal vein occlusion: the Standard Care vs Corticosteroid for Retinal Vein Occlusion (SCORE) study report 5. Arch Ophthalmol. 2009;127(9):1101–14.

16. Brand CS. Management of retinal vascular diseases: a patient-centric approach. Eye (Lond). 2012;26 Suppl 2:S1–16. Review.
17. Kuppermann BD, Blumenkranz MS, Haller JA, et al. Dexamethasone DDS Phase II Study Group. Randomized controlled study of an intravitreous dexamethasone drug delivery system in patients with persistent macular edema. Arch Ophthalmol. 2007;125:309–17.
18. Haller JA, Bandello F, Belfort Jr R, Blumenkranz MS, Gillies M, Heier J, Loewenstein A, Yoon YH, Jacques ML, Jiao J, Li XY, Whitcup SM, OZURDEX GENEVA Study Group. Randomized, sham-controlled trial of dexamethasone intravitreal implant in patients with macular edema due to retinal vein occlusion. Ophthalmology. 2010;117(6):1134–46.
19. Haller JA, Bandello F, Belfort Jr R, Blumenkranz MS, Gillies M, Heier J, Loewenstein A, Yoon YH, Jiao J, Li XY, Whitcup SM, Ozurdex GENEVA Study Group, Li J. Dexamethasone intravitreal implant in patients with macular edema related to branch or central retinal vein occlusion twelve-month study results. Ophthalmology. 2011;118(12):2453–60.
20. Epstein DL, Algvere PV, von Wendt G, Seregard S, Kvanta A. Benefit from bevacizumab for macular edema in central retinal vein occlusion: twelve-month results of a prospective, randomized study. Ophthalmology. 2012;119(12):2587–91.
21. Pielen A, Feltgen N, Isserstedt C, Callizo J, Junker B, Schmucker C. Efficacy and safety of intravitreal therapy in macular edema due to branch and central retinal vein occlusion: a systematic review. PLoS One. 2013;8(10):e78538.
22. Russo V, Barone A, Conte E, Prascina F, Stella A, Noci ND. Bevacizumab compared with macular laser grid photocoagulation for cystoid macular edema in branch retinal vein occlusion. Retina. 2009;29(4):511–5.
23. Wroblewski JJ, Wells 3rd JA, Gonzales CR. Pegaptanib sodium for macular edema secondary to branch retinal vein occlusion. Am J Ophthalmol. 2010;149(1):147–54.
24. Stewart MW. Pharmacokinetics, pharmacodynamics and pre-clinical characteristics of ophthalmic drugs that bind VEGF. Expert Rev Clin Pharmacol. 2014;7(2):167–80.
25. Campochiaro PA, Heier JS, Feiner L, Gray S, Saroj N, Rundle AC, Murahashi WY, Rubio RG, BRAVO Investigators. Ranibizumab for macular edema following branch retinal vein occlusion: six-month primary end point results of a phase III study. Ophthalmology. 2010;117(6): 1102–12.
26. Brown DM, Campochiaro PA, Singh RP, Li Z, Gray S, Saroj N, Rundle AC, Rubio RG, Murahashi WY, CRUISE Investigators. Ranibizumab for macular edema following central retinal vein occlusion: six-month primary end point results of a phase III study. Ophthalmology. 2010;117(6):1124–33.
27. Gerding H, Monés J, Tadayoni R, Boscia F, Pearce I, Priglinger S. Ranibizumab in retinal vein occlusion: treatment recommendations by an expert panel. Br J Ophthalmol. 2015;99(3): 297–304.
28. Singer MA, Awh CC, Sadda S, Freeman WR, Antoszyk AN, Wong P, Tuomi L. HORIZON: an open-label extension trial of ranibizumab for choroidal neovascularization secondary to age-related macular degeneration. Ophthalmology. 2012;119(6):1175–83.
29. Heier JS, Clark WL, Boyer DS, Brown DM, Vitti R, Berliner AJ, Kazmi H, Ma Y, Stemper B, Zeitz O, Sandbrink R, Haller JA. Intravitreal aflibercept injection for macular edema due to central retinal vein occlusion: two-year results from the COPERNICUS study. Ophthalmology. 2014;121(7):1414–20.
30. Ogura Y, Roider J, Korobelnik JF, Holz FG, Simader C, Schmidt-Erfurth U, Vitti R, Berliner AJ, Hiemeyer F, Stemper B, Zeitz O, Sandbrink R, GALILEO Study Group. Intravitreal aflibercept for macular edema secondary to central retinal vein occlusion: 18-month results of the phase 3 GALILEO study. Am J Ophthalmol. 2014;158(5):1032–8.
31. Campochiaro PA, Clark WL, Boyer DS, Heier JS, Brown DM, Vitti R, Kazmi H, Berliner AJ, Erickson K, Chu KW, Soo Y, Cheng Y, Haller JA. Intravitreal aflibercept for macular edema following branch retinal vein occlusion: the 24-week results of the VIBRANT study. Ophthalmology. 2015;122(3):538–44.
32. Lotery AJ, Regnier S. Patterns of ranibizumab and aflibercept treatment of central retinal vein occlusion in routine clinical practice in the USA. Eye (Lond). 2015;29(3):380–7.

33. Singer M, Tan CS, Bell D, Sadda SR. Area of peripheral retinal nonperfusion and treatment response in branch and central retinal vein occlusion. Retina. 2014;34(9):1736–42.
34. Ford JA, Shyangdan D, Uthman OA, Lois N, Waugh N. Drug treatment of macular oedema secondary to central retinal vein occlusion: a network meta-analysis. BMJ Open. 2014;4(7):e005292.
35. Moisseiev E, Waisbourd M, Ben-Artsi E, et al. Pharmacokinetics of bevacizumab after topical and intravitreal administration in human eyes. Graefes Arch Clin Exp Ophthalmol. 2014;252(2):331–7.
36. Ahn J, Kim H, Woo SJ, et al. Pharmacokinetics of intravitreally injected bevacizumab in vitrectomized eyes. J Ocul Pharmacol Ther. 2013;29(7):612–8.
37. Heier JS, Brown DM, Chong V, et al. Intravitreal aflibercept (VEGF trap-eye) in wet age-related macular degeneration. Ophthalmology. 2012;119:2537–48.
38. Papadopoulos N, Martin J, Ruan Q, et al. Binding and neutralization of vascular endothelial growth factor (VEGF) and related ligands by VEGF Trap, ranibizumab and bevacizumab. Angiogenesis. 2012;15:171–85.
39. Stewart MW, Rosenfeld PJ. Predicted biological activity of intravitreal VEGF Trap. Br J Ophthalmol. 2008;92:667–8.
40. Bakall B, Folk JC, Boldt HC, et al. Aflibercept therapy for exudative age-related macular degeneration resistant to bevacizumab and ranibizumab. Am J Ophthalmol. 2013;156:15–22.
41. Cho H, Shah CP, Weber M, et al. Aflibercept for exudative AMD with persistent fluid on ranibizumab and/or bevacizumab. Br J Ophthalmol. 2013;97:1032–5.
42. Campochiaro PA, Hafiz G, Mir TA, Scott AW, Solomon S, Zimmer-Galler I, Sodhi A, Duh E, Ying H, Wenick A, Shah SM, Do DV, Nguyen QD, Kherani S, Sophie R. Scatter photocoagulation does not reduce macular edema or treatment burden in patients with retinal vein occlusion: the relate trial. Ophthalmology. 2015;122(7):1426–37.

Chapter 8
Cystoid Macular Edema in Retained Lens Fragments After Cataract Surgery

Motasem Al-latayfeh

Introduction

Cystoid macular edema is a well-known complication of retained lens fragments after cataract surgery. It occurs in 11–28 % of cases [1, 2]. It is one of the causes of visual loss after uneventful cataract surgery also. It has been reported to occur in 2–3 % after phacoemulsification [3–5]. Retained lens fragment (RLF) is a serious event in cataract surgery that occurs in about 1 % of cases. It frequently requires both medical and surgical intervention to minimize complications and visual loss. In this chapter, we will discuss the pathophysiology of CME in RLF and proper medical and surgical management.

Incidence and Etiology

RLF is an uncommon complication of cataract surgery. It has been reported to occur in 0.18–1.1 % of cases [6–8]. Certain factors affect the incidence of RLF including the surgical technique that has been used to remove the cataractous lens (extracapsular extraction vs. phacoemulsification), surgeon's experience, type of cataract such as posterior polar cataract, and hard nucleus [6, 9–11].

The size and nature of the dropped lens varies depending on the stage during phacoemulsification when the posterior capsule rupture (PCR) occurs. It may vary from a dropped whole nucleus if PCR occurred during initial hydrodissection, to only soft cortical matter if PCR occurred later during irrigation aspiration. The size

M. Al-latayfeh, MD
Department of Opthalmology, Hashemite University, Zarqa, Jordan
e-mail: motasem974@gmail.com

S. Schaal, H.J. Kaplan (eds.), *Cystoid Macular Edema*,
DOI 10.1007/978-3-319-39766-5_8

and the nature of the dropped lens pieces will affect the level of induced inflammation, the potential complications, and the management plan.

CME has been reported to occur in 11–28 % of RLF and is a major reason for reduced visual acuity [1, 2] although CME is well known to occur even after uneventful phacoemulsification [12]. It is believed that the inflammatory mediators released in response to cataract surgery play a major role in the formation of CME [13].

Pathophysiology of Lens-Induced Immune Response

The anterior chamber of the eye is immunologically privileged, and lens proteins are sequestered from the host immune system by the lens capsule [14]. However, recently it has been shown that crystallin lens proteins are present within the anterior chamber [15] in other ocular tissues and in serum [16]. Nevertheless, the immune system is normally tolerant to lens crystallins via various immunoregulatory mechanisms [14, 17]. However, tolerance to these proteins is abrogated by inflammatory mediators released during cataract surgery [18] that induces an immediate autoimmune reaction [18–20]. An intense immune reaction ensues, involving macrophages, that breaches the blood retinal barrier resulting in cystoid macular edema (CME) [21, 22]. Rupture of the anterior vitreous face may contribute to the development of CME [23, 24].

Clinical Presentation

Patients with RLF present postoperatively with reduced visual acuity from several possible causes – anterior uveitis, elevated intraocular pressure, corneal edema, and CME [1, 2, 5, 10, 25–29]. Clinically significant CME may occur immediately after surgery or within several weeks, although 80 % of patients show spontaneous resolution [30].

Clinical examination will reveal intraocular inflammation with lens fragments floating in the vitreous cavity or lying on the retinal surface. Fundus fluorescein angiography will frequently show a typical petalloid pattern although optical coherence tomography is most helpful in demonstrating the anatomical presence of CME with multiple intraretinal cysts [31–33]. Retinal detachment has been reported to be present in 3.8–45 % of cases, most frequently secondary to unsuccessful attempts by the cataract surgeon to recover the dislocated fragments [34–37]. Among other complications are retained lens fragments in the anterior chamber, as well as posterior to the iris presenting as an iris mass [39–41].

Management of CME Secondary to RLF

Medical Management

Medical treatment of CME may include the use of topical nonsteroidal anti-inflammatory drugs (NSAIDs) or corticosteroids [44]. Prophylactic use of NSAID agents has been shown to be effective in reducing the incidence of pseudophakic CME [42, 43]. However, since intraocular inflammation is the major cause of RLF, CME aggressive corticosteroid therapy is important both topically and systemically [44].However, surgical removal of the dislocated lens fragments via pars plana vitrectomy will remove the inciting proteins and lens fragments, as well as quell the inflammation.

Surgical Management

Dislocation of lens fragments during cataract surgery can be the result of several factors – a hard nucleus, posterior polar cataract, weak zonules (as in pseudoexfoliation or various genetic syndromes [Marfans, Ehlers-Danlos]), high myopia, but is most frequently associated with a poorly dilated pupil. In difficult cases, the surgeon may need to stabilize the lens capsule and detect/manage posterior capsular tears if they occur during the operation.

The main goals of intraoperative management is to maintain anterior chamber depth, prevent vitreous prolapse, avoid dislocation of lens material into the vitreous cavity, and finish the case as safely and quickly as possible with or without intraocular lens implantation [45–48].

From a vitreoretinal perspective, the anterior segment surgeon should minimize the manipulation of posteriorly dislocated lens fragments in the vitreous cavity to avoid the creation of vitreous traction resulting in retinal tears, detachment, and/or vitreous hemorrhage.

Conservative Management Versus Pars Plana Vitrectomy

The ultimate goal in the management of RLF cases is to ensure a good visual outcome. Pars plana vitrectomy surgery has been shown to be effective in resolution of corneal edema, control of intraocular pressure, and preservation of good vision [9, 10, 26]. In 2009, Barr and Schaal reported a retrospective case series of 42 patients divided into three groups: group 1 (12 patients) had early vitrectomy (<1 week), group 2 (15 patients) late vitrectomy (>1 week), and group 3 (15 patients) only medical treatment. At 1 year, there was no statistically significant difference in final visual acuity between the three groups (group 1, 20/25; group 2, 20/28; group 3, 20/38, $p=0.52$) or intraocular pressure [1].

Although there are no established guidelines to determine when to treat cases conservatively, their results suggested that if there isn't a rapid response to medical therapy, vitrectomy surgery should be performed.

Other reports also did not find any relationship between timing of vitrectomy and final visual outcome [34, 35, 49–54].

The most important factor in determining the timing of vitrectomy surgery is the severity of the intraocular inflammation – mild intraocular inflammation may be managed initially by topical or systemic therapy. Persistent inflammation, worsening of visual acuity, increasing intraocular pressure, and severe ocular pain are indications for early vitrectomy.

Technique of Pars Plana Vitrectomy

The most common technique reported by retinal surgeons to remove residual lens matter is three-port 20-gauge pars plana vitrectomy. They allow use of the ultrasonic fragmatome if necessary to remove large nuclear fragments from the vitreous cavity. Some surgeons crush the retained lens pieces between the light pipe and vitrectomy probe which facilitates their removal by the vitrectomy probe without the use of the fragmatome [29, 35, 49]. Some surgeons have used the OZil phaco handpiece instead of the fragmatome and showed very good results [55].

The most important step during vitrectomy surgery for removal of RLF is to perform a complete vitrectomy, including meticulous removal of the vitreous around the lens fragments before removal to prevent traction on the retina. This will reduce the incidence of retinal tears and retinal detachment. Some surgeons suggest the use of perfluorocarbons (a heavy liquid frequently used in vitreoretinal surgery especially in retinal detachment) to separate the lens fragments from the retinal surface and bring them into the mid-vitreous cavity for safer removal by the fragmatome or vitrectomy probe [29, 35, 49, 56, 57].

With the introduction of the small gauge sutureless vitrectomy (23 and 25 gauge), surgeons have began to use small ports for the removal of RLF [58–62]. In 2009, Ho and colleagues reported a case series where 25-gauge vitrectomy was used exclusively to remove lens fragments of various sizes [60]. They reported comparable outcome and rate of complications to 20-gauge vitrectomy [60]. In an era where there is a continuous shift toward less-invasive and sutureless surgeries, small gauge vitrectomy surgery will continue to gain popularity for the removal of RLF.

Outcome of Pars Plana Vitrectomy Surgery for RLF

Pars plana vitrectomy surgery to remove vitreous lens fragments has been shown to be associated with improved visual acuity, reduction of intraocular inflammation, and intraocular pressure; 20/40 or better vision ranged from 44 to 72 % [9, 26, 50].

In a multivariate analysis to identify predictive factors of poor visual outcome (20/200 or worse), the following were shown to be anterior vitrectomy at the time of cataract surgery, absence of sulcus lens, preexisting eye disease, and development of glaucoma [50]. Other factors associated with a poor visual outcome include retinal detachment and CME [28, 35, 37, 38].

Conclusion

CME is a major complication after cataract surgery complicated by RLF. The introduction of modern phacoemulsification techniques resulted initially in an increased incidence of posterior lens fragment dislocation. Management of CME includes aggressive medical therapy with topical and oral NSAIDs and corticosteroids. If severe intraocular inflammation doesn't resolve quickly, pars plana vitrectomy with removal of residual lens material should be performed.

References

1. Schaal S, Barr CC. Management of retained lens fragments after cataract surgery with and without pars plana vitrectomy. J Cataract Refract Surg. 2009;35:863–7.
2. Cohen SM, Davis A, Cukrowski C. Cystoid macular edema after pars plana vitrectomy for retained lens fragments. J Cataract Refract Surg. 2006;32:1521–6.
3. Gulkilik G, Kocabora S, Taskapili M, Engin G. Cystoid macular edema after phacoemulsification: risk factors and effect on visual acuity. Can J Ophthalmol. 2006;41:699–703.
4. Ray S, D'Amico DJ. Pseudophakic cystoid macular edema. Semin Ophthalmol. 2002;17:167–80.
5. Henderson BA, Kim JY, Ament CS, Ferrufino-Ponce ZK, Grabowska A, Cremers SL. Clinical pseudophakic cystoid macular edema. Risk factors for development and duration after treatment. J Cataract Refract Surg. 2007;33:1550–8.
6. Aasuri MK, Kompella VB, Majji AB. Risk factors for and management of dropped nucleus during phacoemulsification. J Cataract Refract Surg. 2001;27:1428–32.
7. Pande M, Dabbs TR. Incidence of lens matter dislocation during phacoemulsification. J Cataract Refract Surg. 1996;22:737–42.
8. Jaycock P, Johnston RL, Taylor H, et al. The Cataract National Dataset electronic multi-centre audit of 55,567 operations: updating benchmark standards of care in the United Kingdom and internationally. Eye (Lond). 2009;23:38–49.
9. Kim JE, Flynn Jr HW, Smiddy WE, et al. Retained lens fragments after phacoemulsification. Ophthalmology. 1994;101:1827–32.
10. Gilliland GD, Hutton WL, Fuller DG. Retained intravitreal lens fragments after cataract surgery. Ophthalmology. 1992;99:1263–7.
11. Schwartz SG, Holz ER, Mieler WF, Kuhl DP. Retained lens fragments in resident-performed cataract extractions. CLAO J. 2002;28:44–7.
12. Stark Jr WJ, Maumenee AE, Fagadau W, et al. Cystoid macular edema in pseudophakia. Surv Ophthalmol. 1984;28(Suppl):442–51.
13. Flach AJ. The incidence, pathogenesis and treatment of cystoid macular edema following cataract surgery. Trans Am Ophthalmol Soc. 1998;96:557–634.
14. Streilein JW. Ocular immune privilege: the eye takes a dim but practical view of immunity and inflammation. J Leukoc Biol. 2003;74:179–85.

15. Sandberg HO, Closs O. The alpha and gamma crystallin content in aqueous humor of eyes with clear lenses and with cataracts. Exp Eye Res. 1979;28:601–10.
16. Andley UP. Crystallins in the eye: function and pathology. Prog Retin Eye Res. 2007;26:78–98.
17. Taylor AW, Kaplan HJ. Ocular immune privilege in the year 2010: ocular immune privilege and uveitis. Ocul Immunol Inflamm. 2010;18:488–92.
18. Marak Jr GE. Phacoanaphylactic endophthalmitis. Surv Ophthalmol. 1992;36:325–39.
19. Oprescu M. The etiopathology of phacoantigenic uveitis and phacolytic glaucoma. Oftalmologia. 1992;36:207–13.
20. Wilkinson CP, Green WR. Vitrectomy for retained lens material after cataract extraction: the relationship between histopathologic findings and the time of vitreous surgery. Ophthalmology. 2001;108:1633–7.
21. Yanoff M, Fine BS, Brucker AJ, Eagle Jr RC. Pathology of human cystoid macular edema. Surv Ophthalmol. 1984;28(Suppl):505–11.
22. Yeo LM, Charteris DG, Bunce C, Luthert PJ, Gregor ZJ. Retained intravitreal lens fragments after phacoemulsification: a clinicopathological correlation. Br J Ophthalmol. 1999;83:1135–8.
23. Hitchings RA. Aphakic macular oedema: a two-year follow-up study. Br J Ophthalmol. 1977;61:628–30.
24. Irvine AR, Bresky R, Crowder BM, Forster RK, Hunter DM, Kulvin SM. Macular edema after cataract extraction. Ann Ophthalmol. 1971;3:1234–5.
25. von Lany H, Mahmood S, James CR, et al. Displacement of nuclear fragments into the vitreous complicating phacoemulsification surgery in the UK: clinical features, outcomes and management. Br J Ophthalmol. 2008;92:493–5.
26. Margherio RR, Margherio AR, Pendergast SD, et al. Vitrectomy for retained lens fragments after phacoemulsification. Ophthalmology. 1997;104:1426–32.
27. Tommila P, Immonen I. Dislocated nuclear fragments after cataract surgery. Eye (Lond). 1995;9(Pt 4):437–41.
28. Romero-Aroca P, Fernandez-Ballart J, Mendez-Marin I, Salvat-Serra M, Baget-Bernaldiz M, Buil-Calvo JA. Management of nucleus loss into the vitreous: long term follow up in 63 patients. Clin Ophthalmol. 2007;1:505–12.
29. Oruc S, Kaplan HJ. Outcome of vitrectomy for retained lens fragments after phacoemulsification. Ocul Immunol Inflamm. 2001;9:41–7.
30. Bonnet S. Repercussions of cataract surgery on the development of cystoid macular edema in the diabetic patient. Bull Soc Belge Ophtalmol. 1995;256:127–9.
31. Guex-Crosier Y. The pathogenesis and clinical presentation of macular edema in inflammatory diseases. Doc Ophthalmol. 1999;97:297–309.
32. Kusbeci T, Eryigit L, Yavas G, Inan UU. Evaluation of cystoid macular edema using optical coherence tomography and fundus fluorescein angiography after uncomplicated phacoemulsification surgery. Curr Eye Res. 2012;37:327–33.
33. Cagini C, Fiore T, Iaccheri B, Piccinelli F, Ricci MA, Fruttini D. Macular thickness measured by optical coherence tomography in a healthy population before and after uncomplicated cataract phacoemulsification surgery. Curr Eye Res. 2009;34:1036–41.
34. Ho SF, Zaman A. Clinical features and outcomes of pars plana vitrectomy in patients with retained lens fragments after phacoemulsification. J Cataract Refract Surg. 2007;33:2106–10.
35. Scott IU, Flynn Jr HW, Smiddy WE, et al. Clinical features and outcomes of pars plana vitrectomy in patients with retained lens fragments. Ophthalmology. 2003;110:1567–72.
36. Fastenberg DM, Schwartz PL, Shakin JL, Golub BM. Management of dislocated nuclear fragments after phacoemulsification. Am J Ophthalmol. 1991;112:535–9.
37. Greven CM, Piccione K. Delayed visual loss after pars plana vitrectomy for retained lens fragments. Retina. 2004;24:363–7.
38. Yang CS, Lee FL, Hsu WM, Liu JH. Management of retained intravitreal lens fragments after phacoemulsification surgery. Ophthalmologica. 2002;216:192–7.
39. Teo L, Chee SP. Retained lens fragment in the anterior segment as a cause of recurrent anterioruveitis. Int Ophthalmol. 2010;30:89–91.

40. Oliveira C, Liebmann JM, Dodick JM, Topilow H, Cykiert R, Ritch R. Identification of retained nucleus fragment in the posterior chamber using ultrasound biomicroscopy. Am J Ophthalmol. 2006;141:964–6.
41. Olsen TW, Lim JI, Grossniklaus HE. Retained lens material masquerading as a growing, pigmented iris tumor. Arch Ophthalmol. 1996;114:1154–5.
42. Flach AJ. Topical nonsteroidal antiinflammatory drugs in ophthalmology. Int Ophthalmol Clin. 2002;42:1–11.
43. Kim SJ, Flach AJ, Jampol LM. Nonsteroidal anti-inflammatory drugs in ophthalmology. Surv Ophthalmol. 2010;55:108–33.
44. Shelsta HN, Jampol LM. Pharmacologic therapy of pseudophakic cystoid macular edema: 2010 update. Retina. 2011;31:4–12.
45. Stewart MW. Managing retained lens fragments: raising the bar. Am J Ophthalmol. 2009;147:569–70.
46. Schutz JS, Mavrakanas NA. Posterior-assisted levitation in cataract surgery. Curr Opin Ophthalmol. 2010;21:50–4.
47. Arbisser LB, Charles S, Howcroft M, Werner L. Management of vitreous loss and dropped nucleus during cataract surgery. Ophthalmol Clin North Am. 2006;19:495–506.
48. Olsson RB, Ritland JS, Bjornsson OM, Syrdalen P, Eide N, Overgard R. A retrospective study of patients with retained nuclear fragments after cataract extraction. Acta Ophthalmol Scand. 2000;78:677–9.
49. Borne MJ, Tasman W, Regillo C, Malecha M, Sarin L. Outcomes of vitrectomy for retained lens fragments. Ophthalmology. 1996;103:971–6.
50. Ho LY, Doft BH, Wang L, Bunker CH. Clinical predictors and outcomes of pars plana vitrectomy for retained lens material after cataract extraction. Am J Ophthalmol. 2009;147:587–94.
51. Bessant DA, Sullivan PM, Aylward GW. The management of dislocated lens material after phacoemulsification. Eye (Lond). 1998;12(Pt 4):641–5.
52. Kageyama T, Ayaki M, Ogasawara M, Asahiro C, Yaguchi S. Results of vitrectomy performed at the time of phacoemulsification complicated by intravitreal lens fragments. Br J Ophthalmol. 2001;85:1038–40.
53. Stefaniotou M, Aspiotis M, Pappa C, Eftaxias V, Psilas K. Timing of dislocated nuclear fragment management after cataract surgery. J Cataract Refract Surg. 2003;29:1985–8.
54. Merani R, Hunyor AP, Playfair TJ, et al. Pars plana vitrectomy for the management of retained lens material after cataract surgery. Am J Ophthalmol. 2007;144:364–70.
55. Chiang A, Garg SJ, Alshareef RA, et al. Removal of posterior segment retained lens material using the OZil phacoemulsification handpiece versus Fragmatome during pars plana vitrectomy. Retina. 2012;32:2119–26.
56. Millar ER, Steel DH. Small-gauge transconjunctival vitrectomy with phacoemulsification in the pupillary plane of dense retained lens matter on perfluorocarbon liquids after complicated cataract surgery. Graefes Arch Clin Exp Ophthalmol. 2013;251:1757–62.
57. Boscher C, Lebuisson DA, Lean JS, Nguyen-Khoa JL. Vitrectomy with endoscopy for management of retained lens fragments and/or posteriorly dislocated intraocular lens. Graefes Arch Clin Exp Ophthalmol. 1998;236:115–21.
58. El Batarny AM. Transconjunctival sutureless 23-gauge vitrectomy for vitreoretinal diseases: outcome of 30 consecutive cases. Middle East Afr J Ophthalmol. 2008;15:99–105.
59. Fine HF, Iranmanesh R, Iturralde D, Spaide RF. Outcomes of 77 consecutive cases of 23-gauge transconjunctival vitrectomy surgery for posterior segment disease. Ophthalmology. 2007;114:1197–200.
60. Ho LY, Walsh MK, Hassan TS. 25-Gauge pars plana vitrectomy for retained lens fragments. Retina. 2010;30:843–9.
61. Kiss S, Vavvas D. 25-gauge transconjunctival sutureless pars plana vitrectomy for the removal of retained lens fragments and intraocular foreign bodies. Retina. 2008;28:1346–51.
62. Baker PS, Spirn MJ, Chiang A, et al. 23-Gauge transconjunctival pars plana vitrectomy for removal of retained lens fragments. Am J Ophthalmol. 2011;152:624–7.

Part III
Surgical Management of CME

Chapter 9
Surgical Management of Macular Edema Associated with Uveitis

Alexander L. Grigalunas and Pauline T. Merrill

Uveitis is a significant cause of vision loss in the working-age population in the developed world [1–3]. The most common cause of vision loss in uveitis patients is macular edema (ME) [1, 4]. Initial management of uveitic ME is primarily medical, as reviewed in another chapter of this volume. In some cases, however, maximum-tolerated medical therapy may be inadequate, and compliance with medical regimens may also be an issue. Surgical approaches may provide an alternative or adjunctive means of controlling uveitis and uveitic ME.

Primary vitrectomy for uveitis has been demonstrated to remove vitreous haze, potentially to improve control of inflammation, and to assist in diagnosis. Vitreous haze may limit vision as well as limit the ability of the treating ophthalmologist to adequately examine, diagnose, and treat posterior uveitis. Vitrectomy clears the vitreous cavity of opacities. An adherent vitreomacular interface may also play a role in the development of ME [5]. Hikichi and Trempe (1993) noted that in patients who develop uveitic ME, 78 % did not have a posterior vitreous detachment. Vitrectomy also removes inflammatory modulators contained within the vitreous while prospectively reducing the time inflammatory factors are retained within the vitreous cavity [6]. Additionally, the removed vitreous gel is replaced with aqueous humor, which has anti-inflammatory properties [7]. In cases in which the underlying cause of uveitis is in question, a diagnostic vitrectomy may also have the secondary effect of decreasing macular edema.

Uveitic ME is often associated with additional structural complications affecting the posterior segment. Vitrectomy may be indicated for epiretinal membrane (ERM), vitreomacular traction (VMT), traction or rhegmatogenous retinal detachment (RD), and vitreous hemorrhage. The vitrectomy itself along with correction of the structural complications may have a beneficial effect on macular edema.

A.L. Grigalunas, MD • P.T. Merrill, MD (✉)
Department of Ophthalmology, Rush University Medical Center,
1725 W. Harrison Street, Ste 915, Chicago, IL 60612, USA
e-mail: pauline.merrill@gmail.com

S. Schaal, H.J. Kaplan (eds.), *Cystoid Macular Edema*,
DOI 10.1007/978-3-319-39766-5_9

A surgical approach proven effective in randomized prospective studies is the fluocinolone acetonide (FlAc) intravitreal implant. This sustained-release steroid implant provides an Food and Drug Administration (FDA) approved treatment with dramatic effect on uveitic ME.

In this chapter, we review the background, techniques, outcomes, and complications of primary vitrectomy, vitrectomy for structural complications, and fluocinolone implant for uveitis with associated ME.

Primary Vitrectomy in Uveitis

Not long after the introduction of pars plana vitrectomy in the 1970s [8–10], Diamond and Kaplan described combined lensectomy–vitrectomy for complicated cataracts secondary to uveitis in 15 eyes [11]. The majority of eyes showed significant improvement in visual acuity. While lower postoperative acuity was associated with cystoid macular edema in six eyes, the outcome was noted to be superior to eyes undergoing lens extraction without vitrectomy. In 1981, Algvere et al. reported the use of therapeutic vitrectomy in 14 patients with chronic uveitis, ten of whom showed visual improvement [12]. In the same year Engel et al. described the utility of vitrectomy for diagnosis in ocular inflammation [13]. Focusing specifically on the effect of vitrectomy on inflammation-related ME, in 1992 Dugel et al. reported angiographic improvement in ME in 9 of 11 eyes [14].

Technique

Inflammation should be controlled preoperatively, as large amounts of preoperative inflammatory activity have been significantly linked with increased postoperative inflammation in patients with uveitis undergoing vitrectomy ($p<0.02$) [15]. Patients may be placed on high-dose systemic oral steroids (i.e., 1 mg/kg prednisone) starting 1–2 days prior to surgery in order to minimize the risk of increased postoperative inflammation. A standard three-port vitrectomy is employed. Smaller gauge techniques may help to minimize increased iatrogenic inflammation, but 20-gauge vitrectomy may facilitate concomitant procedures such as pars plana lensectomy. If endolaser is performed, care must be taken, as excessive laser may also exacerbate postoperative inflammation by increasing vascular permeability [16, 17].

Complete removal of the vitreous may improve long-term outcomes [18]. Triamcinolone may be used intraoperatively to visualize and facilitate complete removal of vitreous from the macular interface as well as the anterior hyaloid [19, 20]. Upon completion of the core vitrectomy, triamcinolone is injected into the vitreous cavity, highlighting the residual vitreous cortex and hyaloid. A silicone-tipped needle or internal limiting membrane (ILM) forceps may be used to remove adherent posterior hyaloid. Triamcinolone may be left in the vitreous cavity to decrease postoperative inflammation [21].

The role of removal of the ILM for uveitic ME remains unclear. In their report on vitrectomy of 42 eyes, Wiechens et al. (2001) removed the ILM in 15 eyes. While ME improved in 60 % of eyes overall, there was no difference between eyes with and without ILM removal [22]. Gutfleisch et al. (2007) studied 19 patients with uveitic ME who underwent vitrectomy with ILM peeling and concurrent intravitreal triamcinolone [23]. Postoperatively, angiographic ME improved in 58 % of patients. The authors noted, however, that ILM peeling in uveitic ME is difficult and may cause tissue damage; they do not recommend ILM peeling unless there is VMT present. Cho and D'Amico's series (2012) of 24 patients with chronic ME undergoing 25-gauge vitrectomy with ILM peel included four with uveitis [24]. There was slight nonsignificant improvement in visual acuity and macular thickness as measured by spectral domain optical coherence tomography (SD-OCT) in these patients (429 μm to 407 μm; $p=0.92$).

For diagnostic vitrectomy, as much undiluted vitreous should be obtained as possible to send for laboratory evaluation including cultures, PCR testing, cytology, and flow cytometry. Approximately 1 cc of undiluted vitreous may be safely obtained by standard vitrectomy techniques. Additional undiluted vitreous can be obtained via techniques such as infusion of air or heavy liquids. Using perfluoron as originally described by Quiroz-Mercado for large-volume vitreous biopsy [25], one may safely obtain 3–5 cc of undiluted vitreous [26].

Outcomes

While there are no large, randomized, controlled, prospective studies of vitrectomy for uveitic ME, since the early studies referenced above, there have been numerous small studies suggesting potential benefit. Becker and Davis reviewed 44 articles on vitrectomy for uveitis from 1981 to 2005, which included a total of 1762 eyes [27]. Overall, there was a reduction in the median percentage of eyes with ME from 36 % preoperatively to 18 % post-vitrectomy. Improvements in visual acuity and inflammation control were also suggested, but the highest evidence grade of the articles reviewed was CII-3: "at least fair evidence that the service can improve health outcomes but … the balance of benefits and harms is too close to justify a general recommendation" [28].

To date, there have been two small randomized, controlled, prospective trials comparing the effect of vitrectomy versus medical therapy in uveitic ME. Tranos et al. (2006) studied 23 patients with recalcitrant uveitic ME and no other macular pathology who were randomized into a vitrectomy group and a systemic medical therapy group [29]. Vision improved by two or more lines in 50 % of the eyes undergoing vitrectomy versus 18 % in the medical group. Angiographic improvement of ME was observed in 33 % of the vitrectomized eyes compared to 14 % in the control group. Quinones et al. (2010) randomized 20 eyes with recalcitrant intermediate uveitis to vitrectomy or immunomodulatory therapy; three eyes in each group had ME [30]. All three in the surgical group showed resolution of ME, while two of three in the medical group showed improvement in ME. In both of these small studies, differences did not reach statistical significance.

A number of reports have focused on the effect of vitrectomy for uveitic ME in specific anatomic locations or diagnoses. In 1992, Kaplan suggested that vitrectomy may provide an alternative to systemic immunosuppression in intermediate uveitis [31]. Since then, intermediate uveitis has been the most common diagnosis in reports of vitrectomy for uveitis, with generally positive results for both macular edema and vision [27].

Following vitrectomy for refractory uveitic ME in 53 patients, Wiechens et al. (2003) reported a resolution or reduction in ME in 59 % of patients with intermediate uveitis, 57 % with juvenile idiopathic arthritis (JIA) associated uveitis, and 41 % with multifocal choroiditis. There was a concurrent two-line improvement in Snellen visual acuity in 50 %, 71.4 %, and 41.7 %, respectively [32]. In a later report focusing predominantly on juvenile intermediate uveitis, ME was significantly reduced in 8 of 10 eyes post-vitrectomy [33].

In sarcoid uveitis, Kiryu et al. (2001) demonstrated resolution of medication-resistant ME in 14 (78 %) of 18 patients who underwent vitrectomy [34]. Half of the eyes also had peeling of ERM or adherent posterior vitreous cortex. Interestingly, in both the vitrectomy only and the membrane-peeling groups, seven of nine eyes showed improvement in ME.

Sullu et al. (2005) performed vitrectomy for posterior segment complications of Behçet's disease in 20 eyes, including five with ME [35]. They noted complete improvement of ME in three eyes (60 %) after vitrectomy.

Llorenç et al. (2011) showed improvement in ME following vitrectomy in 16 eyes with human leukocyte antigen HLA-A29-positive birdshot chorioretinopathy [36]. Nine eyes had preoperative ME with a mean macular thickness of 537.8 μm by HD-OCT. Four of the nine eyes also had ERM; all nine had either ERM peeling or Brilliant Blue-assisted ILM peeling. ME improved postoperatively in eight of nine eyes (89 %), with a final mean macular thickness of 218.7 μm ($p=0.0039$).

Considerations

Patients with chronic uveitis and ME may develop fixed retinal cysts, enlarged foveal avascular zones, and/or thinning of intraretinal layers. Patients with such findings may not be good candidates for primary vitrectomy, as surgical management is unlikely to correct the underlying pathology.

Vitrectomy for Other Complications of Uveitis

Uveitis may lead to additional vitreoretinal pathology associated with ME including ERM, retinal detachment, vitreous opacities, and vitreous hemorrhage, all of which may be amenable to surgical treatment. Both inflammation and steroid treatment contribute to increased cataract formation in patients with uveitis. Many of these structural complications may benefit from treatment by vitrectomy combined with other indicated procedures.

ERM

The prevalence of ERM has been reported as 40–48 % in patients with uveitis [37–39]. Nicholson et al. (2014) reported on a large cohort of uveitis patients with ERM evaluated by SD-OCT [39]. Among the 598 patients, 246 had ERM in at least one eye. Multivariate analysis suggested that ERM is associated with approximately one line of visual acuity loss in these patients. Central retinal thickness of greater than 350 μm in conjunction with an ERM conferred a significant decrease in visual acuity compared to patients with central retinal thicknesses between 200 μm and 350 μm.

Results of ERM peeling in patients with uveitic ME have suggested some benefit. Dev et al. (1999) studied five eyes with ERM and ME diagnosed clinically or via angiography with chronic idiopathic pars planitis who underwent ERM peel with vitrectomy [40]. Four of five eyes had visual acuity improvement and reduction or elimination of ME. Kiryu et al. (2003) showed resolution of ME by fluorescein angiography (FA) in four of seven eyes with sarcoid uveitis that underwent ERM peel with vitrectomy [41]. Visual improvements, however, were not significant. Tanawade et al. (2014) showed improvement in vision in five eyes with ERM and concurrent uveitic ME and six eyes with concurrent ERM, VMT, and uveitic ME that underwent ERM peeling with or without ILM peeling [42]. Nine of eleven eyes showed resolution of ME and VMT on OCT at 3 months postoperatively.

Retinal Detachment

The incidence of rhegmatogenous RD in patients with uveitis has been reported as high as 3 % [43]. As these are often complex retinal detachments, vitrectomy is usually indicated. There is little in the literature, however, regarding ME in uveitis patients undergoing vitrectomy for retinal detachment. Yu and Chung (1994) repaired seven traction retinal detachments (TRDs) and eleven combined traction/rhegmatogenous detachments in patients with chronic uveitis [44]. While the exact number was not reported, the authors did state that many of these eyes had preoperative ME. Postoperative ME was seen in two patients in the TRD group and one patient in the combined group. Recurrence of TRD occurred in two patients and combined RD in six patients.

Vitreous Opacities/Vitreous Hemorrhage

A significant cause of decreased vision in uveitis may be non-clearing vitreous opacities and/or vitreous hemorrhage (VH). In a series of six eyes with pars planitis undergoing vitrectomy for VH, Potter et al. (2001) reported two eyes with preoperative ME [45]. Vision in both eyes improved; final acuity in one was 20/20, with the other 20/100 likely due to ME.

Ieki et al. (2004) performed vitrectomy for non-clearing vitreous opacity in 11 eyes, 5 of which had preoperative treatment-resistant ME [46]. After 6 months, all five eyes had either resolution or improvement of ME as determined by FA. Three of these eyes gained two or more Snellen visual acuity lines and achieved visual acuity of 20/40 or better, while the other two eyes had stable visual acuity at the final visit.

Vitrectomy has also been reported to reduce ME in juvenile uveitis with vitreous opacities. Trittibach et al. (2006) reported on 29 eyes that underwent vitrectomy for vitreous opacities ($n=25$), VH ($n=3$), and retinal detachment ($n=1$) [33]. ME was reduced in eight of ten eyes that had preoperative ME ($p=0.021$). Overall, LogMAR visual acuity improved from an average of 0.91–0.33 postoperatively ($p=0.001$).

Cataract

Combined cataract surgery and pars plana vitrectomy may be indicated if significant cataract is present, but the combined surgery may incite new or worsen preexisting ME. In 1979, Diamond and Kaplan studied 25 eyes that underwent combined vitrectomy and pars plana lensectomy without placement of intraocular lens (IOL). They reported resolution of preoperative cystoid macular edema (CME) in 4 of 12 eyes [47]. More recently, Androudi et al. (2005) reported 36 eyes with chronic uveitis that underwent combined phacoemulsification and pars plana vitrectomy [48]. Nine of the eyes (25 %) had preoperative ME confirmed by FA. Postoperatively, six of these nine eyes had persistent edema, while ten new cases of ME were identified. Only four of the ten new cases of ME resolved during the follow-up period.

Complications of Vitrectomy

Acceleration of cataract formation following vitrectomy for uveitis is seen in virtually all phakic patients, and significant cataract development has been reported as high as 100 % [34]. Other relatively common complications following vitrectomy for uveitic ME include increased or decreased intraocular pressure, RD, VH, and ERM. In an early series of 12 eyes undergoing vitrectomy for peripheral uveitis, Mieler et al. (1988) reported a 50 % repeat surgery rate for RD, VH, or cataract; nonetheless final acuity improved an average of five lines [49]. In their review of 44 papers assessing vitrectomy in a total of 1762 eyes, Becker and Davis counted postoperative complications including 112 progressing cataracts, 56 partial and 21 total RDs, 51 secondary glaucomas, 45 cases of hypotony and 15 of phthisis, 36 macular puckers, 22 VHs, 7 hyphemae, and 3 choroidal detachments [27]. In a retrospective review of 74 uveitic eyes that underwent 25-gauge vitrectomy, 56 of which had preoperative ME, Soheilian et al. found ERM formation in 23 %, elevated intraocular pressure in 11 %, irreparable RD in 6.7 %, subretinal neovascular membrane in 2.7 %, macular hole in 5.4 %, phthisis bulbi in 5.4 %, and chronic hypotony in 5.4 % [15]. Nicholson et al. found that ERM formed in patients with uveitis at a significantly greater rate after vitrectomy (16/141) compared with those that did not undergo vitrectomy (6/141) ($p=0.026$) [39]. Vitrectomy with concurrent intravitreal triamcinolone was found to cause ocular hypertension in 9/19 (47 %) of patients [23].

Fluocinolone Acetonide Intravitreal Implant (Retisert)

Background

Local or systemic corticosteroids, with or without concurrent systemic immunomodulating medications, may fail to resolve uveitic ME. Even when effective, local steroid injections often need to be repeated multiple times to achieve control of uveitic ME. The 0.59 mg fluocinolone acetonide (FlAc) intravitreal implant (Retisert; Bausch & Lomb) [50] releases steroid into the vitreous cavity for an average of 30 months and was approved by the FDA for treatment of noninfectious uveitis in 2005. Surgical implantation of a FlAc implant provides an alternative to multiple local steroid injections or systemic therapy.

Technique

Details of the implantation technique have been well described [51–53]. Briefly, the implant is prepared by securing a double-armed 8-0 prolene suture through the anchor strut of the implant with a single knot. After prepping the eye in aseptic fashion, a conjunctival peritomy is performed in an area with healthy appearing conjunctiva, away from underlying pathology such as a snowbank or traction. The surgeon may consider avoiding areas likely to be used for future glaucoma surgeries. Cautery is used to achieve hemostasis. In eyes that have previously undergone vitrectomy, an infusion line is placed to maintain intraocular pressure. A 20-gauge microvitreoretinal (MVR) blade is used to make a 3.5 mm full-thickness sclerotomy along a concentric line 4.0 mm posterior to the limbus. Any prolapsed vitreous may be cut with a vitrector or excised using a Weck-Cel sponge and Westcott scissors. The implant is inserted into the vitreous cavity with the drug-eluting portion facing anteriorly. The previously placed anchor suture is then passed through the sclera on either side of the incision and tied, thereby gently approximating the scleral incision. The tails of the double-armed prolene are then placed under interrupted 9-0 prolene sutures that are used to close the sclerotomy. The interrupted sutures are rotated to bury the knots. The proper position of the implant is confirmed by indirect ophthalmoscopy. Balanced salt solution is injected into the vitreous cavity to normalize the intraocular pressure. The conjunctival peritomy is closed with 6-0 plain gut sutures, and subconjunctival antibiotics are given.

Berger and Mendoza have suggested an alternate suture technique for closer approximation of the sclerotomy [54]. Slow-absorbing 8-0 polyglycolic acid sutures may be used on the inner aspects of the sclerotomy, prior to placing two distal 9-0 prolene permanent sutures. Use of fewer permanent sutures may also reduce the risk of conjunctival erosion.

Outcomes

The first report of long-term safety and efficacy of FlAc implantation to control posterior uveitis was published by Jaffe et al. in 2005 [51]. Thirty-six eyes were randomized to either a 0.59 mg or a 2.1 mg FlAc implant. With follow-up of at least 12 months in 72 % of patients, 24 months in 44 %, and 30 months in 25 %, only two patients were noted to have recurrent inflammation, both at 29 months or later. Visual acuity stabilized or improved in 90 % of patients, with the authors speculating that the improved vision was primarily due to reduced macular edema.

Results of the FlAc implant in a large group of patients were first reported by the multicenter Fluocinolone Acetonide Uveitis Study Group in 2006 [55]. Two hundred and seventy-eight eyes of patients with long-standing noninfectious posterior uveitis that had previously undergone systemic and local therapy were randomized to receive a FlAc implant of 0.59 mg or 2.1 mg and were subsequently followed for 3 years [56]. Patients with bilateral disease had FlAc implanted in the eye with the more severe uveitis.

Recurrence rates in the 0.59 mg dose group were reduced from 62 % over the year before implantation to 4 % at 1 year, 10 % at 2 years, and 20 % at 3 years after implantation. These recurrence rates were also significantly lower than those of the fellow non-implanted eyes (44 %, 52 %, 59 % at 1, 2, and 3 years, respectively) ($p<0.01$). At 3 years after implantation, there was no significant difference in mean visual acuity from baseline values in implanted eyes, while mean vision declined in fellow eyes ($p<0.01$). Macular edema was evaluated based on the area of hyperfluorescence on FA. Reduction in ME in the implanted eyes was seen in 86 % at 1 year and 73 % at 3 years, versus 28 % at 1 year and 28 % at 3 years in fellow non-implanted eyes. The mean area of ME in implanted eyes maintained a statistically significant decrease lower than baseline at 1, 2, and 3 years after implantation ($p<0.01$) [56].

In 2011, the 2-year results from the Multicenter Uveitis Steroid Treatment (MUST) trial were published, including evaluation of ME by OCT. This NIH-sponsored randomized clinical trial compared the safety and efficacy of the FlAc implant to systemic therapy in 255 patients with noninfectious intermediate, posterior, and panuveitis [38]. In this trial, ME was defined as center point macular thickness of greater than 240 microns assessed on Stratus OCT-3. At baseline, the proportion of eyes with ME was similar between the implant group (41 %) and the systemic therapy group (39 %). The implant group showed significantly greater reduction in proportion of eyes with ME compared with the systemic medication group at 6 months (decreased to 20 % and 34 %, respectively, $p=0.002$). At 2 years, both groups still showed improvement from baseline (22 % and 30 %), although the difference between the two groups was no longer statistically significant ($p = 0.071$).

Other reports have also shown significant resolution of ME following FlAc implantation. Shen et al. (2013) reported FlAc implantation, leading to early improvement or resolution of uveitic ME in 12 eyes as measured by change in multiple SD-OCT parameters at 3 months post-implantation (all with $p < 0.05$) [57]. Arcinue et al. (2013) showed reduction in OCT central retinal thickness in 16 eyes, from 340 μm preoperatively to 248 μm 1 year after FlAC implantation [58].

FlAc implantation results in weaning and discontinuation of systemic corticosteroids needed to control posterior inflammation and ME in up to 77 % of cases [58]. Jaffe et al. reported that at 34 weeks post-implantation, use of systemic medication to control uveitis decreased from 52.9 to 12.1 %, and periocular injections were reduced from 63.0 to 2.2 % [55].

Several studies have looked at FlAc in specific uveitic entities. Rush et al. (2011) investigated outcomes of FlAc implantation in 36 eyes of patients with HLA-A29-positive birdshot chorioretinopathy. They found a reduction in ME from 36 % of eyes at baseline to 6% at 12 months ($p = 0.006$) as measured by FA [59].

Mahajan et al. (2009) reported a case series of patients with sympathetic ophthalmia (SO) who underwent FlAc implantation. They showed a reduced need for systemic corticosteroids to control intraocular inflammation while improving or stabilizing visual acuity [60]. The authors believe patients' improved visual acuities were due to the reduction of ME.

A study by Hu et al. (2011) of two patients with immune recovery uveitis showed resolution of ME without reactivation of cytomegalovirus (CMV) with simultaneous use of ganciclovir and: highly-active antiretroviral therapy (HAART) with a FlAc implant [61]. Caution must be exercised, however, as there are reports of PCR-proven herpetic necrotizing retinitis [62], CMV endotheliitis [63], and CMV retinitis [64] following FlAc implantation in immunocompetent as well as immunocompromised patients.

Complications

The most striking complication of FlAc implantation is increased intraocular pressure. At 34 weeks after FlAc implantation, 59 % of patients had a rise greater than or equal to 10 mmHg [55]. Two years after FlAc implantation, 61 % of patients required treatment for elevated intraocular pressures ($p < 0.0001$), and 17 % developed glaucoma ($p = 0.0008$). At 3 years, 67 % of eyes with the FlAc implant had an increase in IOP greater than or equal to 10 mmHg [56]. The MUST investigators found a fourfold increase in incidence of IOP elevation greater than 10 mmHG, absolute IOP greater than 30 mmHG, and the need for medical and surgical treatments for elevated IOP [38]. They noted that despite intervention to lower IOP, glaucoma developed in 17 % in the implant group compared with 4 % in the systemically treated group ($p = 0.001$).

Virtually all phakic eyes receiving a FlAc implant will develop visually significant cataract within a few years. The MUST investigators found an 80 % increased risk for the need for cataract surgery with FlAc when compared to systemic therapy alone at 2 years [38]. At 3 years, Callanan et al. (2008) found that 93 % of phakic eyes required cataract surgery, compared to 20 % of fellow eyes ($p<0.01$) [56]. Most of the cataracts were removed between 24 weeks and 2 years post-implantation. Cataract formation may be especially concerning in pediatric populations still at risk for amblyopia [65].

Other complications are much less frequent. ERM formation may occur in cases without a preexisting ERM [57]. Transient hypotony occurs in nearly 10 % of patients following implantation [55]. Endophthalmitis has been reported following implantation in 0.4–4.5 %, with MUST data showing an incidence of 1.3 % [38, 55, 66]. Vitreous banding from the posterior pole to the FlAc implant has also been reported to occur [67]. Scleral melt following FlAc implantation has been reported in one patient [68].

Several studies have addressed the need for a second FlAc implantation due to recurrent inflammation, occurring on average 32.5 months [69] to 38 months [70] after initial FlAc implantation. Removal or exchange of the implant may be associated with additional complications. Dissociation of the drug-eluting cup from the implant strut has been reported to occur in as many as 40.7 % of explantation cases, rarely resulting in retinal tear and suprachoroidal hemorrhage [71]. Dissociation of the components is thought to occur the longer the implant has been in place, secondary to hydration of the adhesive between the implant strut and the drug-eluting cup, and has been particularly noted in earlier-generation implants. On average, dissociation during removal or exchange occurred 46.7 months after initial implantation. Intact implants that were removed or exchanged had been in the eye 32.5 months on average. If explantation is required, the sclerotomy should be enlarged to 4 mm to allow for reduced shearing forces on the implant during removal. Use of an infusion line may be helpful as well.

Spontaneous late dissociation of the implant into the vitreous cavity not associated with surgical explantation has been reported to occur in 5.4 % of implants, occurring on average at 71.1 months post-implantation [72]. In these cases, bimanual removal with an infusion cannula and soft-tipped extrusion cannula may be used to remove the dissociated portion of the implant. Late spontaneous dissociation with dislocation of the implant into the anterior chamber resulting in corneal endothelial damage has been reported in two patients with prior vitrectomy [73]. A corneal incision was used to retrieve the dissociated portion.

Cost may also be a complicating factor in FlAc implantation. The MUST trial research group (2014) investigated the cost-effectiveness of the implant versus systemic therapy for noninfectious uveitis and found that implant therapy has a higher cost over 3 years in patients with bilateral disease ($69,300 implant vs $52,500 systemic) with modest, nonstatistically significant gain in quality of life years [74]. In unilateral disease, the 3-year cost was more comparable between the two groups ($38,800 implant vs $33,400 systemic). While the implant favored quality of life years in the implant group in unilateral cases, it did not reach statistical significance

($p = 0.12$). The authors concluded that in most cases, the implant was reasonably cost-effective compared to systemic therapy for patients with unilateral uveitis but not for those with bilateral disease.

Conclusions

Following vitrectomy in uveitis patients, there is an overall trend in the literature toward decreased ME, improved visual acuity, and reduction of medications. A large, prospective, randomized clinical trial is needed to confirm these findings. Until such a trial is performed, primary vitrectomy for persistent uveitic ME should be assessed on a case-by-case basis. When uveitic ME is associated with other complications such as ERM, VH, or RD, vitrectomy may have the added benefit of improving the ME.

The FlAc implant has proven to be effective in resolving uveitic ME in a majority of cases. The risks associated with implantation and long-term steroid exposure in the implanted eye are significant and must be deliberated in each case. For many patients, FlAc implantation provides a viable alternative to systemic therapy for ME in chronic uveitis.

References

1. Tomkins-Netzer O, Talat L, Bar A, Lula A, Taylor S, Joshi L, Lightman S. Long-term clinical outcome and causes of vision loss in patients with uveitis. Ophthalmology. 2014;121(12):2387–92.
2. Nussenblatt R. The natural history of uveitis. Int Ophthalmol. 1990;14(5–6):303–8.
3. Durrani O, Tehrani N, Marr J, et al. Degree, duration, and causes of visual loss in uveitis. Br J Ophthalmol. 2004;88(9):1159–62.
4. Lardenoye E, van Kooij B, Rothva A. Impact of macular edema on visual acuity in uveitis. Ophthalmology. 2006;113(8):1446–9.
5. Schepens CL, Avila MP, Jalkh AE, Trempe CL. Role of the vitreous in cystoid macular edema. Surv Ophthalmol. 1984;28 Suppl:499–504.
6. Hikichi T, Trempe CL. Role of the vitreous in the prognosis of peripheral uveitis. Am J Ophthalmol. 1993;116(4):401–5.
7. Streilein JW, Stein-Streilein J. Anterior chamber associated immune deviation (ACAID): regulation, biological relevance, and implications for therapy. Int Rev Immunol. 2002;21:123–52.
8. Machemer R, Parel JM, Norton EW. Vitrectomy: a pars plana approach. Technical improvements and further results. Trans Am Acad Ophthalmol Otolaryngol. 1972;76:462–6.
9. Peyman G, Huamonte F. A disposable vitrectomy instrument: the vitrophage. Can J Ophthalmol. 1975;10(2):281–5.
10. O'Malley C, Heintz RM. Vitrectomy with an alternative instrument system. Ann Ophthalmol. 1975;7:585–8. 591–4.
11. Diamond J, Kaplan H. Lensectomy and vitrectomy for complicated cataract secondary to uveitis. Arch Ophthalmol. 1978;96:1798–804.
12. Algvere P, Alank H, Kickhoff K, Lahde Y, Saari K. Pars plana vitrectomy in the management of intraocular inflammation. Acta Ophthalmol (Copenh). 1981;59:727–36.

13. Engel H, Green W, Michels R, Rice T, Erozan Y. Diagnostic vitrectomy. Retina. 1981;1:121–49.
14. Dugel P, Rao N, Ozler S, et al. Pars plana vitrectomy for intraocular inflammation-related cystoid macular edema unresponsive to corticosteroids. A preliminary study. Ophthalmology. 1992;99(10):1535–41.
15. Soheilian M, Ramezani A, Soheilian R. 25-gauge vitrectomy for complicated chronic endogenous/autoimmune uveitis: predictors of outcomes. Ocul Immunol Inflamm. 2013;21(2):93–101.
16. Larsson L, Nuija E. Increased permeability of the blood-aqueous barrier after panretinal photocoagulation for proliferative diabetic retinopathy. Acta Ophthalmol Scand. 2001;79(4):414–6.
17. Moriarty A, Spalton D, Shilling J, Ffytche T, Bulsara M. Breakdown of the blood-aqueous barrier after argon laser panretinal photocoagulation for proliferative diabetic retinopathy. Ophthalmology. 1996;103(5):833–8.
18. Heiligenhaus A, Bornfeld N, Foerster MH, Wessing A. Long-term results of pars plana vitrectomy in the management of complicated uveitis. Br J Ophthalmol. 1994;78:549–54.
19. Peyman G, Cheema R, Conway M, Fang T. Triamcinolone acetonide as an aid to visualization of the vitreous and the posterior hyaloid during pars plana vitrectomy. Retina. 2000;20:554–5.
20. Sakamoto T, Miyazaki M, Hisatomi T, et al. Triamcinolone-assisted pars plana vitrectomy improves the surgical procedures and decreases the postoperative blood-ocular barrier breakdown. Graefes Arch Clin Exp Ophthalmol. 2002;240:423–9.
21. Sonoda KH, Enaida H, Ueno A, et al. Pars plana vitrectomy assisted by triamcinolone acetonide for refractory uveitis: a case series study. Br J Ophthalmol. 2003;87(8):1010–4.
22. Wiechens B, Nölle B, Reichelt JA. Pars-plana vitrectomy in cystoid macular edema associated with intermediate uveitis. Graefes Arch Clin Exp Ophthalmol. 2001;239(7):474–81.
23. Gutfleisch M, Spital G, Mingels A, et al. Pars plana vitrectomy with intravitreal triamcinolone: effect on uveitic cystoid macular oedema and treatment limitations. Br J Ophthalmol. 2007;91(3):345–8.
24. Cho M, D'Amico DJ. Transconjunctival 25-gauge pars plana vitrectomy and internal limiting membrane peeling for chronic macular edema. Clin Ophthalmol. 2012;6:981–9.
25. Quiroz-Mercado H, Rivera-Sempertequi J, Macky T, et al. Performing vitreous biopsy by perfluorocarbon-perfused vitrectomy. Am J Ophthalmol. 2005;140(6):1161–3.
26. Merrill P, Duval R. Use of PFO for large-volume vitreous biopsy. https://www.youtube.com/watch?v=sTh5hCR3v50. Accessed 1 Jan 2015.
27. Becker M, Davis J. Vitrectomy in the treatment of uveitis. Am J Ophthalmol. 2005;140(6):1096–105.
28. United States Preventive Service Task Force. Grade definitions – US preventive service task force. www.uspreventiveservicestaskforce.org/Page/Name/grade-definitions#grade-definitions-prior-to-may-2007. Accessed 1 Jan 2015.
29. Tranos P, Scott R, Zambarakji H, Ayliffe W, Pavesio C, Charteris DG. The effect of pars plana vitrectomy on cystoid macular oedema associated with chronic uveitis: a randomized controlled pilot study. Br J Ophthalmol. 2006;90(9):1007–10.
30. Quinones K, Choi J, Yilmaz T, et al. Pars plana vitrectomy versus immunomodulatory therapy for intermediate uveitis: a prospective, randomized pilot study. Ocul Immunol Inflamm. 2010;18(5):411–7.
31. Kaplan H. Surgical treatment of intermediate uveitis. Dev Ophthalmol. 1992;23:185–9.
32. Wiechens B, Reichelt JA, Urbat C, Nölle B. Pars plana vitrectomy in cystoid macular edema of different forms of chronic uveitis. Ophthalmologe. 2003;100(1):33–43.
33. Trittibach P, Koerner F, Sarra GM, Garweg JG. Vitrectomy for juvenile uveitis: prognostic factors for the long-term functional outcome. Eye (Lond). 2006;20(2):184–90.
34. Kiryu J, Kita M, Tanabe T, Yamashiro K, Miyamoto N, Ieki Y. Pars plana vitrectomy for cystoid macular edema secondary to sarcoid uveitis. Ophthalmology. 2001;108(6):1140–4.
35. Sullu Y, Alotaiby H, Beden U, Erkan D. Pars plana vitrectomy for ocular complications of Behçet's disease. Ophthalmic Surg Lasers Imaging. 2005;36(4):292–7.

36. Llorenç V, Keller J, Pelegrin L, Adán A. Pars plana vitrectomy for vitreo-retinal complications of birdshot chorioretinopathy. Ocul Immunol Inflamm. 2011;19(5):346–52.
37. Markomichelakis NN, Halkiadakis I, Pantelia E, et al. Patterns of macular edema in patients with uveitis: qualitative and quantitative assessment using optical coherence tomography. Ophthalmology. 2004;111(5):946–53.
38. Multicenter Uveitis Steroid Treatment (MUST) Trial Research Group. Randomize comparison of systemic anti-inflammatory therapy versus fluocinolone acetonide implant for intermediate posterior, and panuveitis: the multicenter uveitis steroid treatment trial. Ophthalmology. 2011;118(10):1916–26.
39. Nicholson BP, Zhou M, Rostamizadeh M, Mehta P, Agrón E, Wong W, Wiley H, Nussenblatt R, Sen N. Epidemiology of epiretinal membrane in a large cohort of patients with uveitis. Ophthalmology. 2014;121(12):2393–8.
40. Dev S, Mieler W, Pulido J, Mittra R. Visual outcomes after pars plana vitrectomy for epiretinal membranes associated with pars planitis. Ophthalmology. 1999;106(6):1086–90.
41. Kiryu J, Kita M, Tanabe T, et al. Pars plana vitrectomy for epiretinal membrane associated with sarcoidosis. Jpn J Ophthalmol. 2003;47(5):479–83.
42. Tanawade R, Tsierkezou L, Bindra M, Patton N, Jones N. Visual outcomes of pars plana vitrectomy with epiretinal membrane peel in patients with uveitis. Retina. 2015;35(4):736–41.
43. Kerkhoff F, Lamberts Q, van den Biesen P, Rothova A. Rhegmatogenous retinal detachment and uveitis. Ophthalmology. 2003;110(2):427–31.
44. Yu HG, Chung H. Results of vitreous surgery for posterior complications of chronic uveitis. Korean J Ophthalmol. 1994;8(1):20–5.
45. Potter MJ, Myckatyn SO, Maberley AL, Lee AS. Vitrectomy for pars planitis complicated by vitreous hemorrhage: visual outcome and long-term follow-up. Am J Ophthalmol. 2001;131(4):514–5.
46. Ieki Y, Kiryu J, Kita M, et al. Pars plana vitrectomy for vitreous opacity associated with ocular sarcoidosis resistant to medical treatment. Ocul Immunol Inflamm. 2004;12(1):35–43.
47. Diamond JG, Kaplan HJ. Uveitis: effect of vitrectomy combined with lensectomy. Ophthalmology. 1979;86(7):1320–9.
48. Androudi S, Ahmed M, Fiore T, et al. Combined pars plana vitrectomy and phacoemulsification to restore visual acuity in patients with chronic uveitis. J Cataract Refract Surg. 2005;31(3):472–8.
49. Mieler W, Will B, Lewis H, Aaberg T. Vitrectomy in the management of peripheral uveitis. Ophthalmology. 1988;95(7):859–64.
50. Fluocinolone acetonide ophthalmic—Bausch & Lomb: fluocinolone acetonide Envision TD implant. Drugs R D. 2005; 6(2):116–9.
51. Jaffe GJ, McCallum RM, Branchaud B, Skalak C, Butuner Z, Ashton P. Long-term follow-up results of a pilot trial of a fluocinolone acetonide implant to treat posterior uveitis. Ophthalmology. 2005;112:1192–8.
52. Bausch + Lomb. Procedure for Eye Implantation – Retisert®. http://www.retisert.com/surgical-procedure. Accessed 28 Nov 2014.
53. Implantation and removal procedures. Retinal physician. 2011. http://www.retinalphysician.com/articleviewer.aspx?articleID=105433.
54. Berger BB, Mendoza W. Sclerotomy closure for Retisert implant. Retina. 2013;33(2):436–8.
55. Jaffe GJ, Martin D, Callanan D, et al. Fluocinolone acetonide implant (Retisert) for noninfectious posterior uveitis: thirty-four week results of a multicenter randomized clinical study. Ophthalmology. 2006;113:1020–7.
56. Callanan D, Jaffe G, Martin D, Pearson P, Comstock T. Treatment of posterior uveitis with a fluocinolone acetonide implant: three-year clinical trial results. Arch Ophthalmol. 2008;126(9):1191–201.
57. Shen BY, Punjabi OS, Lowder CY, et al. Early treatment response of fluocinolone (Retisert) implantation in patients with uveitic macular edema. Retina. 2013;33(4):873–8.

58. Arcinue CA, Cerón OM, Foster CS. A comparison between the fluocinolone acetonide (Retisert) and dexamethasone (Ozurdex) intravitreal implants in uveitis. J Ocul Pharmacol Ther. 2013;29(5):501–7.
59. Rush RB, Goldstein DA, Callanan DG, Meghpara B, Feuer WJ, Davis JL. Outcomes of birdshot chorioretinopathy treated with an intravitreal sustained-release fluocinolone acetonide-containing device. Am J Ophthalmol. 2011;151(4):630–6.
60. Mahajan VB, Gehrs KM, Goldstein DA, Fischer DH, Lopez JS, Folk JC. Management of sympathetic ophthalmia with the fluocinolone acetonide. Ophthalmology. 2009;116(3): 552–7.
61. Hu J, Coassin M, Stewart JM. Fluocinolone acetonide implant (Retisert) for chronic cystoid macular edema in two patients with AIDS and a history of cytomegalovirus retinitis. Ocul Immunol Inflamm. 2011;19(3):206–9.
62. Ramaiya KJ, Rao PK. Herpetic necrotizing retinitis following fluocinolone acetonide intravitreal implant. Ocul Immunol Inflamm. 2011;19(1):72–4.
63. Park UC, Kim SJ, Yu HG. Cytomegalovirus endotheliitis after fluocinolone acetonide (Retisert) implant in a patient with Behçet uveitis. Ocul Immunol Inflamm. 2011;19(4):282–3.
64. Takakura A, Tessler H, Goldstein D, et al. Viral retinitis following intraocular or periocular corticosteroid administration: a case series and comprehensive review of the literature. Ocul Immunol Inflamm. 2014;22(3):175–82.
65. Patel CC, Mandava N, Oliver SCN, et al. Treatment of intractable posterior uveitis in pediatric patients with the fluocinolone acetonide intravitreal implant (Retisert). Retina. 2012;32(30): 537–42.
66. Pavesio C, Zierhut M, Bairi K, et al. Evaluation of an intravitreal fluocinolone acetonide implant versus standard systemic therapy in noninfectious posterior uveitis. Ophthalmology. 2010;117:567–75.
67. Galor A, Marolis R, Kaiser P, Lowder C. Vitreous band formation and the sustained-release, intravitreal fluocinolone (Retisert) implant. Arch Ophthalmol. 2007;125(6):836–8.
68. Georgalas I, Koutsandrea C, Papaconstantinou D, Mpouritis D, Petrou P. Scleral melt following Retisert intravitreal fluocinolone implant. Drug Des Devel Ther. 2014;8:2373–5.
69. Taban M, Lowder CY, Kaiser PK. Outcome of fluocinolone acetonide implant (Retisert) reimplantation for chronic noninfectious posterior uveitis. Retina. 2008;28(9):1280–8.
70. Jaffe GJ. Reimplantation of a fluocinolone acetonide sustained drug delivery implant for chronic uveitis. Am J Ophthalmol. 2008;145(4):667–75.
71. Nicholson BP, Singh RP, Sears JE, Lowder CY, Kaiser PK. Evaluation of fluocinolone acetonide sustained release implant (Retisert) dissociation during implant removal and exchange surgery. Am J Ophthalmol. 2012;154(6):969–73.
72. Itty S, Martel J, Jaffe G. Spontaneous dislocation of the pellet from the strut in the fluocinolone acetonide sustained release implant (Retisert). Invest Ophthalmol Vis Sci. 2013;54:2946.
73. Chang PY, Kresch Z, Samson CM, Gentile RC. Spontaneous dissociation of fluocinolone acetonide sustained release implant (Retisert) with dislocation into the anterior chamber. Ocul Immunol Inflamm. 2014;Early online:1–4.
74. The MUST Trial Research Group. Cost-effectiveness of fluocinolone acetonide implant versus systemic therapy for noninfectious intermediate, posterior, and panuveitis. Ophthalmology. 2014;121(10):1855–62.

Chapter 10
Surgical Management of Diabetic Macular Edema

Katherine E. Talcott and Dean Eliott

Introduction

Diabetic macular edema (DME) is a common cause of visual loss from diabetic retinopathy and is typically caused by leakage of fluid from abnormal retinal capillaries and microaneurysms [1, 2]. The Early Treatment Diabetic Retinopathy Study (ETDRS) demonstrated the utility of laser photocoagulation, presumably by decreasing vascular permeability [3]. In addition, mechanical causes at the vitreoretinal interface are believed to contribute in select patients [4–7].

Treatment options for DME include medical and ophthalmic interventions. Systemic glycemic and hypertensive control reduces the onset and progression of diabetic retinopathy in both type 1 and type 2 diabetes [8]. Additionally, there are a number of ophthalmic treatments. The ETDRS showed that macular focal and grid laser photocoagulation reduced the risk of visual loss due to DME by 50 %, but only 3 % of patients had improvement of ≥3 lines of visual acuity by the end of the study [3]. Other treatments for DME include intravitreal steroids, such as triamcinolone, dexamethasone, and fluocinolone [9–11]. Intravitreal injection of anti-vascular endothelial growth factor (VEGF) agents, such as pegaptanib, bevacizumab, ranibizumab, and aflibercept, has become a mainstay of treatment [12].

In addition to these treatment options, surgical intervention targeting vitreoretinal interface abnormalities in select DME cases is becoming increasingly recognized. Various groups have reported results of vitrectomy with or without epiretinal membrane (ERM) peeling and with or without internal limiting membrane (ILM)

K.E. Talcott, MD
Department of Ophthalmology, Massachusetts Eye & Ear Infirmary,
Harvard Medical School, 243 Charles St., Boston, MA 02114, USA

D. Eliott, MD (✉)
Retina Service, Department of Ophthalmology, Massachusetts Eye & Ear Infirmary,
Harvard Medical School, 243 Charles St., Boston, MA 02114, USA
e-mail: Dean_Eliott@meei.harvard.edu

S. Schaal, H.J. Kaplan (eds.), *Cystoid Macular Edema*,
DOI 10.1007/978-3-319-39766-5_10

peeling in select cases of DME. In this chapter, our aim is to examine the utility of surgical intervention in DME patients, and more specifically through cases with vitreoretinal interface abnormalities. To review the literature, it is useful to categorize by vitreoretinal interface abnormalities as indicated below.

Rationale for Surgical Intervention

The vitreous has been implicated as a cause of DME due to several mechanisms, all of which lead to increased vascular permeability. The vitreous can cause traction, including anterior-posterior, oblique, and tangential, on Müller cells that results in cell hypertrophy, proliferation, and vascular leakage [13, 14].This traction can also lead to distortion of intraretinal vessels, leading to vascular leakage and disturbances of macular microcirculation [15–18].

Vitrectomy may help relieve this traction and may also help to remove growth factors such as VEGF, interleukin-6 (IL-6), and platelet-derived growth factor (PDGF) which are secreted in diabetic retinopathy and can promote macular edema [19–21]. Vitrectomy can also potentially suppress the release of inflammatory cytokines such as basic fibroblast growth factor that are induced by mechanical stresses. Finally, vitrectomy increases vitreous cavity oxygen tension with resultant improved oxygenation of the posterior segment [22–27].

In a 1988 observational study supporting this, Nasrallah et al. observed a lower prevalence of posterior vitreous detachment (PVD) in the eyes with DME compared to eyes without edema [28]. Later, Lewis et al. in 1992 reported resolution of macular edema in 80 % of cases after vitrectomy for DME associated with posterior hyaloid traction [6]. Additionally, spontaneous resolution of edema in 55 % of eyes with posterior vitreous separation, compared with 25 % of eyes without complete PVD, was observed by Hikichi et al. in 1997 [29].

Evidence for Surgical Intervention

Attached Vitreous with Taut Posterior Hyaloid

Diffuse macular edema, as compared to focal edema from microaneurysms, is characterized by poorly demarcated leakage due to generalized disruption of the blood-retinal barrier and is sometimes associated with a taut posterior hyaloid. Identification of a taut posterior hyaloid in an eye with DME and diffuse leakage has been associated with favorable outcomes after vitrectomy [6, 7, 30]. As mentioned above, Lewis et al. described ten DME patients with diffuse macular edema refractory to laser photocoagulation. These patients did not have a PVD and instead had biomicroscopic evidence of a taut posterior hyaloid. After vitrectomy with removal of the posterior hyaloid membrane, nine patients had reduced edema. Visual acuity (VA) improved by two or more lines in six of ten patients [6]. Subsequently, Harbour et al. described ten

DME eyes that underwent vitrectomy for a taut posterior hyaloid diagnosed clinically. VA improved in four eyes (total ranging from 2–6 lines) and remained stable in the remaining eyes [30]. Other studies have looked at combining vitrectomy with an ILM peel for patients with an attached hyaloid and diffuse DME. Gandorfer et al. evaluated this combined surgical approach in 12 eyes, of which 10 had an attached hyaloid. Retinal thickening resolved or decreased in all eyes and VA improved by at least two lines in 11 eyes [31]. Taken together, these studies suggest a beneficial role for vitrectomy in patients with diffuse DME with presence of a taut posterior hyaloid.

Vitrectomy appears to be beneficial in cases of diffuse DME with a taut posterior hyaloid by relieving tangential tension. In diffuse DME, permeability of the inner blood-retinal barrier has been seen on fluorescein angiography (FA) and breakdown of the outer blood-retinal barrier has been implicated in animal models [32, 33]. Condensation and contraction of the hyaloid membrane is thought to cause tangential vitreomacular traction and increase the permeability of the retinal vasculature [7]. More recently, optical coherence tomography (OCT) imaging suggests that these tangential tractional forces can lead to a subclinical macular detachment. Kaiser et al. reviewed OCT imaging on nine DME eyes with posterior hyaloid traction, finding retinal thickening in all patients and shallow macular traction detachment in eight of the eyes. They suggest that resolution of the detachment with vitrectomy may explain the improved VA in these patients [4]. Regardless of the mechanisms, these studies support vitrectomy with posterior hyaloid elevation and removal for DME cases with a taut posterior hyaloid. Figure 1 offers an illustrative example of a diabetic patient with a taut posterior thickened hyaloid, macular edema on OCT, and diffuse macular leakage on FA. After subsequent vitrectomy with posterior hyaloid elevation, fundus changes and macular edema improved at the third postoperative month.

Attached Vitreous with Vitreomacular Traction

Vitreomacular traction (VMT) is associated with foveal distortion, and eyes with this condition often respond favorably to surgical intervention. Best visualized by OCT, VMT is defined as vitreofoveal attachment and traction with perifoveal vitreoretinal separation [29, 34, 35]. Figure 2 offers an illustrative example of a diabetic patient with DME and VMT where the posterior hyaloid is attached at the fovea but the perifoveal hyaloid is elevated.

The Diabetic Retinopathy Clinical Research Network (DRCRnet) Vitrectomy Study was a large prospective study that examined vitrectomy for DME in eyes with at least moderate vision loss and VMT [36]. The study included 87 eyes with VMT based on the "investigator's evaluation," baseline VA 20/63 to 20/400, and OCT central subfield thickness >300 μm. Surgical intervention beyond vitrectomy was not standardized. Membrane peel (ERM) was performed in 61 % and ILM peeling in 54 % of cases. At 6 months postoperatively, median OCT thickness decreased by 160 μm and 68 % of eyes had ≥50 % reduction in macular thickness. VA improved by ≥10 letters in 38 % of eyes but deteriorated by ≥10 letters in 22 % of eyes [36]. After separation of vitreofoveal traction, improvement of macular edema was

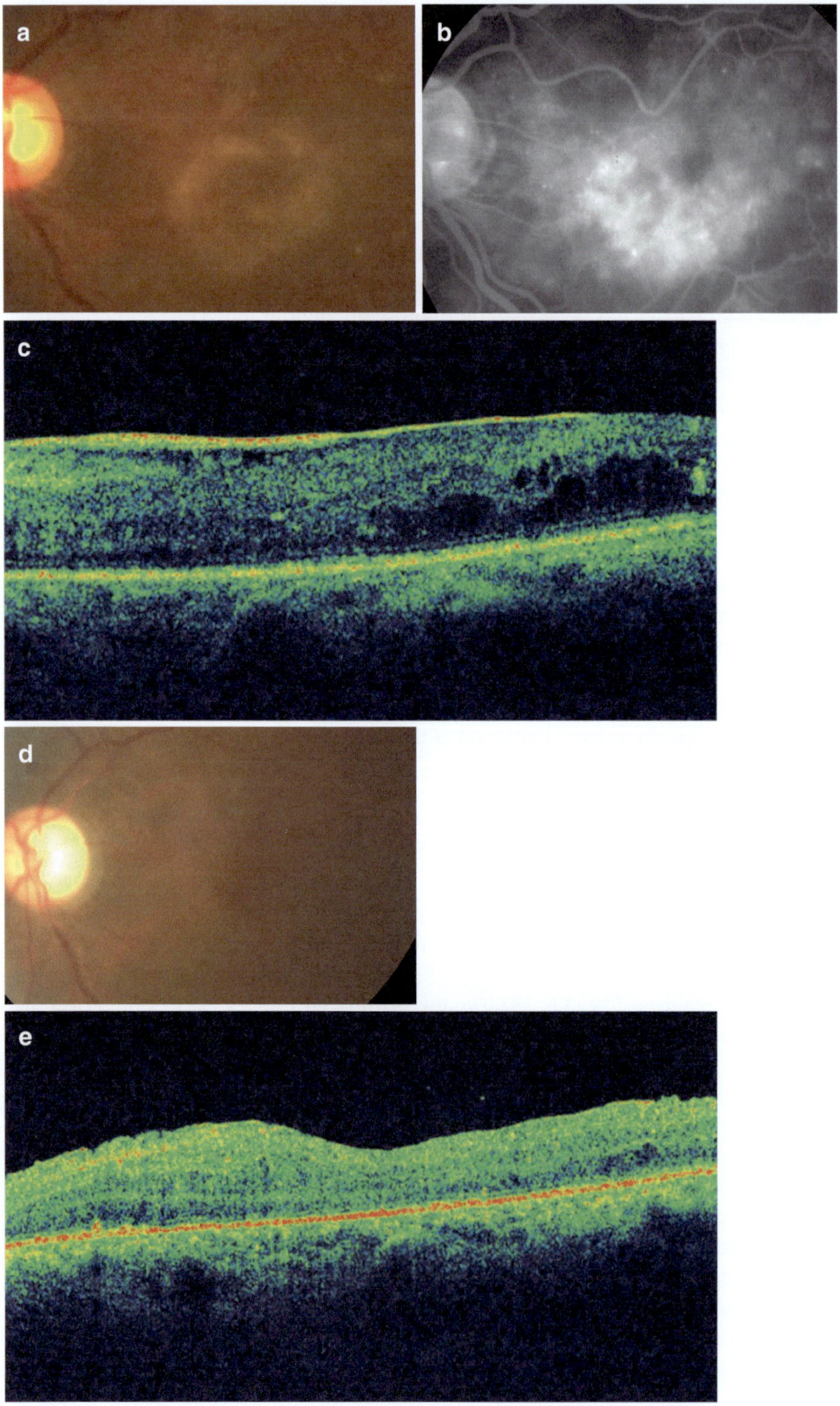
a
b
c
d
e

Fig. 1 Improvement of diffuse DME after vitrectomy and posterior hyaloid elevation in a patient with taut posterior hyaloid. (**a**) Preoperative fundus photograph. (**b**) Late frame of preoperative FA showing diffuse leakage. (**c**) Preoperative OCT showing thick hyaloid and macular edema. (**d**) Postoperative fundus photograph. (**e**) OCT at postoperative month 3 after vitrectomy and posterior hyaloid elevation with significant improvement

detected on OCT (Fig. 2). Based on this study, vitrectomy for DME associated with VMT appears beneficial; however, the study has several shortcomings. There was no control group, and VMT was defined by clinical judgment rather than a standardized definition. Finally, surgical interventions were not standardized [36]. Taken together, these results suggest that vitrectomy with posterior hyaloid elevation and removal can be beneficial in the setting of DME with VMT.

Attached Vitreous and No Observable Traction

In addition to cases with a taut posterior hyaloid or VMT, there is also support in the literature for vitrectomy in some patients with an attached hyaloid but no observable traction. Ikeda et al. described three DME eyes without clinical evidence of traction in the pre-OCT era that underwent vitrectomy. The cystoid changes had disappeared by 5 days postoperatively in all eyes. The diffuse macular edema had resolved within 2 weeks and VA was maintained or improved [37]. Otani et al. subsequently evaluated 13 DME eyes with retinal swelling on OCT before and after vitrectomy. At 6 months postoperatively, the mean foveal thickness decreased significantly from 630 to 350 μm. The best corrected visual acuity (BCVA) improved by more than two lines in 38 % of eyes and remained the same in 54 % [38]. Additionally, La Heij et al. found resolution of macular edema in all patients after a median period of 3 months and improvement of VA (median improvement of five lines) after vitrectomy in 21 eyes with DME with an attached hyaloid but no known traction [39]. Taken together, these three studies suggest that DME may improve in patients with an attached hyaloid, even without known traction.

There are several reasons that these patients with an attached hyaloid without traction may benefit from vitrectomy. First, there may be subclinical traction from the posterior hyaloid that may not be detected clinically, as Ikeda et al. and La Heij did not use OCT. In addition, vitrectomy may serve to increase vitreous oxygen tension. Regardless, these results on DME are less impressive than those involving patients with known traction but may be considered, especially in refractory cases.

Detached Vitreous (PVD)

Based on the above studies, traction appears to be a significant cause of diffuse retinal leakage in DME that can improve with vitrectomy. If the hyaloid is detached and there is no other known etiology to cause traction, such as an epiretinal membrane (ERM), there is less of a rationale for surgery. Several studies have examined this.

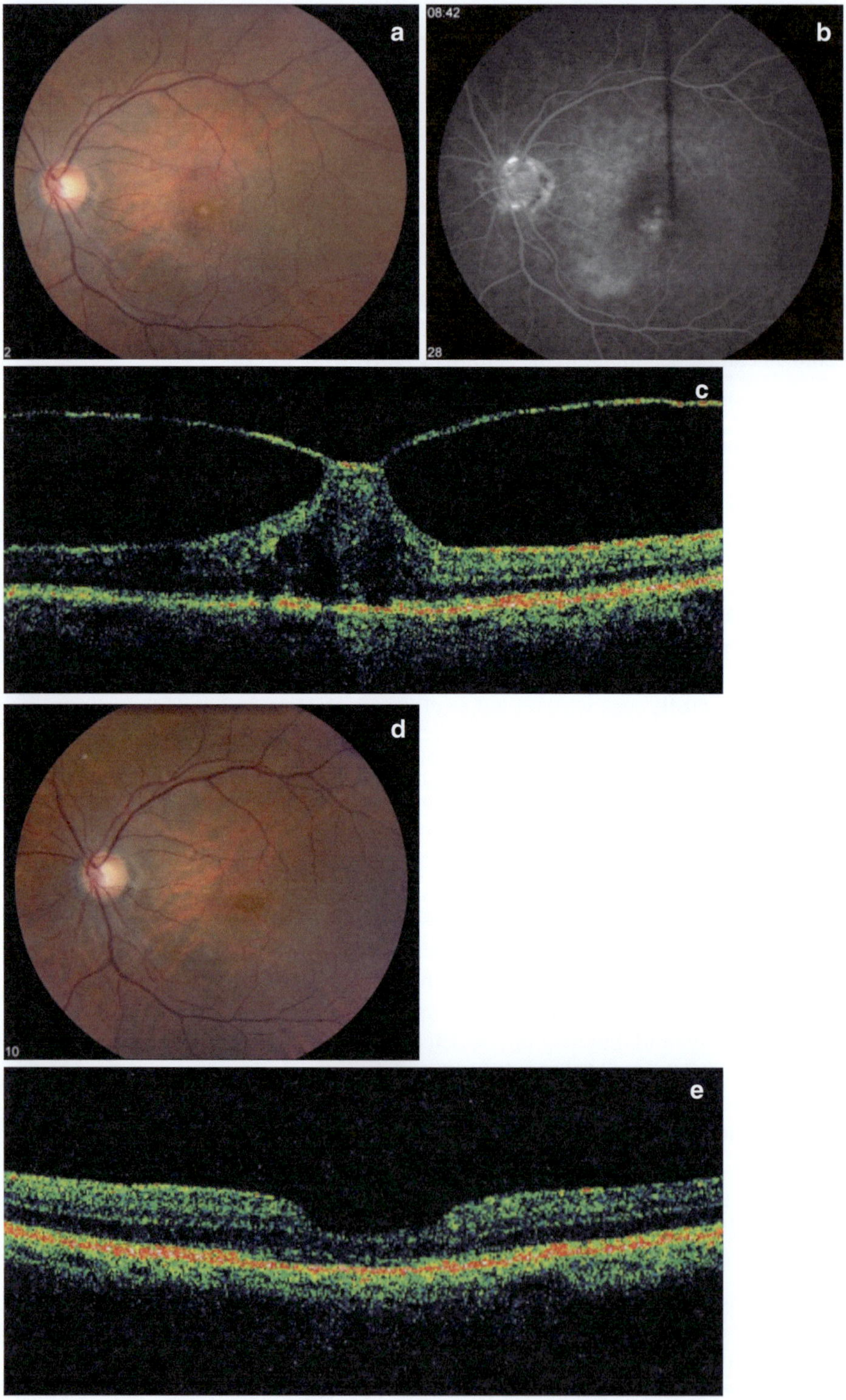
a
2
08:42
b
28
c
d
10
e

Fig. 2 Improvement of DME after vitrectomy and posterior hyaloid elevation in a diabetic patient with vitreofoveal traction. (**a**) Preoperative fundus photograph. (**b**) Preoperative fluorescein angiogram. (**c**) Preoperative OCT showing posterior hyaloid attachment at fovea with surrounding perifoveal hyaloid detachment and DME. (**d**) Postoperative fundus photograph. (**e**) OCT showing resolution of vitreofoveal traction and DME after vitrectomy without ILM peeling

Ikeda et al. in 2000 described five DME eyes that had a detached hyaloid without ERM on exam and confirmed intraoperatively. After vitrectomy, four eyes had resolution of the DME and all had improved VA. This was attributed to removal of cytokines and an increase in vitreous oxygen tension after surgery [37]. Other studies have failed to replicate these findings. Massin et al. evaluated eight eyes with diffuse DME and detached hyaloid without ERM before and after vitrectomy using OCT. While retinal thickness decreased from 522 to 428 μm after surgery, median VA actually worsened from 20/100 to 20/200 [5]. These studies suggest that vitrectomy is generally not indicated for mild DME in patients with a detached hyaloid without traction.

Detached Vitreous (PVD) with Epiretinal Membrane

Like a taut posterior hyaloid or VMT, an epiretinal membrane (ERM) can also exert traction on the retina and contribute to DME. ERM peeling has been suggested as an adjunct to vitrectomy in select cases of DME where an ERM is present. Although the majority of studies examining surgical intervention for DME have focused on cases of traction from the posterior hyaloid, some groups have looked at the utility of ERM peeling in eyes with DME. For instance, a subgroup of DME patients examined by Yamamoto et al. had a PVD and ERM before undergoing vitrectomy and membrane peel. This subgroup of five patients had significant improvement in postoperative mean VA, and the final VA improved by two or more lines in 60 % of eyes. Although mean foveal thickness decreased from 448 to 238 μm, this difference was not statistically significant [40]. Figure 3 offers an illustrative example of diabetic patient with a PVD and ERM on OCT; foveal contour improved following vitrectomy and membrane peel. Vitrectomy with membrane peel could be considered in select cases. The same criteria should be used as for nondiabetic ERM. Surgery should be considered for symptomatic visual loss associated with obvious ERM.

The Role of Internal Limiting Membrane Peeling During Diabetic Vitrectomy

Rationale for Surgical Intervention

As an adjunct to vitrectomy, peeling the ILM has been recommended in select cases of DME. The ILM may thicken in DME due to cellular proliferation and deposition of

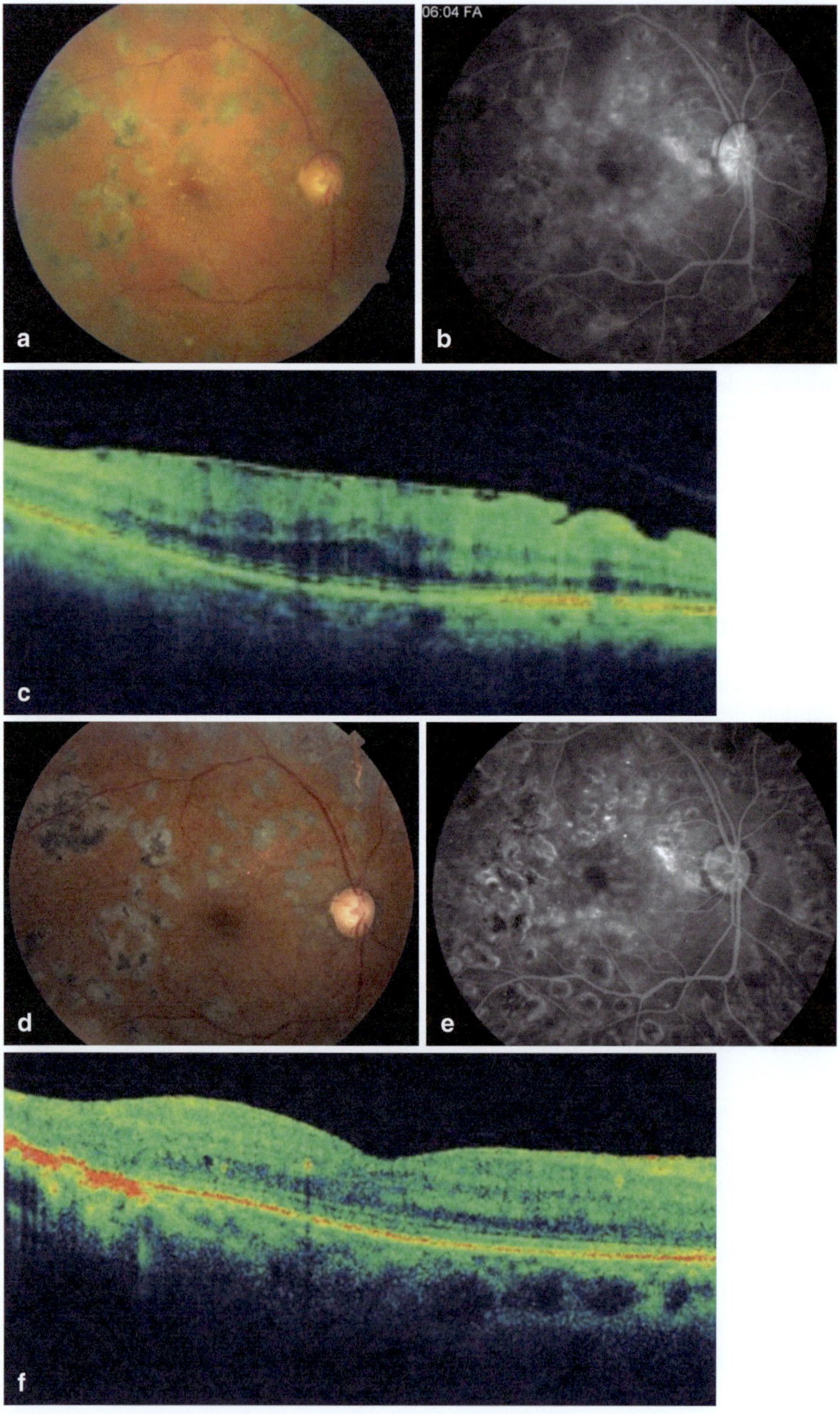
06:04 FA
a
b
c
d
e
f

Fig. 3 Improvement of macular edema and foveal contour after vitrectomy and ERM peel in diabetic patient with ERM and PVD. (**a**) Preoperative fundus photograph. (**b**) Preoperative fluorescein angiogram. (**c**) Preoperative OCT showing PVD and ERM. (**d**) Postoperative fundus photograph. (**e**) Postoperative fluorescein angiogram. (**f**) OCT showing resolution of vitreofoveal traction and DME after vitrectomy without ILM peeling

extracellular matrix. This leads to decreased water movement between the vitreous and retina, build-up of proteins in the interstitial space, decreased diffusion of proteins to the vitreous space, and macular edema [41, 42]. Removal of this thickened ILM eliminates a possible barrier to cytokines and oxygen [43, 44]. It can also help to ensure complete removal of residual cortical vitreous [41, 45]. Similar to a taut posterior hyaloid or VMT, tangential traction can also be exerted by an ILM. ILM peeling can also ensure complete removal of epiretinal cells. This may limit postoperative ERM formation by removing the scaffold for proliferating cells [46]. For these reasons, ILM peeling has been proposed as an adjunct to vitrectomy in select cases of DME.

In order to better understand how ILM peeling is beneficial, several studies have thoroughly investigated changes in pathology and imaging. Gentile et al. described two cases of diffuse DME after vitrectomy that demonstrated a taut ILM. After repeat vitrectomy with ILM peeling, macular edema and VA improved. The ILM was analyzed with immunostaining and revealed an inner monolayer of cytokeratin-positive (retinal pigment epithelial (RPE) cells) and/or glial fibrillary acidic protein-positive cells with smooth muscle actin (SMA) immunoreactivity. As SMA indicates myofibroblast differentiation and the contractile ability of the RPE and glial cells, these changes likely caused tangential traction which was relieved by ILM peeling [47]. The tangential traction that can be exerted by the ILM was also imaged in a study by Abe et al. They performed a retrospective case series of 26 DME eyes imaged with OCT to identify both traction seen on tomography and fine folds seen on three dimensional imaging. After ILM peeling, the fine folds resolved, even in those eyes without traction on tomography. Surgically obtained specimens confirmed that the fine folds involved the ILM [48]. This suggests that ILM peeling can help resolve tangential traction in DME, even when not obvious on standard tomography.

Evidence for Surgical Intervention

Peeling of the ILM has been proposed as a helpful adjuvant to vitrectomy for DME but results in the literature are mixed. Kamura et al. evaluated 34 DME eyes treated with ILM peeling during vitrectomy compared to eyes treated with vitrectomy alone and found that VA improved significantly after vitrectomy regardless of ILM peeling and without a significant difference between the groups [49]. Bahadir et al. examined 17 DME eyes that underwent ILM peeling during vitrectomy, and comparing them to eyes with vitrectomy alone found a significant improvement in postoperative VA in both groups, but no difference between them [50]. Rosenblatt et al. reviewed 26 eyes with refractory DME without traction that were treated with vitrectomy and ILM peel. There was a statistically significant improvement of mean VA (50 % of eyes gained at least two lines of VA) and mean foveal thickness (311 μm from 575 μm) [51]. Patel et al. evaluated ten eyes with diffuse refractory DME which underwent vitrectomy and ILM peeling compared to vitrectomy alone, finding that ILM peeling was associated with a significant improvement in foveal thickness and macular volume, but not with change in VA [52]. Additionally, Recchia et al. examined ten patients after vitrectomy and ILM removal with diffuse DME refractory to laser, finding both improvement in central macular thickness and VA [53]. Finally, Yanyali et al. treated 12 DME eyes with vitrectomy and ILM peel compared to controls treated with laser in this prospective study, finding a significant improvement in mean foveal thickness and VA in the surgical group but not in the laser group [54]. In a later study, Yanyali et al. reviewed 27 DME eyes that underwent vitrectomy with ILM peeling, finding a significant decrease in foveal thickness and improvement in VA [55]. In summary, the majority of these studies report some additional benefit with ILM peeling; however, restoration of foveal anatomy was more common than improvement in VA. In practice, employment of ILM peeling for diffuse DME appears mixed, as in the DRCRnet Vitrectomy Study that showed 54 % of surgeons elected to peel the ILM [36].

Prognostic Factors

Several prognostic factors for favorable outcomes after surgical intervention for DME have been identified, perhaps most importantly preoperative VA and early surgical intervention. Pendergast et al. showed a strong correlation between preoperative and postoperative VA. They examined 55 DME eyes that underwent vitrectomy with stripping of a taut posterior hyaloid and found that eyes with preoperative BCVA of 20/200 or worse responded less favorable to vitrectomy. Eyes with preoperative BCVA of 20/100 or better improved by a median of 60 % compared to 18 % the eyes with VA of 20/200 or worse [7]. Harbour et al. examined ten DME patients who underwent vitrectomy for a taut posterior hyaloid and found that the three eyes with rapid deterioration of vision from DME followed by prompt surgical intervention (less than 1 month) experienced the most improvement in final BCVA [30].

Other studies have used OCT to delineate prognostic factors for DME and surgical intervention by identifying markers for photoreceptor damage that would limit visual potential. Maheshwary et al. found a statistically significant correlation between percentage disruption of the IS/OS junction and VA in 62 DME eyes using OCT [56]. Additionally, Chhablani et al. found that external limiting membrane (ELM) integrity correlated with postoperative outcome in their study of 34 eyes with resistant DME treated with vitrectomy [57]. Finally, Nishijima et al. identified hyperreflective foci in the outer retina that were predictive of photoreceptor damage and poor vision in their study of 32 DME eyes that underwent vitrectomy [58].

Additionally, other ocular and systemic prognostic factors have been identified. Longer axial length was found to be associated with better VA after vitrectomy by Wakabayashi et al. in 51 eyes with DME that underwent vitrectomy [59]. Better glycemic control also correlated with better outcomes. Yamada et al. examined 44 diabetic eyes that underwent vitrectomy with ILM peeling for DME and found that the postoperative macular thickness was significantly thicker with higher glycosylated hemoglobin levels [60]. These studies suggest that there are retinal, ocular, and systemic factors that can help identify patients who could benefit from surgical intervention for DME.

Summary

When considered by categories of vitreoretinal interface problems, the utility of vitrectomy in select DME cases becomes clearer. Vitrectomy has been shown to be beneficial in most DME cases where a taut posterior hyaloid or vitreomacular traction is present. It is beneficial in select cases where the posterior hyaloid is attached, even if there is no observable traction. When separation of the posterior hyaloid has occurred, vitrectomy can be beneficial in select cases where an ERM is present.

Favorable anatomic results are more common than visual results when vitrectomy and other surgical interventions are performed in select cases of DME. As discussed, VA can improve 5–15 letters postoperatively but may worsen in some cases. Despite this limited improvement in VA, OCT results are often more impressive. Foveal thickness usually decreases postoperatively by 100–250 μm on OCT or greater than 50 % reduction of retinal thickening. The fact that improvement on OCT does not translate to significant visual results may reflect that vitrectomy is often performed for refractory DME cases with long-standing edema with irreversible macular damage.

In summary, eyes with observable vitreous and/or epiretinal traction are most likely to improve after vitrectomy. Eyes with refractory edema and no observable traction, however, are less likely to improve. Unfortunately, improvement in retinal thickening is often more impressive than improvement in VA even in these select cases. However, vitrectomy and other surgical interventions may be beneficial for select cases of DME, especially when surgical intervention is undertaken early, before photoreceptor damage has occurred.

References

1. Cogan DG, Toussaint D, Kuwabara T. Retinal vascular patterns. IV Diabetic retinopathy. Arch Ophthalmol. 1961;66:366–78.
2. O'Doherty M, Dooley I, Hickey-Dwyer M. Interventions for diabetic macular oedema: a systematic review of the literature. Br J Ophthalmol. 2008;92(12):1581–90.
3. Photocoagulation for diabetic macular edema. Early Treatment Diabetic Retinopathy Study report number 1. Early Treatment Diabetic Retinopathy Study research group. Arch Ophthalmol. 1985;103(12):1796–806.
4. Kaiser PK, Riemann CD, Sears JE, Lewis H. Macular traction detachment and diabetic macular edema associated with posterior hyaloidal traction. Am J Ophthalmol. 2001;131(1):44–9.
5. Massin P, Duguid G, Erginay A, Haouchine B, Gaudric A. Optical coherence tomography for evaluating diabetic macular edema before and after vitrectomy. Am J Ophthalmol. 2003;135(2):169–77.

6. Lewis H, Abrams GW, Blumenkranz MS, Campo RV. Vitrectomy for diabetic macular traction and edema associated with posterior hyaloidal traction. Ophthalmology. 1992;99(5):753–9.
7. Pendergast SD, Hassan TS, Williams GA, Cox MS, Margherio RR, Ferrone PJ, et al. Vitrectomy for diffuse diabetic macular edema associated with a taut premacular posterior hyaloid. Am J Ophthalmol. 2000;130(2):178–86.
8. The effect of intensive treatment of diabetes on the development and progression of long-term complications in insulin-dependent diabetes mellitus. The Diabetes Control and Complications Trial Research Group. N Engl J Med. 1993;329(14):977–86.
9. Yilmaz T, Weaver CD, Gallagher MJ, Cordero-Coma M, Cervantes-Castaneda RA, Klisovic D, et al. Intravitreal triamcinolone acetonide injection for treatment of refractory diabetic macular edema: a systematic review. Ophthalmology. 2009;116(5):902–11; quiz 12–3.
10. Lam DS, Chan CK, Mohamed S, Lai TY, Lee VY, Liu DT, et al. Intravitreal triamcinolone plus sequential grid laser versus triamcinolone or laser alone for treating diabetic macular edema: six-month outcomes. Ophthalmology. 2007;114(12):2162–7.
11. Martidis A, Duker JS, Greenberg PB, Rogers AH, Puliafito CA, Reichel E, et al. Intravitreal triamcinolone for refractory diabetic macular edema. Ophthalmology. 2002;109(5):920–7.
12. Nicholson BP, Schachat AP. A review of clinical trials of anti-VEGF agents for diabetic retinopathy. Graefes Arch Clin Exp Ophthalmol. 2010;248(7):915–30.
13. Schubert HD. Cystoid macular edema: the apparent role of mechanical factors. Prog Clin Biol Res. 1989;312:277–91.
14. Bringmann A, Wiedemann P. Involvement of Muller glial cells in epiretinal membrane formation. Graefes Arch Clin Exp Ophthalmol. 2009;247(7):865–83.
15. Wolfensberger TJ, Gregor ZJ. Macular edema–rationale for therapy. Dev Ophthalmol. 2010;47:49–58.
16. Smiddy WE, Green WR, Michels RG, de la Cruz Z. Ultrastructural studies of vitreomacular traction syndrome. Am J Ophthalmol. 1989;107(2):177–85.
17. Augustin A, Loewenstein A, Kuppermann BD. Macular edema. General pathophysiology. Dev Ophthalmol. 2010;47:10–26.
18. Lindqvist N, Liu Q, Zajadacz J, Franze K, Reichenbach A. Retinal glial (Muller) cells: sensing and responding to tissue stretch. Invest Ophthalmol Vis Sci. 2010;51(3):1683–90.
19. Noma H, Funatsu H, Mimura T, Harino S, Hori S. Vitreous levels of interleukin-6 and vascular endothelial growth factor in macular edema with central retinal vein occlusion. Ophthalmology. 2009;116(1):87–93.
20. Praidou A, Klangas I, Papakonstantinou E, Androudi S, Georgiadis N, Karakiulakis G, et al. Vitreous and serum levels of platelet-derived growth factor and their correlation in patients with proliferative diabetic retinopathy. Curr Eye Res. 2009;34(2):152–61.
21. Praidou A, Papakonstantinou E, Androudi S, Georgiadis N, Karakiulakis G, Dimitrakos S. Vitreous and serum levels of vascular endothelial growth factor and platelet-derived growth factor and their correlation in patients with non-proliferative diabetic retinopathy and clinically significant macula oedema. Acta Ophthalmol. 2011;89(3):248–54.
22. Williamson TH, Grewal J, Gupta B, Mokete B, Lim M, Fry CH. Measurement of PO2 during vitrectomy for central retinal vein occlusion, a pilot study. Graefes Arch Clin Exp Ophthalmol. 2009;247(8):1019–23.
23. Stefansson E, Novack RL, Hatchell DL. Vitrectomy prevents retinal hypoxia in branch retinal vein occlusion. Invest Ophthalmol Vis Sci. 1990;31(2):284–9.
24. Holekamp NM, Shui YB, Beebe DC. Vitrectomy surgery increases oxygen exposure to the lens: a possible mechanism for nuclear cataract formation. Am J Ophthalmol. 2005;139(2): 302–10.
25. Siegfried CJ, Shui YB, Holekamp NM, Bai F, Beebe DC. Oxygen distribution in the human eye: relevance to the etiology of open-angle glaucoma after vitrectomy. Invest Ophthalmol Vis Sci. 2010;51(11):5731–8.
26. Giblin FJ, Quiram PA, Leverenz VR, Baker RM, Dang L, Trese MT. Enzyme-induced posterior vitreous detachment in the rat produces increased lens nuclear pO2 levels. Exp Eye Res. 2009;88(2):286–92.

27. Quiram PA, Leverenz VR, Baker RM, Dang L, Giblin FJ, Trese MT. Microplasmin-induced posterior vitreous detachment affects vitreous oxygen levels. Retina. 2007;27(8):1090–6.
28. Nasrallah FP, Jalkh AE, Van Coppenolle F, Kado M, Trempe CL, McMeel JW, et al. The role of the vitreous in diabetic macular edema. Ophthalmology. 1988;95(10):1335–9.
29. Hikichi T, Fujio N, Akiba J, Azuma Y, Takahashi M, Yoshida A. Association between the short-term natural history of diabetic macular edema and the vitreomacular relationship in type II diabetes mellitus. Ophthalmology. 1997;104(3):473–8.
30. Harbour JW, Smiddy WE, Flynn Jr HW, Rubsamen PE. Vitrectomy for diabetic macular edema associated with a thickened and taut posterior hyaloid membrane. Am J Ophthalmol. 1996;121(4):405–13.
31. Gandorfer A, Messmer EM, Ulbig MW, Kampik A. Resolution of diabetic macular edema after surgical removal of the posterior hyaloid and the inner limiting membrane. Retina. 2000;20(2):126–33.
32. Krupin T, Waltman SR, Szewczyk P, Koloms B, Farber M, Silverstein B, et al. Fluorometric studies on the blood-retinal barrier in experimental animals. Arch Ophthalmol. 1982;100(4):631–4.
33. Kirber WM, Nichols CW, Grimes PA, Winegrad AI, Laties AM. A permeability defect of the retinal pigment epithelium. Occurrence in early streptozocin diabetes. Arch Ophthalmol. 1980;98(4):725–8.
34. Kim BY, Smith SD, Kaiser PK. Optical coherence tomographic patterns of diabetic macular edema. Am J Ophthalmol. 2006;142(3):405–12.
35. Baskin DE. Optical coherence tomography in diabetic macular edema. Curr Opin Ophthalmol. 2010;21(3):172–7.
36. Haller JA, Qin H, Apte RS, Beck RR, Bressler NM, Browning DJ, et al. Vitrectomy outcomes in eyes with diabetic macular edema and vitreomacular traction. Ophthalmology. 2010;117(6):1087–93. e3.
37. Ikeda T, Sato K, Katano T, Hayashi Y. Improved visual acuity following pars plana vitrectomy for diabetic cystoid macular edema and detached posterior hyaloid. Retina. 2000;20(2):220–2.
38. Otani T, Kishi S. Tomographic assessment of vitreous surgery for diabetic macular edema. Am J Ophthalmol. 2000;129(4):487–94.
39. La Heij EC, Hendrikse F, Kessels AG, Derhaag PJ. Vitrectomy results in diabetic macular oedema without evident vitreomacular traction. Graefes Arch Clin Exp Ophthalmol. 2001;239(4):264–70.
40. Yamamoto T, Akabane N, Takeuchi S. Vitrectomy for diabetic macular edema: the role of posterior vitreous detachment and epimacular membrane. Am J Ophthalmol. 2001;132(3):369–77.
41. Matsunaga N, Ozeki H, Hirabayashi Y, Shimada S, Ogura Y. Histopathologic evaluation of the internal limiting membrane surgically excised from eyes with diabetic maculopathy. Retina. 2005;25(3):311–6.
42. Saravia M. Persistent diffuse diabetic macular edema. The role of the internal limiting membrane as a selective membrane: the oncotic theory. Med Hypotheses. 2011;76(6):858–60.
43. Stefansson E. Physiology of vitreous surgery. Graefes Arch Clin Exp Ophthalmol. 2009;247(2):147–63.
44. Hoerauf H, Bruggemann A, Muecke M, Luke J, Muller M, Stefansson E, et al. Pars plana vitrectomy for diabetic macular edema. Internal limiting membrane delamination vs posterior hyaloid removal. A prospective randomized trial. Graefes Arch Clin Exp Ophthalmol. 2011;249(7):997–1008.
45. Gandorfer A, Rohleder M, Grosselfinger S, Haritoglou C, Ulbig M, Kampik A. Epiretinal pathology of diffuse diabetic macular edema associated with vitreomacular traction. Am J Ophthalmol. 2005;139(4):638–52.
46. Schaal S, Tezel TH, Kaplan HJ. Surgical intervention in refractory CME–role of posterior hyaloid separation and internal limiting membrane peeling. Ocul Immunol Inflamm. 2008;16(5):209–10.

47. Gentile RC, Milman T, Eliott D, Romero JM, McCormick SA. Taut internal limiting membrane causing diffuse diabetic macular edema after vitrectomy: clinicopathological correlation. Ophthalmologica. 2011;226(2):64–70.
48. Abe S, Yamamoto T, Kashiwagi Y, Kirii E, Goto S, Yamashita H. Three-dimensional imaging of the inner limiting membrane folding on the vitreomacular interface in diabetic macular edema. Jpn J Ophthalmol. 2013;57(6):553–62.
49. Kamura Y, Sato Y, Isomae T, Shimada H. Effects of internal limiting membrane peeling in vitrectomy on diabetic cystoid macular edema patients. Jpn J Ophthalmol. 2005;49(4):297–300.
50. Bahadir M, Ertan A, Mertoglu O. Visual acuity comparison of vitrectomy with and without internal limiting membrane removal in the treatment of diabetic macular edema. Int Ophthalmol. 2005;26(1–2):3–8.
51. Rosenblatt BJ, Shah GK, Sharma S, Bakal J. Pars plana vitrectomy with internal limiting membranectomy for refractory diabetic macular edema without a taut posterior hyaloid. Graefes Arch Clin Exp Ophthalmol. 2005;243(1):20–5.
52. Patel JI, Hykin PG, Schadt M, Luong V, Fitzke F, Gregor ZJ. Pars plana vitrectomy with and without peeling of the inner limiting membrane for diabetic macular edema. Retina. 2006;26(1):5–13.
53. Recchia FM, Ruby AJ, Carvalho Recchia CA. Pars plana vitrectomy with removal of the internal limiting membrane in the treatment of persistent diabetic macular edema. Am J Ophthalmol. 2005;139(3):447–54.
54. Yanyali A, Nohutcu AF, Horozoglu F, Celik E. Modified grid laser photocoagulation versus pars plana vitrectomy with internal limiting membrane removal in diabetic macular edema. Am J Ophthalmol. 2005;139(5):795–801.
55. Yanyali A, Horozoglu F, Celik E, Nohutcu AF. Long-term outcomes of pars plana vitrectomy with internal limiting membrane removal in diabetic macular edema. Retina. 2007;27(5):557–66.
56. Maheshwary AS, Oster SF, Yuson RM, Cheng L, Mojana F, Freeman WR. The association between percent disruption of the photoreceptor inner segment-outer segment junction and visual acuity in diabetic macular edema. Am J Ophthalmol. 2010;150(1):63–7. e1.
57. Chhablani JK, Kim JS, Cheng L, Kozak I, Freeman W. External limiting membrane as a predictor of visual improvement in diabetic macular edema after pars plana vitrectomy. Graefes Arch Clin Exp Ophthalmol. 2012;250(10):1415–20.
58. Nishijima K, Murakami T, Hirashima T, Uji A, Akagi T, Horii T, et al. Hyperreflective foci in outer retina predictive of photoreceptor damage and poor vision after vitrectomy for diabetic macular edema. Retina. 2014;34(4):732–40.
59. Wakabayashi Y, Kimura K, Muramatsu D, Usui Y, Umazume K, Suzuki J, et al. Axial length as a factor associated with visual outcome after vitrectomy for diabetic macular edema. Invest Ophthalmol Vis Sci. 2013;54(10):6834–40.
60. Yamada Y, Suzuma K, Ryu M, Tsuiki E, Fujikawa A, Kitaoka T. Systemic factors influence the prognosis of diabetic macular edema after pars plana vitrectomy with internal limiting membrane peeling. Curr Eye Res. 2013;38(12):1261–5.

Chapter 11
Surgical Management of CME Associated with Vitreoretinal Interface

Mauricio Maia, Juliana Bottós, Javier Elizalde, Emerson Badaro, and J. Fernando Arevalo

Introduction

Cystoid macular edema (CME) after ocular surgery was first described in 1953 by Irvine and is related to the release of inflammatory mediators such as prostaglandins, leukotrienes, histamine, bradykinins, platelet-activating factor (PAF), and interleukin (IL)-1 [1–4]. The original report described cystoid changes after vitreous incarceration at the corneal wound after intracapsular cataract surgery. However, nowadays, this terminology is used for any macular edema after surgical procedures. A classic feature of this disease is the cystoid macular abnormalities related to swelling of the outer plexiform layer following release of cytokines at the vitreous cavity, which results in the classic hallmark petaloid pattern seen by fluorescein angiogram (FA) (Fig. 1); additionally, new insights have been added by spectral-domain optical coherence tomography (OCT) technology (Fig. 1b). The management of this entity is described in another chapter. The differential diagnosis should include epiretinal membrane, macular hole, age-related macular degeneration,

M. Maia, MD, PhD
Vitreoretinal Surgery Unit, Universidade Federal de Sao Paulo, Brazilian Institute of Fight Against Blindness, 901, Otto Ribeiro Street, Assis/Presidente Prudente, SP, Brazil

J. Bottós, MD • E. Badaro, MD
Vitreoretinal Sector, Department of Ophthalmology, Federal University of São Paulo, UNIFESP, Brazil, 821, Botucatu Street, São Paulo, SP, Brazil

J. Elizalde, MD
Vitreoretinal Surgery Unit, Institut Barraquer, Barcelona, Spain

J.F. Arevalo, MD, FACS (✉)
Retina Division, Department of Ophthalmology, Wilmer Eye Institute, The Johns Hopkins University School of Medicine, 600 N. Wolfe, Street, Maumenee 708, Baltimore, MD 21287, USA
e-mail: arevalojf@jhmi.edu

S. Schaal, H.J. Kaplan (eds.), *Cystoid Macular Edema*,
DOI 10.1007/978-3-319-39766-5_11

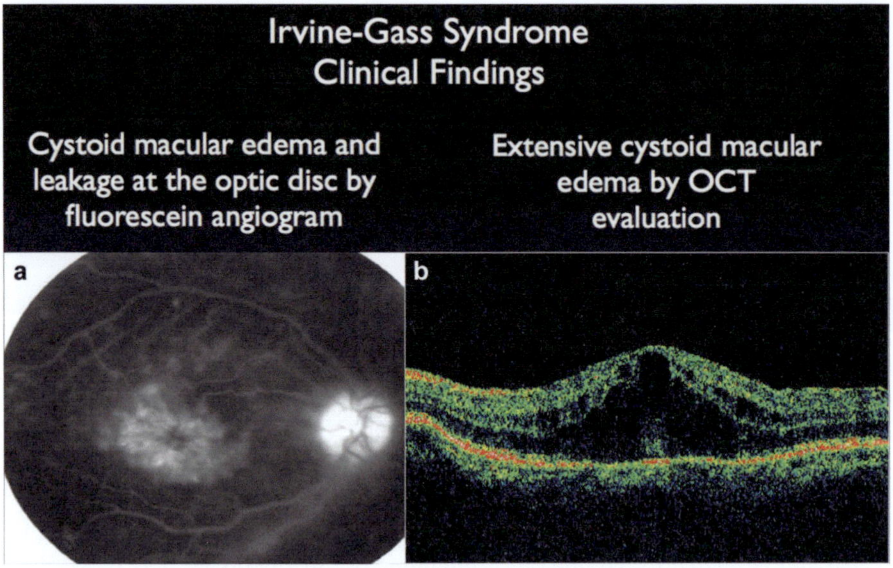

Fig. 1 Clinical findings in Irvine-Gass syndrome. (**a**) Cystoid macular edema due to leakage of fluorescein at the macula; note the petaloid patterns of leakage. (**b**) Optical coherence tomography (OCT) showing the cystic changes due to release of inflammatory mediators

central serous chorioretinopathy, and, most importantly, vitreomacular traction (VMT) syndrome [1–4].

In 1970, Reese et al. described an unusual macular condition in which an incomplete posterior vitreous detachment (PVD) resulted in traction on the macula accompanied by decreased visual acuity (VA) [5]. This condition was confirmed, not by imaging techniques (such as OCT) as they were not yet available at that time, but through the use of histological studies. Therefore, the term vitreomacular traction (VMT) syndrome was coined.

Epidemiology

In observational and interventional studies, the mean age of patients diagnosed with VMT is around 65–75 years, with a predominance of females. The condition is unilateral in approximately 80 % of cases [6].

The prevalence of epiretinal membrane (ERM) increases with age and is approximately 2 % in people over 50 years of age and 20 % in individuals older than 70 years. It can be bilateral in 20–30 % of cases [7, 8].

Idiopathic VMT syndrome can occur in either sex, at any age, and has no racial predilection [8]. The incidence in women seems to be distinctly higher (about 65 %), which may be attributed to the earlier onset of PVD due to premature vitreous liquefaction, likely associated with declining estrogen levels in the postmenopausal period [9].

CME and VMT: Physiopathogenesis

A common physiopathological event in these diseases is vitreous syneresis (Fig. 2a). Increasingly with age, synchysis of the vitreous gel and ultimately syneresis lead to posterior vitreous detachment (PVD), a non-pathological process. PVD is not related to significant problems in most patients; however, if there is an imbalance of vitreal glycosaminoglycans and hyaluronic acid, the vitreoretinal adhesion to the macular area does not weaken; pathological adhesion of the vitreous to the macular area may occur, and abnormal PVD may happen, in a process known as vitreomacular adhesion (VMA) (Fig. 2b) [1, 9, 10], that results in no abnormalities at the macular architecture.

Focal VMA occurs when the perifoveal vitreous cortex is adherent to the macula after detaching from the surrounding retina. This situation typically is asymptomatic non-pathological and causes no discernible retinal changes [2]. Alternatively, VMA may result in abnormalities of the macular anatomy, resulting in the so-called

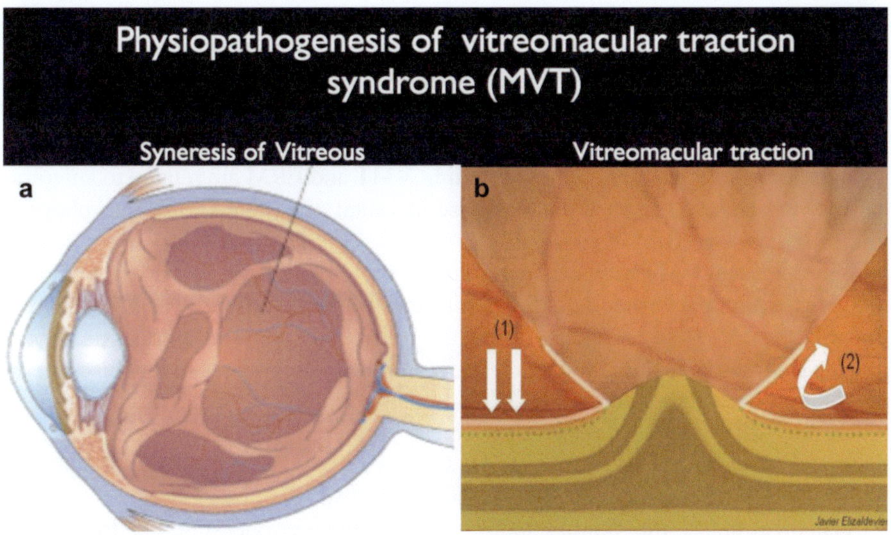

Fig. 2 Physiopathogenesis of vitreomacular traction (VMT) syndrome. (**a**) Natural history of posterior vitreous detachment and vitreous syneresis. (**b**) Proposed mechanism of epiretinal membrane (ERM) proliferation in vitreomacular traction syndrome, according to Johnson [4] and Chang et al. [14]. (*1*) After development of a partial posterior vitreous detachment, small splits within the internal limiting membrane may form, allowing glial cells to gain access to the superficial retina (*arrows*), which serves as a scaffold for ERM proliferation. (*2*) These cells also proliferate on the detached hyaloid face (*arrow*), strongly anchoring the vitreous to the macula

vitreomacular traction (VMT) syndrome (Fig. 2b); this occurs when the forces of macular attachment are strong enough to cause anatomical disturbance of the macular architecture (Fig. 2b).

In VMT, tractional forces on the macula may cause two different pathologies [11] (Fig. 3):

1. A focal configuration of the traction, also named V-shaped macular traction (Fig. 3), which corresponds to less than 1,500 μm of traction: this is related to macular holes (Fig. 4) and cystoid macular edema (Fig. 5).
2. A broad configuration of the traction, also named J-shaped macular traction, which corresponds to more than 1,500 μm of traction: this is related to epiretinal membrane formation and retinal thickening (Fig. 3).

By definition, VMT is always pathologic and symptomatic [1]. Symptoms commonly associated with VMT include metamorphopsia and blurred vision. Asymptomatic VMA is not an indication for treatment and is a normal transient phase in the course of PVD.

Diagnosis

The first step in diagnosis is a complete history from the patient, including type and duration of symptoms, past ocular history (i.e., glaucoma, previous ocular surgeries, trauma, etc.), and past systemic history (i.e., systemic diseases and medications), including the use of drugs potentially related to the development and increase of macular edema (e.g., systemic niacin, topical prostaglandin analogs) [6]. The cardinal symptoms of macular diseases including VMT and ERM are related to anatomical macular changes and include decrease in visual acuity (VA), metamorphopsia, micropsia, and rarely photopsia [6].

Because focal VMT may cause minimal symptoms, it is often diagnosed during OCT evaluation performed in patients for other causes. Chronicity and strong tractional forces in VMT can further distort the retina causing intraretinal cysts or posterior pole tractional retinal detachment. If intraretinal cysts cause a dehiscence in the internal limiting membrane (ILM), a lamellar hole is created, and if a complete break from the ILM to the retinal pigment epithelium (RPE) is formed, a full-thickness macular hole occurs (Fig. 4), seen as in interruption of retinal anatomy with surrounding edema in the macular area [11–13].

Visualization of the fundus should include the peripheral retina to exclude pathology such as retinal tears, vascular lesions, chorioretinitis, and intraocular tumors that could induce macular edema [11].

OCT is useful in assessing the location of cleavage planes for patients in eyes with surgical indication, helps in predicting visual prognosis, and also in postoperative follow-up, assisting, for example, in the detection of recurrent and residual ERMs [14–16]. Analysis of prognostic factors for vision recovery is possible by assessing the structural integrity of the ellipsoid zone (IS/OS junction) and of the external limiting membrane (ELM) [6].

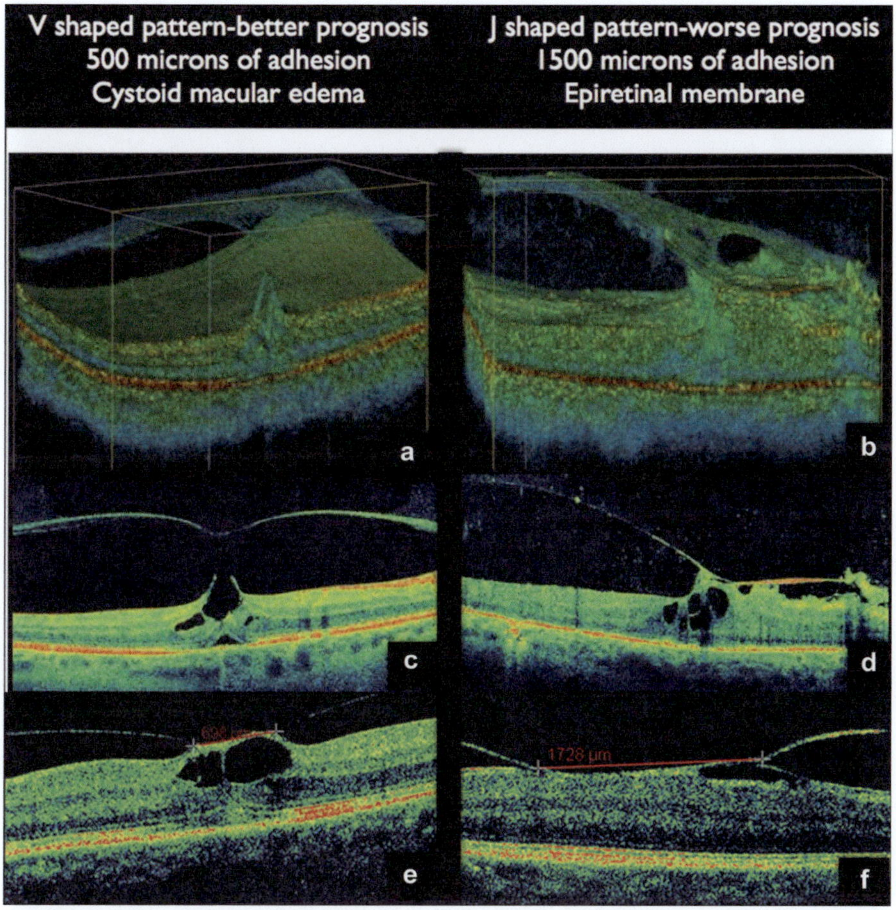

Fig. 3 Distinct HD-OCT images of VMT syndrome based on the morphology and extension of the vitreomacular adhesion. (**a**) V-shaped VMT (focal, less than 1500 um) and cystoid macular edema by 3-dimensional SD-OCT. (**b**) J-shaped VMT (broad, more than 1500 um) and epiretinal membrane by 3-dimensional SD-OCT. (**c**) V-shaped VMT (focal, less than 1500 um) and cystoid macular edema by 3-dimensional SD-OCT. (**d**) J-shaped VMT (broad, more than 1500 um) and epiretinal membrane by 3-dimensional SD-OCT. (**e**) Focal VMT measurement based on the extension of traction. The greatest linear adhesion point 698 μm at the macular area, which better reflects the surgical prognosis in comparison with the morphological classification by preliminary data from 36 eyes that underwent surgery. (**f**) Diffuse VMT measurement based on the extension of traction. The greatest linear adhesion point 1,728 μm at the macular area, which better reflects the surgical prognosis in comparison with the morphological classification by preliminary data from 36 eyes that underwent surgery

The diagnosis of VMT syndrome is often difficult to make through clinical examination alone. Even with thorough fundus contact lens examination, the firm translucent adhesions of the vitreous at the macula may be essentially imperceptible. This explains why this condition was considered to be rare and underdiagnosed [11, 13, 16]. Distinct clinical presentations of VMT have been described

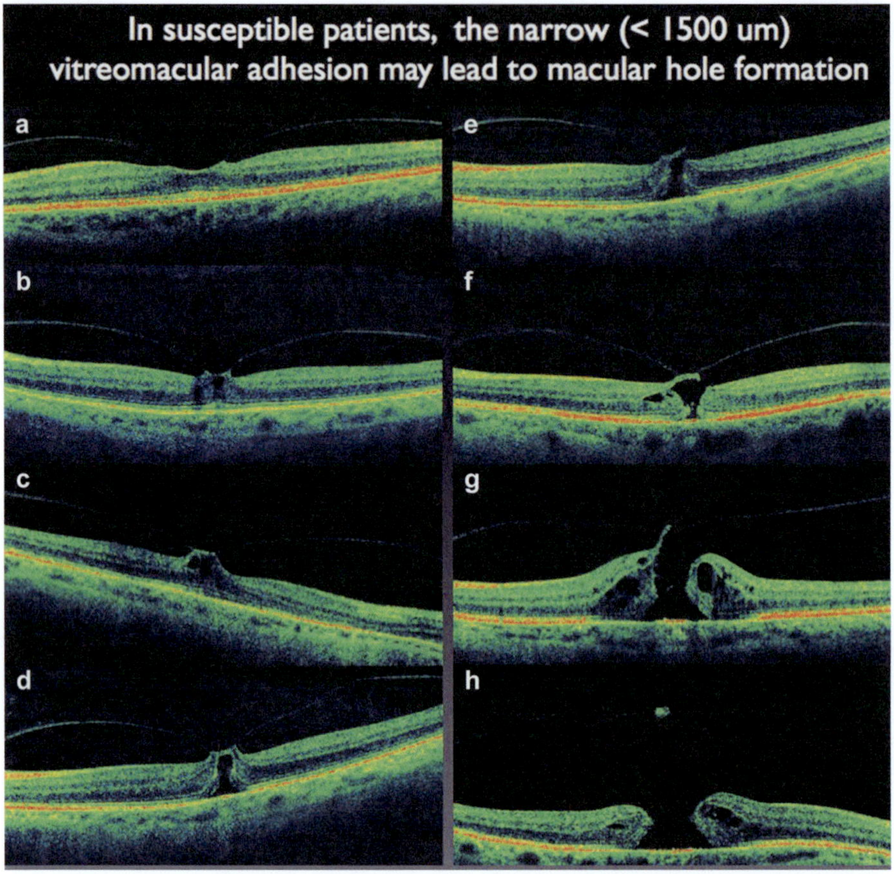

Fig. 4 Evolution of macular hole formation in focal (less than 1500 um) VMT syndrome. HD-OCT images of patients in distinct phases of VMT. (**a**) In some susceptible eyes, there is an abnormal and strong vitreomacular adhesion causing a persistent foveal traction. (**b**) Vitreomacular adhesion changing the foveal anatomy causing the vitreomacular traction (VMT) syndrome. (**c**) VMT and the associated cystoid macular edema. It is still unclear why do some eyes progress to full-thickness macular holes and why do eyes detach the posterior hyaloid and the traction component present regression. (**d**) If the macular traction persists, the cystoid macular edema may progress to a pseudocystic change, and the stage IB macular hole may develop. (**e**) Traction leading to a stage 2 macular hole with eccentric pseudo-operculum and perifoveal detachment which is universally associated with macular holes. (**f**) Traction leading to a more advanced stage 2 macular hole with eccentric pseudo-operculum, cystic changes at the edges of the holes, and a more advanced and perifoveal detachment. (**g**) Progression of traction resulting in a stage 3 macular hole. (**h**) Progression of traction resulting in a stage 4 macular hole

[11, 17, 18]. They include macular surface wrinkling, similar in appearance to ERM. Although in the past this syndrome was considered infrequent and not correlated with other maculopathies, it is now known that ERM may be associated in

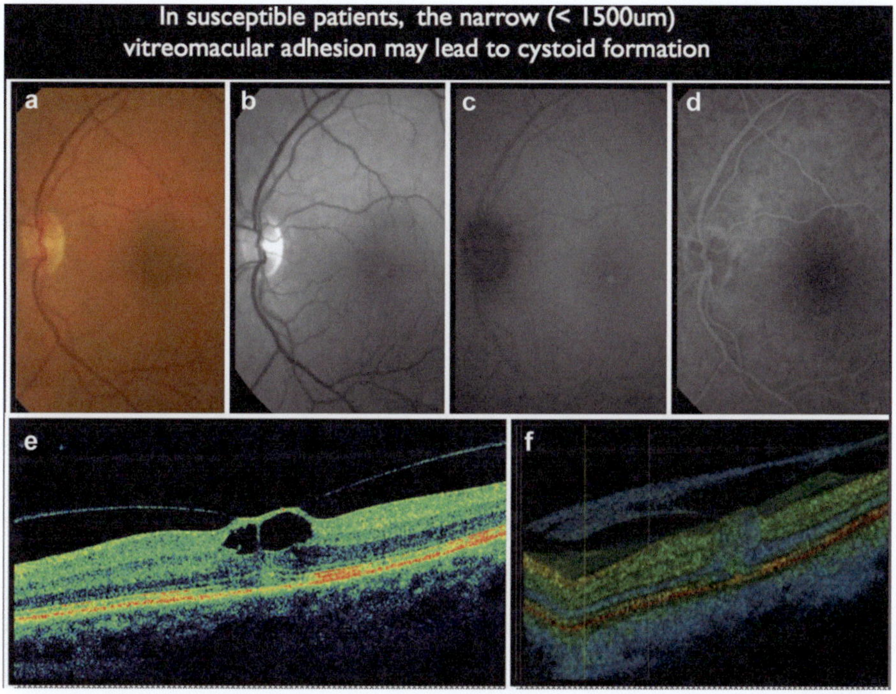

Fig. 5 Fundus photograph. (**a**) Red-free image, (**b**) fundus autofluorescence, (**c**) and fluorescein angiogram (**d**) of a patient with tractional cystoid macular edema. The fundus photograph (**a**) shows a yellow spot that corresponds to the hyperautofluorescent pattern on the autofluorescence image. A corresponding midphase fluorescein angiogram (**d**) shows minimal leakage from the retinal capillaries which are completely different than. High-definition optical coherence tomography (**e**, **f**) shows focal vitreomacular adhesion with a perifoveal vitreous detachment causing tractional cystoid foveal edema. Note that the focal pattern of foveal leakage and no angiographic disk edema related to tractional component (**d**) is completely different than petaloid pattern of edema associated to angiographic edema mediated by cytokines (Fig. 1a); the OCT findings related to the tractional component (**e**–**f**) are also mild in comparison to the edema mediated by cytokines (Fig. 1b)

most cases. A thickened and taut posterior hyaloid membrane may also be noted [19]. Tractional CME is a subtle variant of VMT syndrome, and it may be present in cases of unifocal vitreofoveal traction arising from partial PVD [11].

Classification of CME Related to VMT

The focus of this chapter is to describe the surgical management of CME. For didactic reasons, we will divide CME that may benefit from surgical indications into two

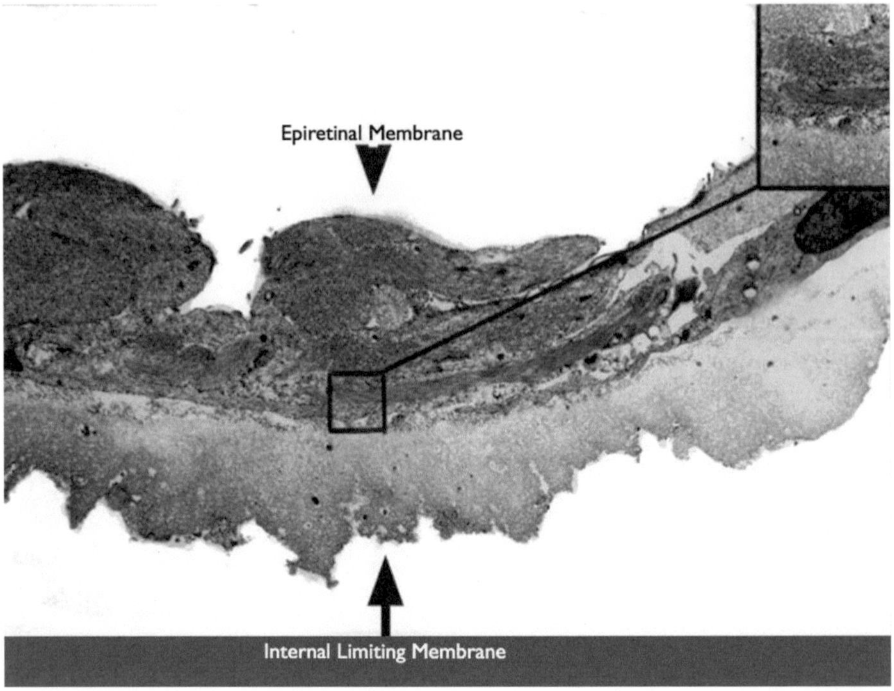

Fig. 6 Epiretinal membrane (ERM) and internal limiting membrane (ILM) analyzed by electron microscopy showing a segment of the ILM (*arrow*) and epiretinal membrane (*arrowhead*). The matrix around the surface is composed of moderate amount of collagen fibrils with native collagen (panel featured above right) (TEM 3800; picture *top right* TEM 24000). The complex interaction of ERM and ILM is the rationale to stain and remove the ILM in all cases related to ERM formation in order to minimize the possibility of ERM recurrence and/or macular edema

different clinical patterns according to the distinct physiopathogenesis, fluorescein angiogram (FA) and OCT findings [11, 13, 16, 20]:

1. CME after cataract surgery related to persistent vitreous base traction and secondary VMT: in these eyes, the common finding is the angiographic papillary edema (extensive FA leakage) associated with a petaloid pattern of leakage at the macula and an important extension of CME by OCT due to chronic release of high amounts of inflammatory mediators which results in a secondary tractional component such as posterior hyaloid traction and/or epiretinal membrane (ERM) formation (Fig. 1) [11, 13, 16, 20].
2. CME related to primary VMT (Figs. 2, 3, 4, and 5): in these eyes, the primary abnormality is an abnormal and incomplete posterior vitreous detachment (PVD) (Fig. 3). The common finding is minimal or no angiographic papillary edema (minimal FA leakage at the optic disk and macula) as well as a focal extension of CME seen on OCT due to a primary tractional component (Figs. 3, 4, and 5) and

minimal release of inflammatory mediators. This results in minimal macular changes on fundus photographs, FA and OCT (Fig. 5). ERM may be also present (Fig. 6) [11, 13, 16, 20].

CME and Secondary Vitreoretinal Interface Disorders (VMT)

CME associated to secondary vitreoretinal interface disorders (VMT) is frequently related to ERM formation in pseudophakic eyes. Surgical intervention is indicated if best-corrected visual acuity (BCVA) is worse than 20/40 and/or metamorphopsia in eyes previously undergoing medical treatment as described before (topical and intravitreal steroids/anti-VEFG) [11, 13, 16, 20].

CME Secondary to VMT

The vitreous is attached to all contiguous structures of the inner eye, including the internal limiting membrane (ILM) of the retina. The concept of VMT is an abnormal adhesion of the vitreous at the macula which may result in morphological macular abnormalities. There are three basic morphological abnormalities that may be observed in such primary VMT (Fig. 5): (1) CME, (2) macular holes, and (3) epiretinal membrane and retinal swelling [11, 13, 16, 20].

In general, surgical intervention in VMT should be performed by pars plana vitrectomy (PPV) if BCVA is worse than 20/40 and/or persistent metamorphopsia with symptoms present for more than 6 months [11, 13, 16, 20].

VMT and Associated Maculopathies Epiretinal Membrane (Broad VMT; Extension > 1,500 μm)

The ERM may play an important role in chronic VMT syndrome [14, 20], mainly in broad adhesions (Fig. 3b) [21]. Partial PVD with vitreal traction can cause small splits within the ILM, allowing glial cells to gain access to the superficial retina (Fig. 2b). In these eyes, epiretinal fibroglial membranes proliferate from the retinal surface onto the back surface of the detached posterior vitreous face. This configuration imparts an increased strength of the vitreomacular adhesion and prolongs the duration of the VMT by preventing the spontaneous separation of the vitreous and the macula (Fig. 2b) [11, 13, 16]. Furthermore, the proliferative epiretinal fibroglial membranes contribute contractile forces by increasing the tangential traction via thickening and tightening of the detached posterior hyaloid and anchoring the posterior hyaloid to the surrounding retinal surface, thus enhancing the anteroposterior traction caused by the VMT adhesion [14, 20] (Fig. 6).

Macular Hole and Tractional Cystoid Macular Edema (Narrow VMT; Extension <1,500 μm)

The vitreoretinal relationship in eyes with tractional CME is similar to that seen in eyes with an early-stage idiopathic macular hole (MH) and 4A-C [15, 20–26]. The smaller the area of the foveal attachment, the greater the point force that is exerted, causing more serious disease [24]. This condition of focal adhesion, also known as vitreofoveal traction syndrome, implies an MH (Fig. 4d–f) and CME formation (4A-C) [9, 20–24]. The strong effect of narrow bands of adhesion can lead to this variant of VMT, also referred as tractional CME (Fig. 5).

Tractional CME must be distinguished from inflammatory diseases such as postoperative pseudophakic CME, retinal vascular diseases, or uveitic CME, which generally exhibits important capillary leakage on fluorescein angiography (Fig. 1a). Otherwise, tractional CME not linked with inflammation shows only minimal leakage if at all [15] (Fig. 5a–d). The reason why vitreofoveal traction leads to MH in some cases (Fig. 4d–f) and tractional CME without hole formation in other cases (Fig. 4a–c), even with time, has yet to be determined [11, 13, 15, 16].

Specific Surgical Indications for CME Associated with VMT

In narrow VMT (less than 1,500 μm), surgical intervention by pars plana vitrectomy (PPV) is indicated if BCVA is worse than 20/40 and/or persistent metamorphopsia is present with symptoms for more than 6 months [11, 13, 16] (Fig. 3).

However, it is reported that incipient eyes with narrow configurations of VMT (<1,500 μm), especially in those with CME associated with VMT, may have spontaneous resolution after complete posterior vitreous detachment (PVD). For this reason, it is especially important that surgical indications in these eyes be very well scrutinized (Figs. 3, 4, and 5) [11, 13, 16]. Normally, in such eyes, surgical consideration requires 6 months of consistently poor or decreased BCVA and vision measurement worse than 20/40 associated with complaint of metamorphopsia [11, 13, 16].

It is very important to be aware that CME is dynamic. It is not clear in the literature why spontaneous resolution of early CME associated with progression of PVD occurs and that a full-thickness macular hole may progress in eyes where tangential traction is more important. This distinct “benign” natural history (Fig. 5) or “more aggressive” outcome (Fig. 4) is probably associated with an unexplained individual trend that is not completely understood [11, 13, 16]. For this reason, surgical intervention in VMT with less than 1,500 microns of macular extension (especially the CME) should be indicated if poor BCVA is persistent for more than 6 months and/or there is an evidence of worsening by OCT and/or metamorphopsia is present.

In cases with less than 250 μm of persistent traction and no ERM is observed, the induction of PVD by ocriplasmin injection or even an intravitreal injection of air/gas may resolve VMT without necessity of surgical intervention [11, 18].

Treatment Options for CME and VMT

In a small number of cases, VMT resolves spontaneously without intervention; therefore, oligosymptomatic cases should be managed conservatively [8]. Asymptomatic ERM should be closely observed.

The primary aim of any intervention in patients with CME secondary to VMT is to release the tractional forces, thus facilitating the restoration of the macular architecture and improvement in BCVA [11, 16].

Pars plana vitrectomy (PPV) is the standard surgical approach for the treatment of VMT and ERM, and if good prognostic factors are present, treatment should be performed [11, 16]. Enhancements in intraocular illumination and wide field non-contact viewing systems have optimized the surgeon's view of the retina. Also, sutureless small gauge sclerotomy and valved trocars associated with the new fluidics of high-speed efficient cutters have reduced perioperative complications [27, 28]; additionally, chromovitrectomy has improved the intraoperative understanding of the vitreoretinal interface [16, 29, 30].

Persistent CME may lead to irreversible visual loss as a result of apoptosis of the photoreceptors [10]. In cases of extensive CME, its resolution is mandatory for the preservation of BCVA. PPV with ILM peeling has been suggested as beneficial for the rapid resolution of the retinal damage and CME in patients with VMT and ERM [8, 16]. The improvement in BCVA continues for more than 6 months, and the mean time to achieve best final vision is about 1 year [10]. Small studies have reported the use pneumatic release of VMT based on the assumption that gas induces a mechanical PVD [11, 16]; however, this is not an option in ERM cases [11, 18, 30].

Pharmacological vitreolysis has been recently advocated as an alternative treatment option for VMT, but the presence of ERM excludes the option of the use of these molecules [18]. Vitreolytic agents break down the peptide bonds in laminin and fribronectin, molecules that maintain adhesion between the posterior vitreous face and ILM. Various vitreolytic agents have been investigated, including collagenase, chondroitinase, hyaluronidase, dispase, nattokinase, plasmin, arginine–glycine–aspartate (RGD) peptides, plasminogen activators, and urea-based molecules [18].

Chromovitrectomy is a modality of treatment that includes the use of vital dyes or crystals to improve visualization of the intraocular tissues during PPV, including vitreous, ERM, and ILM. The ideal vital dyes should be safe for intraocular use, be capable of reliable and selective staining of the intraocular membrasnes, and of rapid elimination from the eye [12].

Many dyes are available for chromovitrectomy, i.e., trypan blue (TB), brilliant blue (BB), indocyanine green (ICG), infracyanine green, and lutein-associated to brilliant blue [12]. ICG is currently used to stain the internal limiting membrane

(ILM) to aid peeling, even though there are serious concerns about retinal toxicity [29]. TB is thought to be the ideal dye for ERM identification, ICG and BB are ideal for ILM peeling, and triamcinolone acetonide (TA) is useful for vitreous identification and complete separation from the ILM [29]. Despite this, the United States Food and Drug Administration has not approved any dyes for use during chromovitrectomy. Currently, BB is not approved for human use in the USA, and other agents such as ICG, TB, and TA are considered off-label drugs to be used during vitreoretinal procedures. However, BB is approved for chromovitrectomy in Europe.

It is unclear if there is an additional benefit from ILM peeling in addition to removal of the VMT and ERM, but it is commonly practiced to ensure complete removal of surface traction and avoid recurrences [6, 15, 16].

After posterior hyaloid removal, the dye should be injected gently into the vitreous cavity filled with fluid (usually balanced salt solution) and left on the retinal surface for the minimal time to allow staining (typically less than 1 min) before being washed out to reduce the possibility of toxic effects [29]. ILM/ERM membrane peeling should be performed, and following completion of vitrectomy, careful checking of the peripheral retina for retinal tears is mandatory [16, 30].

Many cases of VMT maintain good BCVA with mild metamorphopsia and do not require treatment. Some cases can resolve spontaneously with complete PVD, generally with similar favorable anatomic and functional outcomes than surgical treatment [31, 32].

However, other cases manifest poor VA and progressive macular traction which demand surgical treatment. Several investigators reported surgical outcomes associated with VMT syndrome, with improvement of VA in 44–78 % of the cases [16, 31–37]. Melberg and associates [37] obtained visual improvement in only 44 % of the eyes and attributed the limited improvement in BCVA to chronic retinal detachment, premacular fibrosis, CME, and macular schisis. However, the surgical technique was performed more than 20 years ago, and no sutureless PPV, valved trocar, fluidics, and chromovitrectomy were available at that time. Recently, data (2015) from 36 eyes with VMT subjected to PPV, ILM peeling, fluid-air exchange, and combined phaco-PPV associated showed a much better BCVA outcome [16].

Most of the authors did not address the relation between surgical outcomes and the type of vitreous adherence, probably due to it being a small case series [16, 31, 37]. Otherwise, recent studies have shown that specific preoperative OCT patterns of VMT may predict the postoperative visual improvement. Short duration of symptoms, low preoperative macular thickness, and configuration of VMT (V-shaped) shared better visual outcome after surgery [35, 36], while partial posterior vitreous detachment temporal to the fovea (J-shaped) in which prominent CME developed may result in a macular hole or macular atrophy postoperatively [36].

Despite successful relief of posterior hyaloid traction, improvement of signs and symptoms is not always achieved [11]. Usually, patients with focal VMT adhesion and V-shaped pattern have lower preoperative BCVA than those with broad adhesion and J-shaped pattern. It is important to consider that the final VA is similar between both groups, so the improvement of BCVA is higher in focal cases [16]. This also may be a consequence of the degenerative macular changes due to the chronic nature of the broad VMT type, with longer duration of symptoms and prolonged macular thickening [16].

Vitreous surgical techniques include removal of both anteroposterior and tangential tractions. It is important to consider some aspects of the surgical anatomy. In VMT, a "double layer" of preretinal proliferation can be found [16, 29]. The anterior layer may simply represent a thickened posterior hyaloid. Even a double layer of the posterior hyaloid may be found, an anatomical abnormality known as hyaloidosquisis, more frequently observed in highly myopic as well as diabetic eyes, and the use of triamcinolone acetonide are very important in order to identify this anatomical abnormality or other abnormalities of the vitreoretinal interface such as an ERM that may be present [29]. Generally, in these cases, the vitreous is tightly anchored to the foveal center, and its separation is hardly difficult, requiring the peeling of the ERM using no dyes, triamcinolone, or trypan blue before vitreofoveal separation [29]. In a few cases, the ERM and ILM must be peeled "en block" using brilliant blue; in all VMT cases, we suggest to use the triamcinolone for posterior hyaloid identification and, at the end of the surgery, brilliant blue staining for ILM identification and peeling [16, 29].

Surgical Technique for Management of CME Associated with VMT

In both cases (CME secondary to either intraocular surgery due to cytokine release or secondary to VMT), our preferred surgical technique for management of CME is similar: a four-port pars plana vitrectomy (PPV), vitreous base identification, and shaving using preservative-free triamcinolone acetonide (TA) as well as identification of possible retinal tears at the periphery by indentation of vitreous base and removal of all possible tractional components from the iris root/intraocular lens (IOL) [16]. Posterior hyaloid identification and removal (if attached) should be performed using TA. ERM removal should be performed using no dyes (Fig. 7), a higher amount of TA, or even trypan blue if difficulties arise in identification [16].

Despite controversies in the literature, we believe the ILM should be peeled in all cases [16]. Staining with brilliant blue (BB) should be employed (Fig. 8a); however, many techniques may be used to complete this surgical step (Table 1) [29]. It is very common to identify tears at the ILM (Fig. 8b) that are difficult to observe during surgery [30]. These tears work as a scaffold for astrocytes migration and metaplasia to myofibroblasts with contractile properties and result in re-proliferation of the epiretinal tissue and recurrence of the epiretinal membrane (Fig. 6) [11, 16, 30]. The surgeon should complete the ILM peeling over the entire macular area (Fig. 8c–e). During this maneuver, the surgeon may "unroof" the cystic changes, and an iatrogenic

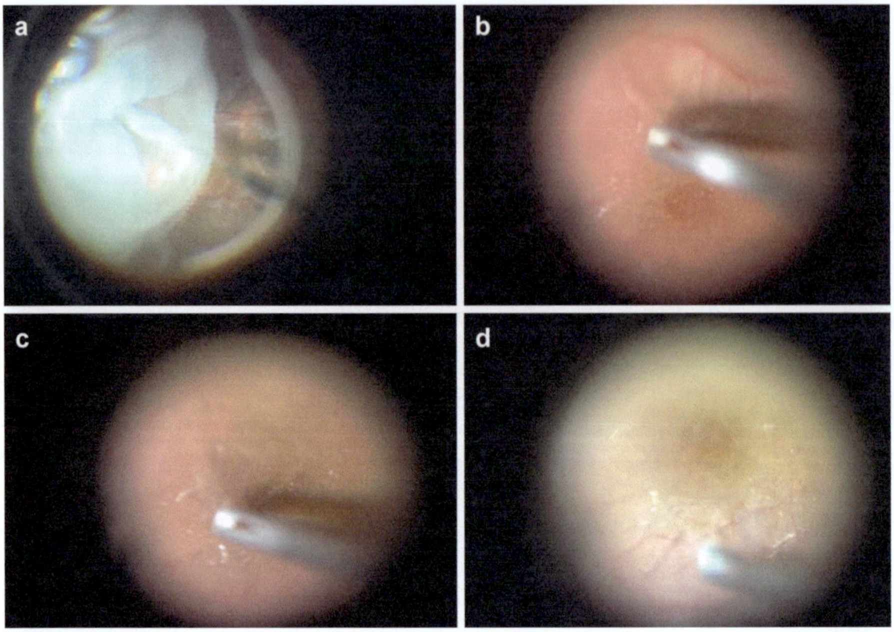

Fig. 7 Chromovitrectomy applied to cystoid macular edema (CME) and ERM formation in Irvine-Gass syndrome after cataract surgery in a proliferative diabetic retinopathy systemic under local as well as systemic control of the disease. The focus is the posterior hyaloid and ERM visualization by deposition of triamcinolone crystals. (**a**) 0.3 ml of preservative-free triamcinolone acetonide (40 mg/ml) injection to identify the vitreoretinal interface after core vitrectomy, posterior hyaloid detachment, and shaving of the vitreous base, (**b**) initial phase of epiretinal membrane (ERM) peeling in an eye with cystoid macular edema, (**c**) intermediate phase of ERM peeling in CME. Note that ERM is thick, and the endgrip forceps must grasp the base of ERM in order to avoid tearing, and (**d**) late phase of ERM peeling in CME. Note that cystic changes are observed in the center of the surgical field. The maneuver to grasp the base of the ERM sometimes is necessary many times for a successful surgical procedure

macular hole may develop [16]; in these cases, fluid-air exchange with filtered air or SF_6 20 % or C_3F_8 15 % should be used as a vitreous substitute following surgeon's preference [16]; prone positioning (3–7 days) is controversial and is not used by our team, except for specific cases, particularly chronic macular holes or persistent iatrogenic holes after surgery. Therefore, fluid-air exchange and air injection at the vitreous cavity (Fig. 8f) are important for the management of CME associated with VMT and should be used in two situations: (1) if the intraoperative manipulation of the macular area is very intense and/or (2) if intraoperative observation of iatrogenic of macular holes [16]. No prone positioning is required after surgery; however, patients may be aware that BCVA will be worse than before the surgical procedure for around 5–7 days (until the intravitreal air/gas bubble is reabsorbed). We particularly advise patients not be placed in prone positioning, and the use of C_3F_8 15 % if macular hole is present along with a history of more than 1 week of decrease in BCVA, even though this is still a controversial subject in the literature [16].

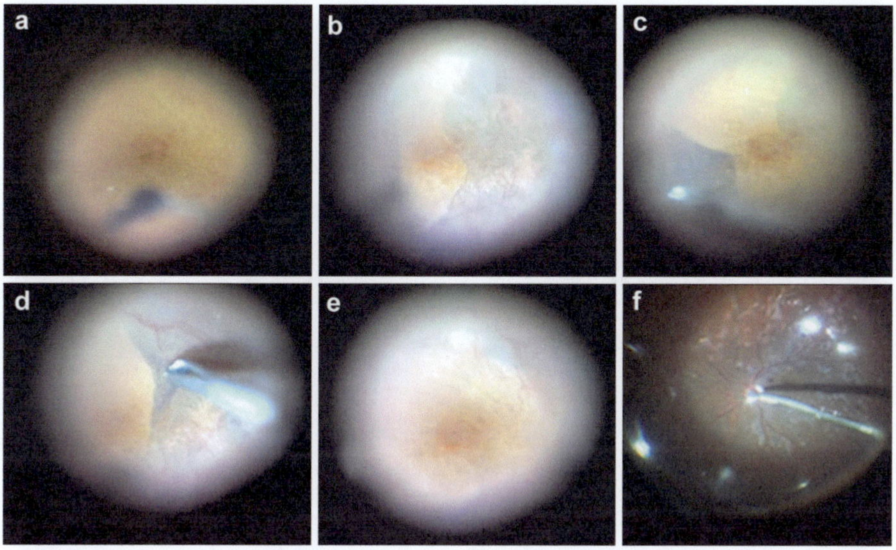

Fig. 8 Chromovitrectomy applied to cystoid macular edema (CME) and ERM formation in Irvine-Gass syndrome after cataract surgery in a proliferative diabetic retinopathy under local as well as systemic control of the disease. The focus is the internal limiting membrane (ILM) identification. (**a**) 0.1 ml of brilliant blue (0.5 mg/ml) injection to identify the ILM after epiretinal membrane (ERM) peeling, (**b**) note the brilliant blue staining of the ILM. A tear at the ILM is observed (unstained retina) just after ERM peeling to the tight adhesion of the previous ERM through the ILM, (**c**) initial phase of ILM peeling in CME. The ILM is also thick, and the endgrip forceps must grasp the base of the ILM tissue in order to avoid tearing, (**d**) final phase of ILM peeling in CME. Note that cystic changes are observed in the center of the surgical field. The maneuver to grasp the base of the ERM sometimes is necessary many times for a successful surgical procedure because the ILM is very friable, (**e**) final aspect of the macula with the cystic changes after ILM peeling, and (**f**) fluid-air exchange and filtered air injection at the vitreous cavity were performed. No prone positioning was indicated

Complications of PPV

PPV for VMT or ERM is a safe procedure, with low rates of complications. Intraoperative complications include vitreous hemorrhage, retinal surface damage, and peripheral iatrogenic retinal breaks [27–30]. Most can be successfully managed if promptly identified intraoperatively. Complications after PPV include formation or progression of preexisting cataract, corneal decompensation, development or recurrence of ERM, retinal detachment, glaucoma, development of a macular hole, macular ischemia, rubeosis iridis, and neovascular glaucoma [6, 11].

Vitrectomy can be incomplete, leaving remnants of vitreous cortex on the ILM, with consequences such as persistent traction and/or renewed proliferation of cells at the vitreoretinal interface which may lead to later recurrent traction [11, 16, 30]. Superficial retinal hemorrhages are common after ILM peeling, although they do not seem to be visually significant in most cases [16].

Table 1 Comparison of substances currently used in chromovitrectomy [24]

Substance	Dilution/osmolarity	Affinity for intraocular structures	Avoiding RPE/retina toxicity	High cost	Chemical properties
Triamcinolone acetonide 40 mg/ml 4 %	No dilution	Vitreous	Use a preservative-free solution	+	Triamcinolone is a synthetic nonsoluble steroid (C24H31FO6; 434 daltons)
Trypan blue 1.2 mg/ml 0.12 %	No dilution or mix with glucose 1.2 mg/ml (0.12 %)/310 mOsm	ERM	Use with no dilution or mix 0.3 ml with 0.1 ml glucose 5 % for better ERM identification	+	Trypan blue is an anionic hydrophilic azo dye (C34H24N6Na4O14S4; 960 daltons)
Patent blue 2.5 mg/ml 0.25 %	No dilution or mix with glucose 2.5 mg/ml (0.25 %)/290 mOsm	ERM	Use with no dilution or mix 0.3 ml with 0.1 ml glucose 5 % for better ERM identification	++	Patent blue is a triarylmethane dye (C27H31N2NaO6S2; 582 daltons)
Brilliant blue 0.25 mg/ml 0.025 %	No dilution/280 mOsm	ILM	Use with dilution	+++	Brilliant blue is a blue anionic aminotriarylmethane compound (C47H48N3S2O7Na; 854 daltons)
Indocyanine green 5 mg, 0.5 %; 25 mg, 2.5 %; 50 mg, 5.0 %	Less than 0.5 mg/ml (0.05 %) Dissolve in small amount of distilled water Dilution: use large amount of BSS	ILM	Add 1 ml distilled water to 1 vial 5 mg Take 0.1 ml of the solution and mix with 0.9 ml BSS	++++	Indocyanine green is a tricarbocyanine dye (C43H47N2NaO6S2; 775 daltons) and contains 3–5 % iodine
Infracyanine green 5 mg, 0.5 %, 25 mg, 2.5 %	Less than 0.5 mg/ml (0.05 %) Dissolve in glucose 5 %/290 mOsm	ILM	Add 1 or 2 ml glucose 5 % to 1 vial of 5 mg	+++++	Infracyanine green has the same chemical formula as ICG but contains no sodium iodine

BSS balanced salt solution, *ERM* epiretinal membrane, *ICG* indocyanine green, *ILM* internal limiting membrane, *RPE* retinal pigment epithelium

Interaction of light from endoillumination source and vital dye may increase or decrease the risk of toxicity. Light-induced retinal toxicity by the endoilluminator is dependent on factors such as the duration of use, type, power, and wavelength of light source [29]. Photosensitizing dyes could enhance phototoxicity by increasing levels of free radicals, creating a photoproduct that could be harmful to retinal cells. We suggest shifting light absorbance from one site of the retina to another [16].

CME and VMT Syndrome: New Concepts

A joint study (Barraquer Institute, Barcelona, Spain, and Federal University of Sao Paulo, Sao Paulo, Brazil) analyzed a variety of vitreomacular traction (VMT) morphologies to establish a major classification that could reflect the preoperative predictive factors of postoperative visual and anatomic outcomes [16]. In this series, 36 eyes submitted to vitrectomy and internal limiting membrane (ILM) peeling were categorized with a VMT pattern (V- or J-shaped) and diameter (focal $\leq$ 1,500 μm or broad > 1,500 μm) based on optical coherence tomography [16].

Different classifications of VMT were compared. Despite similar postoperative best-corrected visual acuity (BCVA) values ($P = 0.393$), cases with focal VMT had greater visual improvement ($P = 0.027$); however, the BCVA improvements did not differ between the groups regarding the classic VMT morphologic patterns: V-shaped and J-shaped ($P = 0.235$) [16].

This study concluded that postoperative outcomes and macular disorders are closely related to VMT size. The adhesion diameter (focal or broad VMT) and not the classic VMT morphologic pattern (V- or J-shaped) may better predict the postoperative anatomic and functional outcomes, and this is used in clinical practice [16].

Conclusions

VMT syndrome is implicated in the pathophysiology of a number of macular disorders, with variable anatomical and function outcomes which underscore the complexity of the disease. These macular changes are intimately related to the VMT configuration, which led to proposals for classification of this syndrome, based on OCT findings [11, 13, 16].

Moreover, the size and strength of the remaining vitreomacular attachment may define the specific maculopathy. Focal VMT usually leads to MH formation, tractional CME, and foveal retinal detachment, while broad VMT is widely associated with ERM, diffuse retinal thickening, and poorer recovery of foveal depression [11, 13, 16].

Future Perspectives

There are several unanswered questions in relation to vitreomacular adhesion. One of the most interesting ones is relating to the role of pharmacologic vitreolysis; positive results from trials have made ocriplasmin a promising pharmacologic agent for the treatment of VMT [18]. Its indication, however, is limited to selected cases and not for ERM. Ongoing studies that should be launched soon will certainly help address safety issues and results by specifying the patients that could benefit from this approach [18].

The field of vital dyes used for chromovitrectomy is extensive and is constantly undergoing improvement [12, 29]. New vital dyes associated with lutein have been tested as well as other dyes in different concentrations and methodologies, with multiple experimental studies and clinical trials underway [12].

References

1. Duker JS, Kaiser PK, Binder S, de Smet MD, Gaudric A, Reichel E, et al. The International Vitreomacular Traction Study Group classification of vitreomacular adhesion, traction, and macular hole. Ophthalmology. 2013;120(12):2611–9.
2. Stalmans P, Duker JS, Kaiser PK, Heier JS, Dugel PU, Gandorfer A, et al. Oct-based interpretation of the vitreomacular interface and indications for pharmacologic vitreolysis. Retina. 2013;33(10):2003–11.
3. Trese MT, Chandler DB, Machemer R, Macular pucker I. Prognostic criteria. Graefe's archive for clinical and experimental ophthalmology = Albrecht von Graefes Archiv fur klinische und experimentelle Ophthalmologie. 1983;221(1):12–5.
4. Vane J, Botting R. Inflammation and the mechanism of action of anti-inflammatory drugs. FASEB J. 1987;1(2):89–96.
5. Reese AB, Jones IS, Cooper WC. Vitreomacular traction syndrome confirmed histologically. Am J Ophthalmol. 1970;69(6):975–7.
6. Steel DH, Lotery AJ. Idiopathic vitreomacular traction and macular hole: a comprehensive review of pathophysiology, diagnosis, and treatment. Eye. 2013;27 Suppl 1:S1–21.
7. Odrobina D, Michalewska Z, Michalewski J, Dziegielewski K, Nawrocki J. Long-term evaluation of vitreomacular traction disorder in spectral-domain optical coherence tomography. Retina. 2011;31(2):324–31.
8. McDonald HR, Johnson RN, Schatz H. Surgical results in the vitreomacular traction syndrome. Ophthalmology. 1994;101(8):1397–402; discussion 1403.
9. Yonemoto J, et al. The age of onset of posterior vitreous detachment. Graefes Arch Clin Exp Ophthalmol. 1994;232(2):67–70.
10. Golan S, Loewenstein A. Surgical treatment for macular edema. Semin Ophthalmol. 2014;29(4):242–56.
11. Bottós JM, Elizalde J, Rodrigues EB, Maia M. Current concepts in vitreomacular traction syndrome. Curr Opin Ophthalmol. 2012;23(3):195–201.
12. Maia M, Furlani BA, Souza-Lima AA, Martins DS, Navarro RM, Belfort Jr R. Lutein: a new dye for chromovitrectomy. Retina. 2014;34(2):262–72.
13. Bottós J, Elizalde J, Rodrigues EB, Farah M, Maia M. Classifications of vitreomacular traction syndrome: diameter vs morphology. Eye (Lond). 2014;28(9):1107–12.

14. Schneider EW, Johnson MW. Emerging nonsurgical methods for the treatment of vitreomacular adhesion: a review. Clin Ophthalmol. 2011;5:1151–65.
15. Jackson TL, Nicod E, Simpson A, et al. Symptomatic vitreomacular adhesion. Retina. 2013;33(8):1503–11.
16. Bottós J, Elizalde J, Rodrigues EB, Farah M, Maia M. Classifications of vitreomacular traction syndrome: diameter vs morphology. Eye (Lond). 2014;28(9):1107–12. doi: 10.1038/eye.2014.128. Epub 2014 Jul 4.
17. Smiddy WE, et al. Vitrectomy for macular traction caused by incomplete vitreous separation. Arch Ophthalmol. 1988;106(5):624–8.
18. Stefanini FR, Maia M, Falabella P, et al. Profile of ocriplasmin and its potential in the treatment of vitreomacular adhesion. Clin Ophthalmol. 2014;8:847–56.
19. Chang LK, et al. Ultrastructural correlation of spectral-domain optical coherence tomographic findings in vitreomacular traction syndrome. Am J Ophthalmol. 2008;146(1):121–7.
20. Sebag J. Anatomy and pathology of the vitreo-retinal interface. Eye (Lond). 1992;6(Pt 6):541–52.
21. Smiddy WE, et al. Ultrastructural studies of vitreomacular traction.
22. Smiddy WE, Green WR, Michels RG, de la Cruz Z. Ultrastructural studies of vitreomacular traction syndrome. Am J Ophthalmol. 1989;107(2):177–85.
23. Smiddy WE, Michels RG, Green WR. Morphology, pathology, and surgery of idiopathic vitreoretinal macular disorders. A review. Retina. 1990;10(4):288–96.
24. Spaide RF, et al. Correlation of vitreous attachment and foveal deformation in early macular hole states. Am J Ophthalmol. 2002;133(2):226–9.
25. Smiddy WE, et al. Ultrastructural studies of vitreomacular traction syndrome. Am J Ophthalmol. 1989;107(2):177–85.
26. Johnson MW, Van Newkirk MR, Meyer KA. Perifoveal vitreous detachment is the primary pathogenic event in idiopathic macular hole formation. Arch Ophthalmol. 2001;119(2):215–22.
27. Brant Fernandes RA, Diniz B, Falabella P, Humayun MS, et al. Fluidics comparison between dual pneumatic and spring return high-speed vitrectomy systems. Ophthamo Surg Lasers Imaging Retina. 2015;46(1):68–72.
28. Magalhães Jr O, Maia M, Rodrigues EB, et al. Perspective on fluid and solid dynamics in different pars plana vitrectomy systems. Am J Ophthalmol. 2011;151(3):401–5.
29. Farah ME, Maia M, Rodrigues EB. Dyes in ocular surgery: principles for use in chromovitrectomy. Am J Ophthalmol. 2009;148(3):332–40.
30. Carpentier C, Zanolli M, Wu L, Sepulveda G, et al. Residual internal limiting membrane after epiretinal membrane peeling: results of the Pan-American Collaborative Retina Study Group. Retina. 2013;33(10):2026–31.
31. Kusaka S, et al. Optical coherence tomography in spontaneously resolving vitreomacular traction syndrome. Ophthalmologica. 2001;215(2):139–41.
32. Sulkes DJ, et al. Spontaneous resolution of vitreomacular traction documented by optical coherence tomography. Arch Ophthalmol. 2000;118(2):286–7.
33. Chen TC, et al. Spectral domain optical coherence tomography: ultra-high speed, ultra-high resolution ophthalmic imaging. Arch Ophthalmol. 2005;123(12):1715–20.
34. Witkin AJ, et al. Anatomic and visual outcomes of vitrectomy for vitreomacular traction syndrome. Ophthalmic Surg Lasers Imaging. 2010;41(4):425–31.
35. Sonmez K, et al. Vitreomacular traction syndrome: impact of anatomical configuration on anatomical and visual outcomes. Retina. 2008;28(9):1207–14.
36. Yamada N, Kishi S. Tomographic features and surgical outcomes of vitreomacular traction syndrome. Am J Ophthalmol. 2005;139(1):112–7.
37. Melberg NS, et al. Vitrectomy for vitreomacular traction syndrome with macular detachment. Retina. 1995;15(3):192–7.

Chapter 12
Surgical Management of Cystoid Macular Edema Associated with Retinal Vascular Occlusions

Ahmet M. Hondur and Tongalp H. Tezel

Retinal Arterial Occlusions

Central Retinal Artery Occlusion

Central retinal artery occlusion leads to a sudden blockage of blood supply to inner retina, resulting in severe vision loss. It is an ophthalmic emergency and widely accepted to be the ocular analogue of acute ischemic cerebral stroke. The risk factors are similar to cerebral stroke and ischemic heart disease [1].

The incidence of acute central retinal artery occlusion is 0.85/100,000 per year. It accounts for 1.13 cases in 10,000 ophthalmological outpatient visits and 57 % of all acute retinal artery obstructions [2, 3].

Although central retinal artery occlusion clinically resembles ischemic cerebral stroke, there are several etio-pathogenic differences. Nearly 80 % of cerebral strokes are ischemic in nature and occur due to the stagnation of blood flow within a cerebral artery secondary to a thrombus or embolus. The remaining 20 % are hemorrhagic strokes and as the name implies develops secondary to a cerebral hemorrhage. Analysis of thrombi retrieved from cerebral arteries of patients with acute ischemic stroke revealed that most thrombi were composed of fibrin and platelets. This observation provides the basis for thrombolytic treatment in ischemic stroke [4].

On the other hand, 74 % of the emboli that cause central retinal artery occlusion are made of cholesterol (Hollenhorst plaques) and only 15.5 % of them are

A.M. Hondur, MD
Department of Ophthalmology, School of Medicine, Gazi University, Besevler, Ankara 06500, Turkey
e-mail: ahondur@gazi.edu.tr

T.H. Tezel, MD (✉)
Department of Ophthalmology, Columbia University College of Physicians and Surgeons, Edward S. Harkness Eye Institute, Columbia University Medical Center, 635 West 165th Street, Box 38, New York 10032, NY, USA

S. Schaal, H.J. Kaplan (eds.), *Cystoid Macular Edema*,
DOI 10.1007/978-3-319-39766-5_12

fibrin-platelet in nature. The remaining 10.5 % are calcific emboli [5]. Hence, only a small percentage of retinal arterial emboli may respond to thrombolytic treatment.

In spite of its embolic etiology, visible emboli can only be seen in 20–40 % of eyes with central retinal artery occlusion [6, 7]. This may be due to the fact that the embolus usually blocks the central retinal artery where it pierces the dural sheath of the optic nerve. The lumen of the artery is at its narrowest at this site, however, it cannot be seen clinically [8]. Fragmentation and distal migration may also cause emboli to not be clinically visible [6].

Transient occlusion of central retinal artery has also been described. Such transient events have been attributed to the dislodging of emboli, vasospasm of the central retinal artery, or transient compromise of the blood flow due to nocturnal hypotension [9–11].

Clinically central retinal artery occlusion can be subgrouped into four different entities [12]:

(i) Non-arteritic permanent central retinal artery occlusion
(ii) Non-arteritic transient central retinal artery occlusion
(iii) Non-arteritic central retinal artery occlusion with cilioretinal sparing
(iv) Arteritic central retinal artery occlusion

There is a "presumed" critical period after the occlusion of the central retinal artery beyond which permanent visual loss occurs. If blockage is removed within this period and blood supply is restored, full visual recovery is possible. Classical knowledge obtained from experiments in old atherosclerotic hypertensive rhesus monkeys indicates that no detectable damage occurs in the retina within the first 97 min after clamping central retinal artery. However, retinal damage becomes massive and irreversible after 240 min [13].

Partial recovery of central vision beyond the described experimental critical period has been reported in patients with non-arteritic permanent central retinal artery occlusion [12, 14, 15]. A simple explanation can be incomplete closure of central retinal artery in such cases [16]. However, discrepancies between the animal model and human disease can also be explained by the failure of central artery clamping to mimic all aspects of central retinal artery occlusion in patients. A recent case series revealed that immediate vitrectomy with or without manual dislodging of the embolus may improve all patients' central visual acuity by more than three Snellen lines and result in 20/40 or better visual acuity in 44 % of the patients. Rapid alleviation of the cytotoxic retinal edema and increased oxygenation of the retinal penumbra were proposed to explain the visual recovery [17]. This study demonstrates that in patients with central retinal artery occlusion, retinal cell death does not solely occur as a result of acute ischemia but also due to secondary events that follow the ischemic episode, such as cytotoxic cell edema. Inner retinal edema develops in all cases with total occlusion with disorganization of inner retinal layers in 77 % of the patients (Fig. 1). The amount of inner retinal edema is a major factor determining the functional outcome of central retinal artery occlusion and plays a more important role than the time to presentation [18]. This indicates that apart from

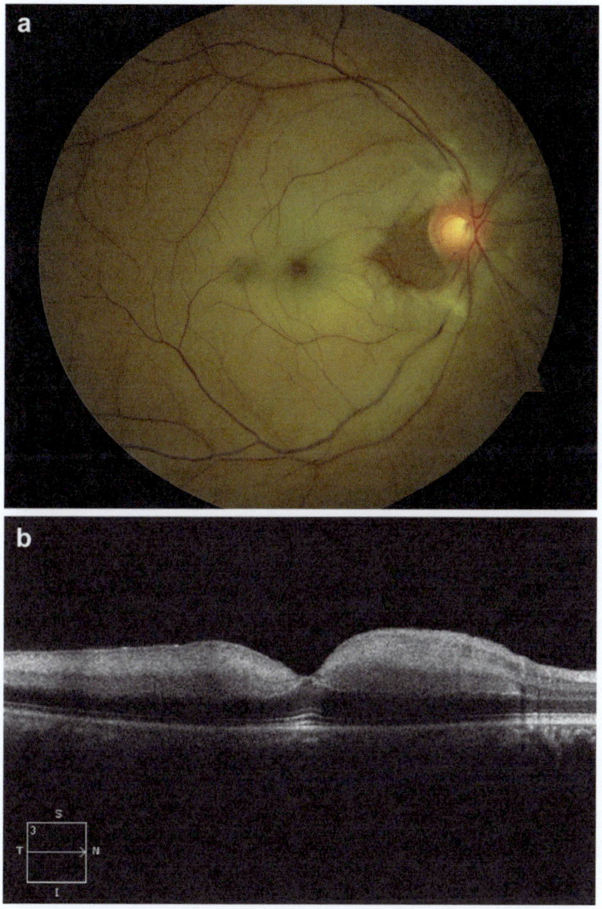

Fig. 1 Forty-seven-year-old patient with central retinal artery occlusion. The patient's visual acuity is at light perception level. (**a**) Fundus exam revels typical whitening of the retina and cherry-red spot. (**b**) A HD-OCT scan reveals hyperreflectivity of the inner retina due to the edema and opacification of the inner retinal layers and cessation of the axoplasmic transport

acute ischemia, there are several secondary events that play a role in inner retinal neuronal loss. In order to comprehend the role of vitrectomy, response of retinal neurons to ischemia has to be reviewed. Once the oxygen saturation starts to drop, inner retinal neurons shut down their excessive metabolic activities to adapt to hypoxic environment. They initiate anaerobic metabolism, increase synthesis of neuroprotective proteins and chaperones, and halt several ATP-consuming processes including the visual cycle. This vegetative state can allow retinal neurons to survive in the hypoxic milieu. Maintenance of viability even in a vegetative state also requires a low but continuous flow of oxygen that is required to maintain basic metabolic needs. Diffusion of oxygen through intact choroid is the most possible source for this limited but vital amount of oxygen. A compensatory increase in choroidal blood flow has been observed in central retinal artery occlusion. The biological effect of oxygen diffusion from the choroid is clinically evident with the intact peripheral visual fields in central retinal artery occlusion where oxygen from the choroid can easily diffuse through the thin peripheral retina to supply adequate oxygen for retinal cell survival. However, the retina is thickest at the perifovea and thus does not allow diffused choroidal oxygen to reach levels as high as in the periphery. Also, the relatively crowded arrangement of retinal neurons aggravates compressional cell death once cytotoxic edema develops. For these reasons, visual field defects manifest most commonly as central scotoma in central retinal artery occlusion. If left untreated, prolonged hypoxia eventually shuts down the energy-dependent ionic pumps and leads to sodium and water leakage into the cell. Hydrops of the retinal neurons finally causes cell rupture and death. Restoration of retinal perfusion before cytotoxic cell edema leads to irreversible neuronal loss can preserve the central vision. Thus the surgical treatment of the central retinal artery occlusion should aim to restore retinal oxygenation either by reestablishing retinal blood flow or by removing the vitreous and elevating preretinal oxygen tension with convectional oxygen currents. Increased oxygenation will initiate full metabolic activity, resolve intracellular edema, and help remaining retinal neurons regain their function. Side benefits of vitrectomy may include removal of inflammatory and pro-apoptotic chemokines, and decreased N-methyl-D-aspartate (NMDA) induced cell death with intravitreal injection of triamcinolone acetonide.

Several other surgical approaches have been attempted to restore the blood flow in central retinal artery occlusion after the failure of medical treatments [19, 20]. The surgical goal has traditionally been to destroy, remove, or dislodge the visible embolus. Thus, traditional surgical approaches aim to address only 20–40 % of the non-arteritic central retinal artery occlusions where the embolus is visible [6, 7].

These traditional surgical approaches are:

(i) Local intra-arterial fibrinolysis
(ii) Neodymium:yttrium-aluminum-garnet (Nd:YAG) embolysis and embolectomy
(iii) Surgical embolectomy
(iv) Surgical cannulation of the central retinal artery

Local intra-arterial fibrinolysis involves local infusion of a fibrinolytic agent, such as urokinase or recombinant tissue plasminogen activator (rt-PA), at the site of occlusion via catheterization of the ophthalmic artery. Although several retrospective reports claimed functional outcomes better than natural history, the recent report of the European Assessment Group for Lysis in the Eye (EAGLE) proved otherwise [21]. In this prospective and randomized multicenter study, patients between the ages of 18 and 75 years who had acute central retinal artery occlusion of less than 20 h onset with a presenting visual acuity of less than 0.32 were randomly assigned to receive either intra-arterial 50 mg recombinant tissue plasminogen activator or a conservative therapy including massage of the eye, topical beta-blocker, acetazolamide, aspirin, heparin, and isovolemic hemodilution. The primary end point was best corrected visual acuity at 1 month. The study was halted after the first interim analysis because similar outcomes were seen in both groups, with an increased risk of complications in the local intra-arterial fibrinolysis group, such as stroke, transient ischemic attacks, aphasia, and hemiparesis [22]. The conclusion of the study was to not recommend local intra-arterial fibrinolysis in treatment of acute central retinal artery occlusion.

Opremcak and Benner were the first to describe the use of Nd:YAG laser to break the intraluminal embolus and dislodge it distally to restore the blood flow in branch retinal artery occlusion [23]. Their technique was subsequently modified by Reynard and Hanscom, to make a small arteriotomy through which the embolus leaves the arterial lumen into the vitreous [24].

Later Opremcak and colleagues reported a case series of ten eyes with central retinal artery occlusion treated with Nd:YAG laser and named the technique "transluminal Nd:YAG embolysis and embolectomy," depending on whether the embolus was fragmented or moved to the vitreous, respectively [25]. The median energy employed was 1 mJ, with an average energy per pulse at 2.4 mJ (range, 0.3–9 mJ). Restoration of retinal blood flow was noted in all eyes; however, intraoperative complications as vitreous or subhyaloid hemorrhage were noted in five (50 %) patients, which mostly required pars plana vitrectomy. Visual acuity improved with an average of 4.8 Snellen lines gained including the eyes that underwent vitrectomy. However, this technique was not extensively embraced due to failure to reproduce similar results, limited effectiveness, and high complication rates [26].

After the report of successful surgical removal of a branch retinal artery embolus [27], there have been attempts of surgical embolectomy for central retinal artery occlusion [26, 28]. With this technique, following standard three-port pars plana vitrectomy with removal of posterior hyaloid, the artery is reached and dissected with a microvitreoretinal blade or bent needle tip, and the plaque is dislodged into the vitreous cavity spontaneously or removed with a vitreoretinal forceps. In case of arterial bleeding, hemostasis is obtained by increasing the intraocular pressure. Although bleeding was a common complication, authors noted that occasionally vasospasm closed the incision. This procedure was also performed with transconjunctival sutureless small-gauge pars plana vitrectomy [28]. However, none of the operated eyes improved beyond counting fingers [26, 28]. Currently, a prospective multicenter study has been recruiting patients to determine whether surgical embolectomy results in better functional outcome compared with natural history [29].

Tang and Topping reported a single case treated with surgical cannulation of the central retinal artery [30]. After vitrectomy, they penetrated the central bifurcation of the central retinal artery with a microvitreoretinal blade and cannulated the central retinal artery for a length of 3.5 mm with a 50-gauge nickel titanium flexible stylet. They moved the stylet forward and backward with circular motions and observed emergence of a small clot. An improvement in visual acuity from counting fingers to 20/25 at 4 months was noted.

In a recent study, the effectiveness and safety of vitrectomy with and without manual dislodging of the embolus was reported [17]. In this case series of 18 eyes with non-arteritic central retinal artery occlusion, immediate 25-gauge pars plana vitrectomy with posterior hyaloid separation and manual dislodging of the embolus was performed within 36 ± 25 h (range: 6–72 h) of the onset of the symptoms.

Intraoperative restoration of the retinal blood flow along with rapid disappearance of the macular edema was observed in all patients. Visual acuity improved more than three lines in all eyes. At 2 weeks, eight patients (44.4 %) were able to see 20/40 or better, whereas visual acuity remained below 20/200 in another eight patients (44.4 %). No significant visual acuity changes were observed after the second postoperative week for up to 12 months. Results of this study indicate that immediate vitrectomy can result in partial restoration of foveal vision in central retinal artery occlusion.

Branch Retinal Artery Occlusion

Branch retinal artery occlusion results in less severe loss of vision compared to central retinal artery occlusion. An embolic event with underlying atherosclerosis is almost always the cause apart from arteritic cilioretinal artery occlusion. Central and branch retinal artery occlusions share the same risk factors. Branch retinal artery occlusion represents 38 % of all acute retinal artery obstructions [2].

Actually, the so-called branch retinal arteries are arterioles; hence, the widely used term of "branch retinal artery occlusion" is a misnomer. Their diameter close to the optic disc is about 100 μm, which is typical for an arteriole. In addition, unlike arteries, they possess neither an internal elastic lamina nor a continuous muscular coat. Therefore, they are not affected by giant cell arteritis [31].

Branch retinal artery occlusion has been divided into three subclasses:

(i) Permanent branch retinal artery occlusion
(ii) Transient branch retinal artery occlusion
(iii) Cilioretinal artery occlusion

  (a) Non-arteritic cilioretinal artery occlusion alone
  (b) Non-arteritic cilioretinal artery occlusion with retinal vein occlusion
  (c) Arteritic cilioretinal artery occlusion

Visible emboli in branch retinal arteries can be observed much more often in branch retinal artery occlusion than in patients with central retinal artery occlusion [32, 33].

The visual prognosis in branch retinal artery occlusion is generally favorable, with final visual acuity of 20/40 or better in 80–90 % of eyes [34, 35]. Some degree of macular perfusion through contralateral temporal branch can prolong the critical period for retinal survival and increase the chance for spontaneous visual recovery in branch retinal artery occlusion [26, 36]. Aggressive therapy is required for branch retinal artery occlusion cases involving the fovea [31].

Two surgical treatment modalities for branch retinal artery occlusion have been described:

(i) Surgical embolectomy
(ii) Nd:YAG embolysis and embolectomy

Surgical removal and intravascular fragmentation of an embolus in a branch retinal arteriole was first described by Peyman and Gremillion [27]. Despite the surgical procedure being done 60 h after the onset of the occlusion, visual acuity of their patient improved from counting fingers to 20/200. The gain in visual acuity was also observed in a following case series where six patients underwent surgical embolectomy within 20.5 h (range 4–33 h) of the occlusion [26]. However, these results may not be any better than the natural course of branch retinal artery occlusion [36].

Opremcak and Benner described Nd:YAG laser embolysis in nine patients [23, 25]. Three patients (33 %) experienced dense vitreous hemorrhage that required vitrectomy to clear the blood. Overall, VA improved an average of 4.67 Snellen lines [25]. The functional outcome of this study is also no different than the natural course of the branch retinal artery occlusion. Moreover, serious complications such as subretinal hemorrhage, retinal tears, choroidal neovascularization, and epiretinal proliferation can occur during or after Nd:YAG laser embolysis [37].

Retinal Venous Occlusions

Central and branch retinal vein occlusions are common causes of vision loss in the elderly and the second most common retinal vascular disease after diabetic retinopathy. Their prevalence is 1–2 % in people older than 40 years of age, with branch retinal vein occlusion being four times as common as central retinal vein occlusion [38–40].

Retinal vein occlusions are classified into two major subclasses:

(i) Central retinal vein occlusion
   - (a) Ischemic
   - (b) Nonischemic

(ii) Branch retinal vein occlusion
   - (a) Ischemic
   - (b) Nonischemic

Hemicentral retinal vein occlusion is a rare and a unique condition where one of the two trunks of the central retinal vein is occluded [41]. Its clinical features resemble those of a central retinal vein occlusion. Macular branch vein occlusion is another subset of branch retinal vein occlusion, where a small branch that drains a part of the macula is affected. Macular branch vein occlusion shows different characteristics than branch retinal vein occlusion. It is not associated with subsequent retinal neovascularization; complications such as macular edema and hemorrhages are less common, resolve earlier [42], and respond to vitrectomy better [43].

All retinal vein occlusion have thrombotic etiologies. The pathogenesis of retinal vein occlusion has been described to follow the principles of thrombogenesis, involving hemodynamic changes (stasis, turbulence) and endothelial injury [44].

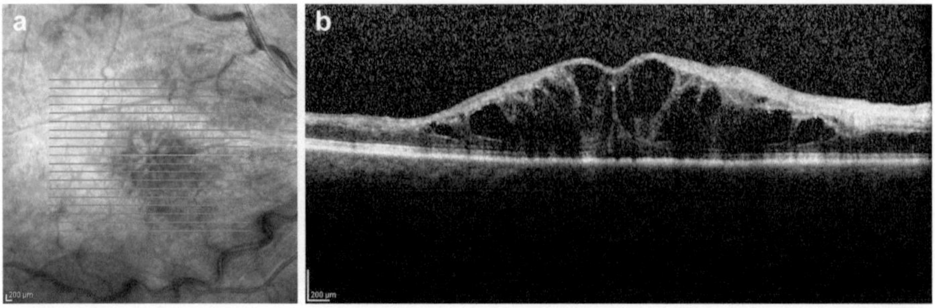

Fig. 2 Seventy-three-year-old male patient with central retinal vein occlusion. (**a**) Posterior segment exam reveals tortuous veins and petaloid appearance of cystoid macular edema. (**b**) Horizontal OCT scan crossing the foveola shows "volcano-style" cystoid macular edema. Note that some of the Muller cell columns have already broken up, allowing lateral spread of the intraretinal fluid indicating the chronicity of the edema

The vein is believed to become narrowed at an arteriovenous crossing point due to compression from the neighboring atherosclerotic artery, where both vessels share the same adventitial sheath. The blood flow in the vein becomes turbulent at the constriction, which inevitably causes endothelial cell damage and death, exposing subendothelial matrix and leading to formation of a clot [45]. Although both branch and central retinal vein occlusions are thrombotic processes, the impact of local and systemic factors in predisposing to these conditions is quite different. For example, increased blood pressure, hyperopia, and atherosclerosis are more common in branch retinal vein occlusion patients, whereas high intraocular pressure seems to play a more important role in the development of central retinal vein occlusion [46]. Such differences also exist in the natural history and therapeutic response of both pathologies [47].

A variety of hematologic risk factors for general venous thrombosis have been observed to occur sporadically in retinal vein occlusions. It was concluded that they do not play a major importance in the pathophysiology of retinal vein occlusion [48, 49].

Retinal vein occlusion results in delay in retinal blood flow through the occluded segment, which in turn leads to macular ischemia and/or edema, two major causes of loss of visual acuity. Increased hydrostatic pressure, ischemia-induced vascular endothelial growth factor upregulation, and inflammation are the major causes of cystoid macular edema in retinal vein occlusion [50, 51]. Moderate to severe macular edema is a part of the clinical picture in 87 % of the central retina vein occlusions (Fig. 2) [52], 51 % of the branch retinal vein occlusions (Fig. 3), and 29 % of the macular branch vein occlusions. It resolves in 51 % of the cases in 2 years [42, 52]. Short duration of macular edema is known to be associated with favorable visual outcome in retinal vein occlusions [53]. Results from various studies have shown that macular edema can be controlled with intraocular injections of anti-vascular endothelial growth factor agents and/or steroid implants [54–56]. Despite good initial response, several intravitreal injections are needed to prevent the recurrence of the macular edema. Pharmacologic therapy also falls short of addressing other

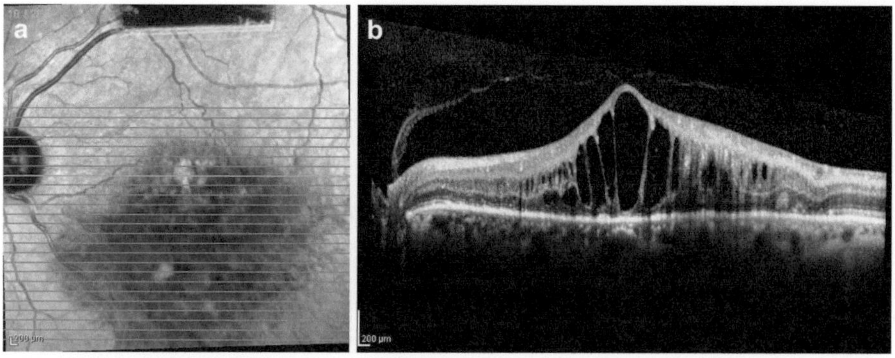

Fig. 3 Seventy-one-year-old male with left inferotemporal branch retinal vein occlusion. (**a**) Occlusion of the inferotemporal retinal vein at the first bifurcation resulted in intraretinal hemorrhages and edema extending toward fovea. (**b**) A cross-sectional HD-OCT reveals acute massive intraretinal fluid buildup at the fovea. Note that posterior hyaloid remained attached at the apex of the cystoid macular edema

comorbidities, such as macular ischemia. Although functional results of several intravitreal anti-vascular endothelial growth factor trials for vein occlusions are favorable, application of these results to daily clinical life may be misleading since in many trials, eyes with characteristics of ischemia such as poor visual acuity and afferent pupil defect were excluded [57, 58].

Central Retinal Vein Occlusion

The prevalence of CRVO is estimated to be 0.80 per 1000 persons (95 % CI: 0.61–0.99) [40]. The surgical approaches described for its treatment can be classified as follows:

(i) Induction of chorioretinal venous anastomosis with intense laser burns
(ii) Surgical establishment of chorioretinal venous anastomosis
(iii) Pars plana vitrectomy
(iv) Radial optic neurotomy (RON) (also called optic nerve sheath decompression)
(v) Retinal vein cannulation and direct injection of recombinant tissue plasminogen activator (also called retinal endovascular lysis)

McAllister and Constable described the technique of laser-induced chorioretinal venous anastomosis for the treatment of nonischemic central retinal vein occlusion, in which a focal laser burn near a tributary vein is performed to rupture the vein wall toward the underlying Bruch's membrane. The aim of this procedure was to produce a functional anastomosis between the occluded vein and choroidal circulation [59, 60]. A chorioretinal anastomosis was achieved in about a third of eyes with nonischemic central retinal vein occlusion. However, no functional anastomosis was achieved in eyes with ischemic central retinal vein occlusion [61]. Difficulty of the technique and low rate of success, coupled with high rate of adverse events such as chorioretinal neovascularization at the treatment site, fibrous tissue proliferation, distal vein closure, macular traction, and vitreous hemorrhage, impeded approval of the technique [62–64]. Also some criticism was raised claiming that the technique conferred no additional benefits when compared to the natural course of nonischemic central retinal vein occlusion [63].

Later, Peyman and colleagues described the surgical method to induce chorioretinal anastomosis [65]. Following a standard three-port pars plana vitrectomy and separation of the posterior hyaloid, they placed multiple slit-like incisions through the Bruch's membrane around major veins in four quadrants. In order to promote chorioretinal vascularization, they inserted Mersilene sutures over these incisions. In their series of five eyes with ischemic central retinal vein occlusion, 10 of 16 anastomoses remained patent. Visual acuity improved in three eyes (60 %) and one eye achieved 20/50 vision. Significant complications included optic atrophy (60 %), occlusion of the retinal veins (40 %), vitreous hemorrhage (80 %), macular traction due to significant epiretinal membrane formation (40 %), and fibrous glial proliferation at chorioretinal incision sites. Absence of iris or angle neovascularization was considered to be a beneficial effect of the surgery.

Kado and colleagues observed increased incidence of posterior vitreous detachment (PVD) in eyes followed with central retinal vein occlusion. They attributed this to the plasma leak into the vitreous from the occluded vessels. High incidence of persistent macular edema in cases with attached posterior hyaloid suggested the role of vitreomacular adhesion in the development of macular edema and pars plana vitrectomy as a surgical remedy to relieve the traction [66]. Potential benefits of vitrectomy also included removal of the cytokines that increase vascular permeability such as vascular endothelial growth factor and an increase in retinal oxygenation [67, 68]. Efficacy of pars plana vitrectomy in central retinal vein occlusion has been reported in many case series. Better visual results have been obtained in eyes with nonischemic central retinal vein occlusion treated earlier [69–75]. Surgical trauma and ischemia-related inner retinal atrophy remained as the two major factors for the failure of visual gain after resolution of the macular edema in these vitrectomized eyes [76].

A false assumption has been considering internal limiting membrane as a barrier for diffusion of intraretinal fluid into vitreous [51]. This idea led to a few attempts to decompress the swollen retina with internal limiting membrane peeling during pars plana vitrectomy [77–79]. As expected, no benefit was seen in peeling the internal limiting membrane, and even a detrimental effect on visual acuity was noted [76, 80–82].

Another surgical approach used to treat central retinal vein occlusion was radial optic neurotomy. This approach was based on the assumption that optic nerve is compressed at the level of lamina cribrosa due to a tight and rigid scleral ring. A radial cut to nasal parapapillary scleral ring was suggested as a remedy to relieve the compression on optic nerve [83]. Despite improvement in visual acuity in some eyes [84–87], this technique was criticized for lacking anatomic basis. Contradicting studies reported the site of occlusion of the vein to be at varying distances posterior to the lamina cribrosa in the optic nerve, rather than at lamina cribrosa as suggested. In histopathological studies lamina cribrosa was found to be a firm, compact, rigid band of collagen tissue instead of an elastic structure that could be decompressed with a radial incision. Also, a common fibrous tissue capsule wrapping the central retinal artery and vein throughout their course at the center of the optic nerve was found to be a more likely structure to compress the central retinal vein rather than the scleral ring outside optic nerve [47, 88–90]. Radial optic neurotomy surgery also carries some serious complications, such as severe immediate intravitreal hemorrhage, choroidovitreal neovascularization, visual field defects, retinal detachment originating from the incision site, neovascular glaucoma, phthisis bulbi, central retinal artery laceration, and optic nerve atrophy [85, 86]. Observing comparable benefits without a radial parapapillary cut indicates that pars plana vitrectomy and subsequent physiological changes, such as increased oxygenation, removal of inflammatory and angiogenic mediators, or relief of traction provide the reported benefits [84].

Retinal endovascular lysis was described by Weiss [91]. In this technique, a beveled bent glass cannula is used to enter manually into the lumen of a peripapillary branch retinal vein followed by injection of recombinant tissue plasminogen activator solution. Weiss and Bynoe also reported positive results in a 28-patient case series, treated at a mean time of 4.9 months (range: 1 week–30 months) after occlusion [92]. However, positive results could not be reproduced in a following study with ischemic eyes [93]. Furthermore, the rationale was later challenged due to the fact that thrombolytic agents would not dissolve an organized thrombus after such a long time [47]. The retrograde flow into the other veins as the thrombolytic is flushed, which was accepted as the intraoperative evidence of successful thrombus lysis, was considered as a sign of unaffected outflow resistance. Development of anti-vascular endothelial growth factor treatment, requirement for sophisticated equipment, long learning curve, and high complication rates including vitreous hemorrhage, retinal detachment, proliferative retinopathy, neovascular glaucoma, and phthisis bulbi remained as major factors for the failure of acceptance of this method [93].

Branch Retinal Vein Occlusion

Branch retinal vein occlusion is the second most common cause of retinal vascular disease after diabetic retinopathy [38–40]. As high as 50–60 % of eyes with branch retinal vein occlusion may achieve a final visual acuity of 20/40 or better without treatment [94, 95]. However, other studies have argued that despite visual acuity generally improving without intervention, clinically significant improvement beyond 20/40 was uncommon in eyes with branch retinal vein occlusion [96]. Although the mean visual acuity in laser-treated eyes improved in the Branch Vein Occlusion Study [97], laser therapy for macular edema was not found to be as efficacious in eyes with a visual acuity of 20/200 or worse, which indicates the need for alternative treatments [98].

The major surgical approaches described for treatment of branch retinal vein occlusion can be classified as follows:

(i) Pars plana vitrectomy with posterior hyaloid detachment
(ii) Arteriovenous dissection/sheathotomy

The mechanism of reduced macular edema by pars plana vitrectomy is similar to that in central retinal vein occlusion. In fact, improvement of the oxygen supply to the ischemic inner retina with pars plana vitrectomy was first demonstrated in a branch retinal vein occlusion model [67]. Increased oxygenation in return could provide arteriolar vasoconstriction and reduced hydrostatic vessel pressure as well as avoid release of mediators of vascular permeability and leakage such as vascular endothelial growth factor. Another mechanism could be relief of traction by removing the posterior hyaloid [99]. In addition, surgical creation of posterior vitreous detachment can accelerate the maturation of collateral vessels [100, 101].

There have been various reports of successful treatment with pars plana vitrectomy for branch retinal vein occlusion associated macular edema [100, 102–104]. A recent prospective multicenter study showed that pars plana vitrectomy had a slight advantage over photocoagulation for the treatment of macular edema secondary to branch retinal vein occlusion [103]. Another study suggested that 25-gauge vitrectomy and intravitreal bevacizumab injection had similar efficacies in improving visual acuity and macular edema in branch retinal vein occlusion at 1-year follow-up [104].

Osterloh and Charles described the technique of surgical arteriovenous dissection or *sheathotomy* for branch retinal vein occlusion [105]. In this procedure, a pars plana vitrectomy is followed by creating an incision in the adventitial sheath at the arteriovenous crossing with separation of the arteriole from the vein. Arteriovenous dissection can be accomplished more easily when the arteriovenous crossing responsible for the occlusion is close to the optic nerve, since the larger vessels are more resistant to surgical trauma and can withstand surgical manipulation more favorably than those located at more distal crossings [106]. Various studies have reported successful treatment of macular edema with sheathotomy in branch retinal vein occlusion [107–111]. Lakhanpal and associates reported successful results after limited arteriovenous crossing manipulation without pars plana vitrectomy using 25-gauge instrumentation in 12 eyes with branch retinal vein occlusion [108].

However, comparative studies of pars plana vitrectomy with or without arteriovenous sheathotomy revealed comparable resolution rates of macular edema and final VA results, suggesting that pars plana vitrectomy alone is responsible for the beneficial effects [100, 102, 112]. Horio and Horiguchi reported that the positive effect of sheathotomy on retinal blood flow was transient, and pars plana vitrectomy was more likely to contribute to the reduction of macular edema [113]. In other studies of arteriovenous sheathotomy, visual improvement was found irrespective of successful dissection of vessels, improvement in circulation, or reperfusion of the preoperative ischemic territory [99, 114–116].

A few studies have reported that addition of internal limiting membrane peeling to arteriovenous dissection may yield better visual results [111, 117], while this was not observed in other studies [118–120].

Intravitreal injection of a thrombolytic agent at the end of pars plana vitrectomy was tested by Christodoulakis and Tsilimbaris in three cases [121]. One patient required a reoperation for intravitreal hemorrhage, and another developed an epiretinal membrane with no major benefit in visual acuity in any of the three eyes. Garcia-Arumi and associates directly injected a thrombolytic agent into the occluded vein after arteriovenous sheathotomy, which resulted in marginally better final visual acuity in cases with intraoperative thrombus release [122]. However, intraoperative thrombus release was observed in only 27.5 % of the cases and was associated with earlier surgery.

Tang and Han studied the histopathological findings after arteriovenous sheathotomy in human cadaver eyes [123]. They reported that complete lysis of the arteriovenous sheath is often difficult because of the tight adhesion and fibrous connections between the arteriole and the vein. They also noted that the common medial wall is only about 15 μm thick and can easily be lacerated during the sheathotomy. In a histopathological study after arteriovenous sheathotomy, remarkable damage in nerve fiber layer, absence of internal limiting membrane, and edema in deeper retinal layers were observed [124]. The connection between the artery and vein was found to be very tight, and the common medial wall separating the lumina of the arteriole and the vein was only 4.5 μm thick, making it almost impossible to dissect without piercing the vessels.

Potential complications of arteriovenous sheathotomy include hemorrhage, retinal tears or detachment, postoperative gliosis with retinal traction, and retinal detachment and nerve fiber layer defects with associated scotoma [106]. Such serious complications raised concerns about the overall value of arteriovenous sheathotomy [125].

Based on best clinical evidence, pars plana vitrectomy with posterior hyaloid detachment appears to be most widely embraced surgical treatment for intractable macular edema due to both central and branch retinal vein occlusions.

References

1. Varma DD, et al. A review of central retinal artery occlusion: clinical presentation and management. Eye (Lond). 2013;27(6):688–97.
2. Brown GC, Shields JA. Cilioretinal arteries and retinal arterial occlusion. Arch Ophthalmol. 1979;97(1):84–92.
3. Rumelt S, Dorenboim Y, Rehany U. Aggressive systematic treatment for central retinal artery occlusion. Am J Ophthalmol. 1999;128(6):733–8.
4. Marder VJ, Chute D, Starkman S, Abolian AM, Kidwell C, Liebeskind D, et al. Analysis of thrombi retrieved from cerebral arteries of patients with acute ischemic stroke. Stroke. 2006;37:2086–93.
5. Arruga J, Sanders MD. Ophthalmologic findings in 70 patients with evidence of retinal embolism. Ophthalmology. 1982;89(12):1336–47.
6. Hayreh SS, Zimmerman MB. Fundus changes in central retinal artery occlusion. Retina. 2007;27(3):276–89.
7. Sharma S, et al. Interobserver agreement in the evaluation of acute retinal artery occlusion. Can J Ophthalmol. 1997;32(7):441–4.

8. Singh S, Das R. The central artery of the retina. I. Origin and course. Br J Ophthalmol. 1960;44:193–212.
9. Hayreh SS, Piegors D, Heistad DD. Serotonin induced constriction of ocular arteries in atherosclerotic monkeys: implications for ischemic disorders of retina and optic nerve head. Arch Ophthalmol. 1997;115:220–8.
10. Hayreh SS, et al. Nocturnal arterial hypotension and its role in optic nerve head and ocular ischemic disorders. Am J Ophthalmol. 1994;117(5):603–24.
11. Hayreh SS, Zimmerman M, Podhajsky P. Incidence of various types of retinal vein occlusion and their recurrence and demographic characteristics. Am J Ophthalmol. 1994;117(4):429–41.
12. Hayreh SS, Zimmerman M. Central retinal artery occlusion: visual outcome. Am J Ophthalmol. 2005;140(3):376–91.
13. Hayreh SS, et al. Central retinal artery occlusion. Retinal survival time. Exp Eye Res. 2004;78(3):723–36.
14. Biousse V, et al. Thrombolysis for central retinal artery occlusion. J Neuroophthalmol. 2007;27(3):215–30.
15. Hsu TK, et al. Embolus-induced branch retinal artery occlusion with a presenting best-corrected visual acuity of <6/12 and visual field defect: yag embolectomy safely restores arteriolar perfusion and/or visual function. Retina Cases Brief Rep. 2013;7(3):210–6.
16. Mangat HS. Retinal artery occlusion. Surv Ophthalmol. 1995;40(2):145–56.
17. Schaal S, Al-Latayfeh M, Barak Y, Tezel T. Restoration of blood flow and vision in central retinal artery occlusion with early vitrectomy. Annual meeting of the American academy of ophthalmology. Chicago, Nov, 2012.
18. Ahn SJ, et al. Retinal and choroidal changes and visual outcome in central retinal artery occlusion: an optical coherence tomography study. Am J Ophthalmol. 2015;159:667–76.
19. Schumacher M, et al. Central retinal artery occlusion: local intra-arterial fibrinolysis versus conservative treatment, a multicenter randomized trial. Ophthalmology. 2010;117(7):1367–75 e1.
20. Fraser SG, Adams W. Interventions for acute non-arteritic central retinal artery occlusion. Cochrane Database Syst Rev. 2009;1:CD001989.
21. Feltgen N, et al. Multicenter study of the European Assessment Group for Lysis in the Eye (EAGLE) for the treatment of central retinal artery occlusion: design issues and implications. EAGLE Study report no. 1. Graefes Arch Clin Exp Ophthalmol. 2006;244(8):950–6.
22. Wolf A, et al. Comparison of superselective intraarterial fibrinolysis with conservative therapy. Use in patients with acute non-arteritic central retinal artery occlusion. Ophthalmologe. 2010;107(9):799–805.
23. Opremcak EM, Benner JD. Translumenal Nd:YAG laser embolysis for branch retinal artery occlusion. Retina. 2002;22(2):213–6.
24. Reynard M, Hanscom TA. Neodymium:yttrium-aluminum-garnet laser arteriotomy with embolectomy for central retinal artery occlusion. Am J Ophthalmol. 2004;137(1):196–8.
25. Opremcak ERA, Ridenour CD, Borkowski LM, Kelley JK. Restoration of retinal blood flow via translumenal Nd:YAG embolysis/embolectomy (TYL/E) for central and branch retinal artery occlusion. Retina. 2008;28(2):226–35.
26. Garcia-Arumi J, et al. Surgical embolus removal in retinal artery occlusion. Br J Ophthalmol. 2006;90(10):1252–5.
27. Peyman GA, Gremillion Jr CM. Surgical removal of a branch retinal artery embolus: a case report. Int Ophthalmol. 1990;14(4):295–8.
28. Matonti F, et al. Surgical embolectomy for central retinal artery occlusion. Can J Ophthalmol. 2013;48(2):e25–7.
29. Arumi GJBS, Leila M, Victori MAZ. Vitreous surgery of arterial and venous retinovascular diseases. In: Sebag J, editor. Vitreous: in health and disease. New York: Springer; 2014. p. 647–61.
30. Tang WM, Topping TM. Vitreous surgery for central retinal artery occlusion. Arch Ophthalmol. 2000;118(11):1586–7.

31. Hayreh SS. Acute retinal arterial occlusive disorders. Prog Retin Eye Res. 2011;30(5): 359–94.
32. Schmidt D, et al. Systemic diseases in non-inflammatory branch and central retinal artery occlusion--an overview of 416 patients. Eur J Med Res. 2007;12(12):595–603.
33. Lim JY, et al. Treatment of branch retinal artery occlusion with transluminal Nd:YAG laser embolysis. Korean J Ophthalmol. 2009;23(4):315–7.
34. Yuzurihara D, Iijima H. Visual outcome in central retinal and branch retinal artery occlusion. Jpn J Ophthalmol. 2004;48(5):490–2.
35. Hayreh SS, Podhajsky PA, Zimmerman MB. Branch retinal artery occlusion: natural history of visual outcome. Ophthalmology. 2009;116(6):1188–94 e1-4.
36. Hayreh SS. Surgical embolus removal in retinal artery occlusion. Br J Ophthalmol. 2007;91(8):1096–7.
37. Mason 3rd JO, Nixon PA, Albert Jr MA. Trans-luminal nd:YAG laser embolysis for branch retinal artery occlusion. Retina. 2007;27(5):573–7.
38. Mitchell P, Smith W, Chang A. Prevalence and associations of retinal vein occlusion in Australia. The Blue Mountains Eye Study. Arch Ophthalmol. 1996;114(10):1243–7.
39. Klein R, et al. The epidemiology of retinal vein occlusion: the Beaver Dam Eye Study. Trans Am Ophthalmol Soc. 2000;98:133–41. discussion 141–3.
40. Rogers S, et al. The prevalence of retinal vein occlusion: pooled data from population studies from the United States, Europe, Asia, and Australia. Ophthalmology. 2010;117(2):313–9. e1.
41. Hayreh SS, Hayreh MS. Hemi-central retinal vein occulsion. Pathogenesis, clinical features, and natural history. Arch Ophthalmol. 1980;98(9):1600–9.
42. Hayreh SS, Zimmerman MB. Fundus changes in branch retinal vein occlusion. Retina. 2015;35:1016–27.
43. Matsumoto M, et al. Retinal blood flow levels measured by laser speckle flowgraphy in patients who received intravitreal bevacizumab injection for macular edema secondary to central retinal vein occlusion. Retina Cases Brief Rep. 2014;8(1):60–6.
44. Wong TY, Scott IU. Clinical practice. Retinal-vein occlusion. N Engl J Med. 2010;363(22): 2135–44.
45. Fekrat S, Finkelstein D. Venous occlusive disease. In: Brown G, Regillo CD, Flynn Jr HW, editors. Vitreoretinal disease: the essentials. New York: Thieme; 1999. p. 117–32.
46. Wong TY, et al. Cardiovascular risk factors for retinal vein occlusion and arteriolar emboli: the atherosclerosis risk in communities & cardiovascular health studies. Ophthalmology. 2005;112(4):540–7.
47. Hayreh SS. Prevalent misconceptions about acute retinal vascular occlusive disorders. Prog Retin Eye Res. 2005;24:493–519.
48. Hayreh SS, Zimmerman M, Podhajsky P. Hematologic abnormalities associated with various types of retinal vein occlusion. Graefes Arch Clin Exp Ophthalmol. 2002;240(3):180–96.
49. Ingerslev J. Thrombophilia: a feature of importance in retinal vein thrombosis? Acta Ophthalmol Scand. 1999;77(6):619–21.
50. Ascaso FJ, Huerva V, Grzybowski A. The role of inflammation in the pathogenesis of macular edema secondary to retinal vascular diseases. Mediators Inflamm. 2014;2014:432685.
51. Scholl S, Kirchhof J, Augustin AJ. Pathophysiology of macular edema. Ophthalmologica. 2010;224 Suppl 1:8–15.
52. Hayreh SS, Zimmerman MB. Fundus changes in central retinal vein occlusion. Retina. 2015;35(1):29–42.
53. Scott IU, et al. Baseline predictors of visual acuity and retinal thickness outcomes in patients with retinal vein occlusion: Standard Care Versus COrticosteroid for REtinal Vein Occlusion Study report 10. Ophthalmology. 2011;118(2):345–52.
54. Haller JA, et al. Randomized, sham-controlled trial of dexamethasone intravitreal implant in patients with macular edema due to retinal vein occlusion. Ophthalmology. 2010;117(6):1134–46 e3.
55. Wu L, et al. Comparison of two doses of intravitreal bevacizumab as primary treatment for macular edema secondary to central retinal vein occlusion: results of the pan American collaborative retina study group at 24 months. Retina. 2010;30(7):1002–11.

56. Prager F, et al. Intravitreal bevacizumab (Avastin) for macular oedema secondary to retinal vein occlusion: 12-month results of a prospective clinical trial. Br J Ophthalmol. 2009;93(4):452–6.
57. Campochiaro PA, et al. Ranibizumab for macular edema following branch retinal vein occlusion: six-month primary end point results of a phase III study. Ophthalmology. 2010;117(6):1102–12 e1.
58. Brown DM, et al. Ranibizumab for macular edema following central retinal vein occlusion: six-month primary end point results of a phase III study. Ophthalmology. 2010;117(6):1124–33 e1.
59. McAllister IL, Constable IJ. Laser-induced chorioretinal venous anastomosis for treatment of nonischemic central retinal vein occlusion. Arch Ophthalmol. 1995;113(4):456–62.
60. McAllister IL, et al. The Central Retinal Vein Bypass Study: a trial of laser-induced chorioretinal venous anastomosis for central retinal vein occlusion. Ophthalmology. 2010;117(5):954–65.
61. Kwok AK, et al. Laser induced chorioretinal venous anastomosis in ischaemic central retinal vein occlusion. Br J Ophthalmol. 2003;87(8):1043–4.
62. Browning DJ, Rotberg MH. Vitreous Hemorrhage complicating laser-induced chorioretinal anastomosis for central retinal vein occlusion. Am J Ophthalmol. 1996;122(4):588–9.
63. Aktan SG, et al. Problems of chorioretinal venous anastomosis by laser for treatment of non-ischemic central retinal vein occlusion. Ophthalmologica. 1998;212(6):389–93.
64. Eccarius SG, Moran MJ, Slingsby JG. Choroidal neovascular membrane after laser-induced chorioretinal anastomosis. Am J Ophthalmol. 1996;122(4):590–1.
65. Peyman GA, Kishore K, Conway MD. Surgical chorioretinal venous anastomosis for ischemic central retinal vein occlusion. Ophthalmic Surg Lasers. 1999;30(8):605–14.
66. Kado M, et al. Vitreous changes and macular edema in central retinal vein occlusion. Ophthalmic Surg. 1990;21(8):544–9.
67. Stefansson E, Novack RL, Hatchell DL. Vitrectomy prevents retinal hypoxia in branch retinal vein occlusion. Invest Ophthalmol Vis Sci. 1990;31(2):284–9.
68. Hikichi T, Konno S, Trempe CL. Role of the vitreous in central retinal vein occlusion. Retina. 1995;15(1):29–33.
69. Tachi N, Hashimoto Y, Ogino N. Vitrectomy for macular edema combined with retinal vein occlusion. Doc Ophthalmol. 1999;97(3–4):465–9.
70. Sekiryu T, et al. Retina tomography after vitrectomy for macular edema of central retinal vein occlusion. Ophthalmic Surg Lasers. 2000;31(3):198–202.
71. Leizaola-Fernandez C, et al. Vitrectomy with complete posterior hyaloid removal for ischemic central retinal vein occlusion: series of cases. BMC Ophthalmol. 2005;5(10):10.
72. Furukawa M, Kumagai K, Ogino N, Uemura A, Larson E. Long-term visual outcomes of vitrectomy for cystoid macular edema due to nonischemic central retinal vein occlusion. Eur J Ophthalmol. 2006;16(6):841–6.
73. Noma H, Mimura T, Shimada K. Changes of macular sensitivity and morphology after pars plana vitrectomy for macular edema with central retinal vein occlusion: a case series. BMC Ophthalmol. 2013;13(2):2.
74. Chuang LH, et al. Vitrectomy and panretinal photocoagulation reduces the occurrence of neovascular glaucoma in central retinal vein occlusion with vitreous hemorrhage. Retina. 2013;33(4):798–802.
75. Noma H, et al. Influence of vitreous factors after vitrectomy for macular edema in patients with central retinal vein occlusion. Int Ophthalmol. 2011;31(5):393–402.
76. Baharivand N, et al. Pars plana vitrectomy and internal limiting membrane peeling for macular edema secondary to retinal vein occlusion. Clin Ophthalmol. 2011;5:1089–93.
77. Mandelcorn MS, Nrusimhadevara RK. Internal limiting membrane peeling for decompression of macular edema in retinal vein occlusion: a report of 14 cases. Retina. 2004;24(3):348–55.
78. Park DH, Kim IT. Long-term effects of vitrectomy and internal limiting membrane peeling for macular edema secondary to central retinal vein occlusion and hemiretinal vein occlusion. Retina. 2010;30(1):117–24.
79. Liang XL, et al. Pars plana vitrectomy and internal limiting membrane peeling for macular oedema secondary to retinal vein occlusion: a pilot study. Ann Acad Med Singapore. 2007;36(4):293–7.

80. Radetzky S, et al. Visual outcome of patients with macular edema after pars plana vitrectomy and indocyanine green-assisted peeling of the internal limiting membrane. Graefes Arch Clin Exp Ophthalmol. 2004;242(4):273–8.
81. DeCroos FC, et al. Pars plana vitrectomy, internal limiting membrane peeling, and panretinal endophotocoagulation for macular edema secondary to central retinal vein occlusion. Am J Ophthalmol. 2009;147(4):627–33 e1.
82. Soheilian M, et al. Visual outcomes in five different approaches for treatment of central retinal vein occlusion. Ophthalmic Surg Lasers Imaging. 2010;41(2):157–65.
83. Opremcak EM, et al. Radial optic neurotomy for central retinal vein occlusion: a retrospective pilot study of 11 consecutive cases. Retina. 2001;21(5):408–15.
84. Aggermann T, et al. A prospective, randomised, multicenter trial for surgical treatment of central retinal vein occlusion: results of the Radial Optic Neurotomy for Central Vein Occlusion (ROVO) study group. Graefes Arch Clin Exp Ophthalmol. 2013;251(4): 1065–72.
85. Arevalo JF, et al. Radial optic neurotomy for central retinal vein occlusion: results of the Pan-American Collaborative Retina Study Group (PACORES). Retina. 2008;28(8):1044–52.
86. Hasselbach HC, et al. Treatment of central retinal vein occlusion by radial optic neurotomy in 107 cases. Graefes Arch Clin Exp Ophthalmol. 2007;245(8):1145–56.
87. Opremcak EM, et al. Radial optic neurotomy for central retinal vein occlusion: 117 consecutive cases. Retina. 2006;26(3):297–305.
88. Hayreh SS, Vrabec F. The structure of the head of the optic nerve in rhesus monkey. Am J Ophthalmol. 1966;61(1):136–50.
89. Hayreh S. Central retinal vein occlusion. Ophthalmol Clin North Am. 1998;11(4):559–90.
90. Hayreh SS. Radial optic neurotomy for central retinal vein occlusion. Retina. 2002;22(6):827. author reply 827.
91. Weiss JN. Treatment of central retinal vein occlusion by injection of tissue plasminogen activator into a retinal vein. Am J Ophthalmol. 1998;126(1):142–4.
92. Weiss JN, Bynoe L. Injection of tissue plasminogen activator into a branch retinal vein in eyes with central retinal vein occlusion. Ophthalmology. 2001;108(12):2249–57.
93. Feltgen N, et al. Retinal endovascular lysis in ischemic central retinal vein occlusion: one-year results of a pilot study. Ophthalmology. 2007;114(4):716–23.
94. Gutman FA, Zegarra H. The natural course of temporal retinal branch vein occlusion. Trans Am Acad Ophthalmol Otolaryngol. 1974;78(2):OP178–92.
95. Magargal LE, et al. Temporal branch retinal vein obstruction: a review. Ophthalmic Surg. 1986;17(4):240–6.
96. Rogers SL, et al. Natural history of branch retinal vein occlusion: an evidence-based systematic review. Ophthalmology. 2010;117(6):1094–101 e5.
97. Group TBVOS. Argon laser photocoagulation for macular edema in branch retinal vein occlusion. Am J Ophthalmol. 1984;98(3):271–82.
98. Rehak J, Rehak M. Branch retinal vein occlusion: pathogenesis, visual prognosis, and treatment modalities. Curr Eye Res. 2008;33(2):111–31.
99. Charbonnel J, et al. Management of branch retinal vein occlusion with vitrectomy and arteriovenous adventitial sheathotomy, the possible role of surgical posterior vitreous detachment. Graefes Arch Clin Exp Ophthalmol. 2004;242(3):223–8.
100. Yamamoto SSW, Yagi F, Takeuchi S, Sato E, Mizunoya S. Vitrectomy with or without arteriovenous adventitial sheathotomy for macular edema associated with branch retinal vein occlusion. Am J Ophthalmol. 2004;138(6):907–14.
101. Chiristoffersen NLB, Larsen M. Pathophysiology and hemodynamics of branch retinal vein occlusion. Ophthalmology. 1999;106:2054–62.
102. Kumagai KFM, Ogino N, Uemura A, Larson E. Long-term outcomes of vitrectomy with or without arteriovenous sheathotomy in branch retinal vein occlusion. Retina. 2007;27: 49–54.
103. Harino S, Bessho K, Kida T. Prospective multicenter study of visual outcomes following three different treatments for macular edema associated with branch retinal vein occlusion: a study by the Japanese BRVO study group. Jpn J Ophthalmol. 2012;56(3):250–61.

104. Sato T, et al. 25-gauge vitrectomy versus intravitreal bevacizumab for macular edema secondary to branch retinal vein occlusion: 1 year follow-up. Ann Acad Med Singapore. 2012;41(7):294–9.
105. Osterloh MD, Charles S. Surgical decompression of branch retinal vein occlusions. Arch Ophthalmol. 1988;106(10):1469–71.
106. Shah GK. Adventitial sheathotomy for treatment of macular edema associated with branch retinal vein occlusion. Curr Opin Ophthalmol. 2000;11(3):171–4.
107. Cahill MT, et al. The effect of arteriovenous sheathotomy on cystoid macular oedema secondary to branch retinal vein occlusion. Br J Ophthalmol. 2003;87(11):1329–32.
108. Lakhanpal RR, Javaheri M, Ruiz-Garcia H, De Juan Jr E, Humayun MS. Transvitreal limited arteriovenous-crossing manipulation without vitrectomy for complicated branch retinal vein occlusion using 25-gauge instrumentation. Retina. 2005;25:272–80.
109. Le Rouic JF, et al. Adventitial sheathotomy for decompression of recent onset branch retinal vein occlusion. Graefes Arch Clin Exp Ophthalmol. 2001;239(10):747–51.
110. Mason 3rd J, et al. Sheathotomy to decompress branch retinal vein occlusion: a matched control study. Ophthalmology. 2004;111(3):540–5.
111. Mester U, Dillinger P. Vitrectomy with arteriovenous decompression and internal limiting membrane dissection in branch retinal vein occlusion. Retina. 2002;22(6):740–6.
112. Figueroa MS, Torres R, Alvarez MT. Comparative study of vitrectomy with and without vein decompression for branch retinal vein occlusion: a pilot study. Eur J Ophthalmol. 2004;14(1):40–7.
113. Horio N, Horiguchi M. Effect of arteriovenous sheathotomy on retinal blood flow and macular edema in patients with branch retinal vein occlusion. Am J Ophthalmol. 2005;139(4): 739–40.
114. Han DP, Bennett S, Williams DF, Dev S. Arteriovenous crossing dissection without separation of the retina vessels for treatment of branch retinal vein occlusion. Retina. 2003;23(2): 145–51.
115. Feltgen N, et al. Arterio-venous dissection after isovolaemic haemodilution in branch retinal vein occlusion: a non-randomised prospective study. Graefes Arch Clin Exp Ophthalmol. 2006;244(7):829–35.
116. Yamaji H, et al. Evaluation of arteriovenous crossing sheathotomy for branch retinal vein occlusion by fluorescein videoangiography and image analysis. Am J Ophthalmol. 2004;137(5):834–41.
117. Asensio Sánchez VM, Rodriguez Bravo I, Botella Oltra G. Adventitial sheathotomy in branch retinal vein occlusion with nonischemic macular edema. Arch Soc Esp Oftalmol. 2004;79(3):347–52.
118. Arai M, et al. Efficacy of vitrectomy and internal limiting membrane removal for macular edema associated with branch retinal vein occlusion. Ophthalmologica. 2009;223(3):172–6.
119. Kumagai K, et al. Long-term visual outcomes after vitrectomy for macular edema with foveal hemorrhage in branch retinal vein occlusion. Retina. 2007;27(5):584–8.
120. Kumagai K, et al. Possible effects of internal limiting membrane peeling in vitrectomy for macular vein occlusion. Jpn J Ophthalmol. 2010;54(1):61–5.
121. Christodoulakis EV, Tsilimbaris MK. The role of vitrectomy assisted rt-PA injection for the management of branch retinal vein occlusion: case report. Semin Ophthalmol. 2007;22(2): 89–93.
122. Garcia-Arumi J, Martinez-Castillo V, Boixadera A, Blasco H, Corcostegui B. Management of macular oedema in branch reti- nal vein occlusion with sheathotomy and recombinant tissue plasminogen activator. Retina. 2004;24(4):530–40.
123. Tang WM, Han DP. A study of surgical approaches to retinal vascular occlusions. Arch Ophthalmol. 2000;118(1):138–43.
124. Feltgen N, et al. Arteriovenous dissection in a living human eye: clinicopathologic correlation. Arch Ophthalmol. 2005;123(4):571–2.
125. Avci R, Inan UU, Kaderli B. Evaluation of arteriovenous crossing sheathotomy for decompression of branch retinal vein occlusion. Eye (Lond). 2008;22(1):120–7.

Chapter 13
Surgical Management of Vitreous Retained Lens Fragments During or Following Phacoemulsification Surgery

Pedro Amat-Peral, Jorge L. Alió y Sanz, and Francisco L. Lugo-Quintás

Introduction

Cataract surgery is presently among the most frequently performed surgical procedures worldwide. Although the technique has developed greatly in recent years, with maneuvers becoming safer and less traumatic, some definitive risks still exist.

One of the most feared complications for eye surgeons is the dislocation of the lens or lens fragments into the vitreous cavity. It is estimated that this complication may occur in 0.3–1.1 % [1] of cases. Fortunately, this decreases significantly and proportionally with improvement in skills as surgeons progress along the learning curve.

Lens dislocation into the vitreous cavity can happen unrelated to surgery, as in the case of ocular trauma, or may be spontaneous as with the Marchesani or Marfan syndrome.

However, far more frequently, lens dislocation occurs intraoperatively as a complication of cataract surgery. Causes of intraoperative lens dislocation are diverse. Dislocation of the whole lens is rare and related to lens instability or infrequently to conditions such as the pseudoexfoliation syndrome. Most of the cases of lens dislocation into the vitreous cavity involve the nucleus or nucleus fragments and are related to rupture of the posterior capsule or zonular dialysis during phacoemulsification surgery (Fig. 1).

P. Amat-Peral, MD, PhD, FEBO • F.L. Lugo-Quintás, MD, PhD
Vitreous-Retina Unit, Vissum, Instituto Oftalmológico de Alicante, C/Cabañal 1, Alicante 03016, Spain

J.L. Alió y Sanz, MD, PhD, FEBO (✉)
Cataract and Refractive Surgery Unit, Vissum, Instituto Oftalmológico de Alicante, C/Cabañal 1, Alicante 03016, Spain

Miguel Hernández University, Alicante, Spain
e-mail: jlalio@vissum.com

S. Schaal, H.J. Kaplan (eds.), *Cystoid Macular Edema*,
DOI 10.1007/978-3-319-39766-5_13

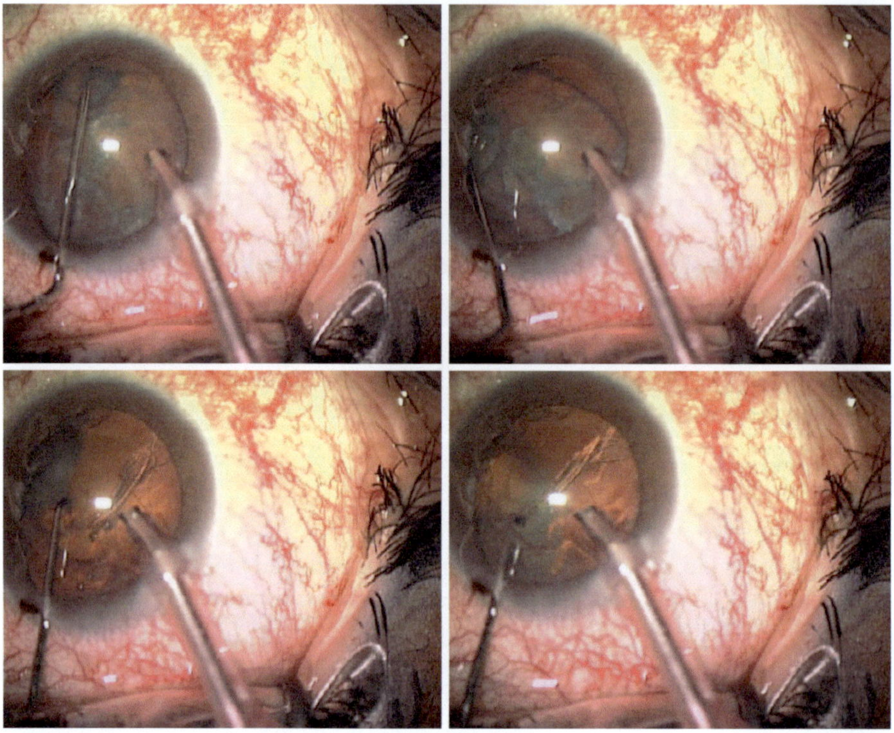

Fig. 1 Process of core dislocation into the vitreous caused by rotating the fragment to the area of rupture; the surgeon has not detected the lack of support maintaining irrigation

Throughout this chapter, we will refer specifically to the complications occurring in cataract surgery and describe how to identify patient risk factors, secondary ocular complications, and appropriate medical and surgical treatment to minimize visual impact and preserve patient quality of life.

Causes for Retained Lens Fragments During or Following Cataract Surgery

It is essential that the surgeon be able to recognize and identify patients with a higher risk of developing this surgical complication to take the appropriate measures and technique modifications to minimize the risk. In a good preoperative evaluation, most of these causes can be detected, including significantly hard cataracts, poor pupillary dilation, capsular pseudoexfoliation, previous trauma causing zonular weakness, and vitrectomized eyes lacking vitreous back support [2].

How Lens Fragments Are Displaced into the Vitreous During Phacoemulsification

Dislocation of lens material during cataract surgery may be essentially due to two mechanisms: posterior capsule rupture (Fig. 1) and dehiscence of the zonules. Tearing of the posterior capsule can occur during the hydrodissection or when the nucleus is phacoemulsified. The latter is more frequent in eyes with variations in anterior chamber depth, especially if high levels of aspiration and power are used, and in previously vitrectomized patients, when the density of the vitreous does not exert posterior support for these changes. Capsular rupture can occur when the core is sculpted too close to the posterior capsule, especially when there is no good visibility. It can also be due to the shift from a dense area of the core to another softer area, where the increase in the suction force can drag nuclear, cortical, and capsular content quickly into the phacoemulsification handpiece opening.

When a posterior capsule tear is detected (Fig. 2), the phacoemulsification technique must be modified to prevent further tearing. The surgeon should avoid rotating the core as it may increase the defect and increase the risk of dislocation (Fig. 1).

Excessive handling and large fluctuations in chamber pressure should be avoided. The surgeon should use a second instrument to hold the nucleus and approach the phaco tip. If it is a large capsular rupture, it can be protected with a sheet slider, raising the upper pole of the nucleus while protecting underneath the aperture and helping extraction by phacoemulsification. Finally, it can be converted to extracapsular extraction of the core with large corneal incision [3].

Maneuvers to perform	Maneuvers to avoid
Remove nuclear fragments that remain in the anterior chamber	Avoid phacoemulsification into the vitreous from the anterior chamber
Use automated vitrectome besides the bimanual technique	Avoid using aggressive maneuvers (like vitreous handles) to rescue lens material that has gone deep into the vitreous
Protect corneal endothelium with viscoelastic fluid	Avoid removing the nucleus by irrigating the vitreous
Aspirate as much of cortical remains as possible	

Complications Related to the Retained Lens Fragments

Lens fragment dislocation is a potentially serious ocular complication with clinical manifestations largely dependent on the amount of dislocated material. While smaller fragments may be generally well tolerated, large amounts can cause severe intraocular inflammation. The intensity of this inflammation as well as the final visual prognosis will depend on the type of lens material, with nuclear fragments causing far more severe symptoms than remnants of epinucleus or cortex. [4].

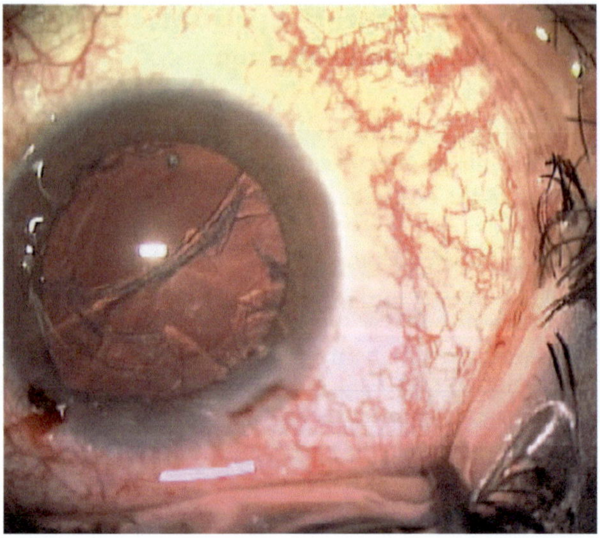

Fig. 2 Posterior capsule rupture

The most common complications include decreased visual acuity, intraocular inflammation, corneal edema, and ocular hypertension. Less frequent complications are retinal detachment, choroidal detachment, vitreous hemorrhage, cystoid macular edema, and endophthalmitis.

A decrease in vision is the most common symptom of this complication with several series reporting visual acuity rates of 20/400 or worse from 41.2 to 89 % [5–7]. Intraocular inflammation is present in most cases with reported rates between 67.1 and 87 % [5–7] and often manifests as corneal edema, secondary glaucoma, or cystoid macular edema. Also known as phacoanaphylactic uveitis, this inflammation is caused by proteins of the lens fragments and may manifest as conjunctival hyperemia with ciliary injection, eye pain, and ocular hypertension. In some cases, this inflammation can be very severe with cell/flare >2+ accompanied by a hypopyon, giving the appearance of a real endophthalmitis. Cases of acute endophthalmitis have been reported that are associated with dislocation of lens fragments and have been demonstrated by positive cultures [8]. Therefore, in cases with the presence of severe intraocular inflammation, culture is required to rule out infection and pursue appropriate treatment.

Corneal edema is another manifestation of lens fragment dislocation and has been estimated as having an incidence of 46–61 % [5, 6]. Corneal edema may be caused by intraocular inflammation as well as by increased intraocular pressure and should be treated rapidly as vitrectomy should ideally be performed with greatest possible corneal transparency.

An increase in intraocular pressure as high as 25–30 mmHg can be seen in about half of these patients [6, 7]. The increase in pressure may be due to either the massive presence of inflammatory cells at the level of trabecula or the remains of lens material. This acute increase in intraocular pressure can cause chronic glaucoma if the inflammation remains persistent.

Retinal detachment is present with an incidence that varies between 3.6 and 21.5 % [1, 9]. It is a feared complication and can be responsible for poor visual prognosis for some patients. This detachment is usually caused by surgical maneuvers in complicated cataract surgery or during subsequent vitrectomy which can cause retinal tears or secondary vitreous traction. Excessive irrigation and the search for material in the vitreous cavity increase the risk of retinal breaks. The lens fragments themselves may directly cause retinal breaks as well as indirectly lead to vitreoretinal traction and neurosensory detachment secondary to inflammation, bleeding, and subsequent cellular proliferation [10].

Cystoid macular edema can appear as a late complication secondary to intraocular inflammation caused by the lens material in approximately 7 % of cases [6].

Evaluation of Patients with Retained Lens Fragments and Management of the Associated Complications

Detailed patient evaluation is important before considering vitrectomy to obtain the best possible results. This preoperative evaluation will depend on the time lag between initial surgery and vitrectomy. If the vitrectomy is immediately following surgical complication, the evaluation will be shallower; however, if a vitreoretinal surgeon or necessary equipment is not available, it is more convenient to delay the surgery and undertake a thorough patient evaluation.

Knowledge of the patient's ocular history helps to determine whether preexisting disease may have caused the complication and determine viability of subsequent surgeries. Eye trauma, high myopia, previous episodes of uveitis, diabetic retinopathy, vitrectomy, sclerectomies, or previous valve implants may complicate surgical removal of fragments or help determine the surgical approach.

When examining the patient, the first thing to be noted is the visual acuity. This will depend on many factors such as the presence of fragments in the visual axis, macular edema, the degree of cellularity in the anterior chamber, and vitritis. Visual acuity is an important prognostic factor because visual acuity of 20/40 or better has been shown to be an indicator of better final visual acuity [9]. The external examination should be performed after and the degree of eye and eyelid inflammation assessed.

When to Operate: Early Versus Delayed Removal

Pars plana vitrectomy for removal of retained lens fragments should be indicated when the displacement of the lens to vitreous cavity occurs spontaneously, secondary to trauma, or following a surgical complication [11–16]. It is also considered when a large part of the crystalline remains have gone into the vitreous cavity and/or persisted in the capsular bag.

Surgery must also be considered to prevent complications attributable to the retention of fragments in the vitreous whether these appear immediately (ocular hypertension, inflammatory reaction), late (cystoid macular edema, retinal detachment), or may affect the visual acuity as in the case of vitreous opacities or symptomatic floaters.

The indication for vitrectomy is not so clear if lens residues are scarce and do not generate pressure or inflammation beyond the early postoperative period [14, 17]. In fact, if the material amount is small, it may gradually be reabsorbed, thus avoiding further surgery.

There is some controversy about determining the optimal timing of vitrectomy to remove the lens fragments. Currently, there are two trends: either to perform the vitrectomy as soon as possible after cataract surgery (early surgery) [18, 19] or do it in a deferred way [9, 15, 16, 20].

Early vitrectomy, immediately after cataract surgery, involves only moderate technical difficulty. In addition, the condition is prevented from worsening and a second procedure is avoided. Wilkinson suggests that the absence of macrophages and other inflammatory markers during the first days after cataract surgery leads us to think that early surgery may prevent further complications [11].

Corneal opacity appears often on the day after surgery and limits the visualization, making it necessary to delay the surgery until the eye is in good condition.

On the other hand, performing vitrectomy when the complication arises makes it necessary to have a vitreoretinal surgeon available with assistants familiar with the technique. In addition, due to the widespread use of topical anesthesia for cataract surgery, either additional peribulbar or retrobulbar anesthesia is required.

Vitrectomy, when deferred, can be performed with the necessary equipment. In addition, the resolution of corneal edema provides transparent media. Moreover, greater hydration of cortex and core debris that occurs over time increases the ease of fragment extraction.

The disadvantages of delaying vitrectomy include delayed resolution of the issue, the need for a second operation, and the increased possibility of a secondary pathology (chronic glaucoma).

Several studies conclude that the time lag before vitrectomy does not significantly influence the final functional outcome [9, 14, 15, 20–22].

However, these findings may be biased by the limited number of cases in the series and the consequent variability.

Although there are studies like those of Kageyama et al. showing that 82 % of patients undergoing vitrectomy at the time of complicated cataract surgery reach a BCVA of 20/40 or greater [12], the literature does not support early vitrectomy as a superior choice.

An initial aggressive drug treatment can aid in delayed vitrectomy by improving corneal edema and acute inflammation, thereby improving visualization and conditions to perform the surgery.

Moreover, other studies conclude that the risk of secondary open-angle glaucoma increases when surgery is delayed by over 1 week [9, 15, 21].

Since it is not always possible to perform vitrectomy the same day as cataract surgery, the most appropriate time to carry it out will depend on the degree of corneal transparency and intraocular inflammation, the patient's general condition, and the availability of instruments and skilled staff.

In general terms, assuming there are no significant complications requiring earlier surgery, the vitrectomy should be performed in the week following failed phacoemulsification [2].

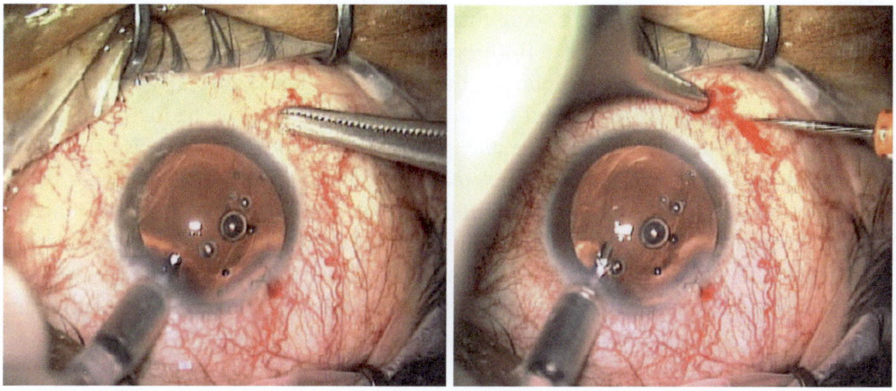

Figs. 3 and 4 Infusing saline through the anterior chamber to avoid hypotonia and to complete correctly the incision maneuvers through trocars

Preoperative Examination

Evaluation depends on when the vitrectomy for extraction of lens remnants is performed. Theoretically, although there is no consensus, this second surgery should ideally occur at the same time as the surgical complication, even though this means a very superficial examination of the patient is undertaken. In this case the surgeon must take into account the intraocular pressure of the eye—usually hypotonus—especially if previously the eye has been manipulated by the cataract surgeon in an attempt to remove the vitreous core. Hypotonia may hinder the incision maneuvers through trocars, which may only incompletely perforate the wall of the globe, causing subretinal fluid infusion. To avoid this, the eye should be filled with viscoelastic fluid through the anterior chamber or a saline infusion through the paracentesis (Figs. 3 and 4).

Because immediate action is not the most frequent due to the difficulty of having a vitreoretinal surgeon available, deferred action is often necessary. In that case a complete clinical record and exploration can be made.

Examination of the Anterior Segment

Slit-lamp examination assesses the degree of corneal transparency when special emphasis is placed on the endothelium and helps determine the choice of location of lens implantation in cases of aphakia. Incisions and degree of cooptation, presence of vitreous incarceration, and remains of suture are problems which also must be solved to avoid further complications. Also important is the evaluation of the cellularity in anterior chamber (Tyndall phenomenon) that can range from slight to a true hypopyon and the presence of blood or fibrin and lens fragments that may be housed in the anterior chamber, trabecular angle, or behind the iris. As discussed above, in cases of suspected endophthalmitis, obtaining microbiological cultures and treatment will be a priority. Both corneal edema and inflammation should be treated but preferably without delaying the removal of lens material. Also pupillary dilation will need to be evaluated because poor mydriasis due to the presence of synechiae complicates the surgery and requires maneuvers to increase the pupil size. Evaluating the structure of the remaining posterior capsule in aphakic cases helps to determine the necessity of implanting the lens either in capsular bag, in sulcus, or sutured. In cases where the lens is implanted, the surgeon should assess the stability of the lens, correct its position if necessary to prevent posterior dislocation, or in cases of instability remove it along with the crystalline remains and defer implantation of an intraocular lens to a later date.

The measurement of intraocular pressure and its pharmacological control in cases of elevation are essential before performing the vitrectomy. Also, the presence of hypotonia can suggest a major complication such as retinal detachment.

Examination of the Posterior Segment

Once the anterior segment is evaluated, a thorough dilated fundus exam should be performed to explore the posterior segment. Through indirect ophthalmoscopy, we can determine the degree of transparency of the vitreous, the presence of bleeding, and size, density, and amount of dislocated lens material. Nuclear fragments cause more inflammation and have a worse prognosis than the remnants of cortex or epinucleus, making composition more important than size. The presence of vitreous hemorrhage is a sign of severity that can be related to inadequate manipulation, direct trauma, or vitreoretinal traction. If the low intensity of media opacity permits indirect ophthalmoscopy, the surgeon must always rule out the presence of retinal breaks that can be treated preemptively with argon laser and the presence of choroidal detachments, most of which can be resolved with conservative treatment. Retinal detachment requires urgent vitrectomy as inflammation caused by the lens fragments in the vitreous cavity increases the risk of developing a proliferative vitreoretinopathy [23]. Finally, the presence of cystic macular edema or Irvine-Gass syndrome, which require early treatment, must be excluded.

Although pars plana vitrectomy itself resolves most symptoms and complications of retained lens fragments, some risks remains. This risk of retinal detachment has been reported in several series ranging from 4 to 10.3 % [24–27].

Moore et al. found an incidence of retinal detachment of 7.3 % before vitrectomy to remove lens fragments and 5.5 % after, with 42 % of these detachments occurring 3 months after surgery and half of them occurring with macular involvement [28]. Due to this, some surgeons recommend performing prophylactic retinal photocoagulation 360° to reduce the risk of subsequent retinal breaks [29].

Complementary Tests

B-Scan Ultrasonography Ultrasound is useful in cases where media opacity obstructs the posterior segment view. It allows assessment of retinal detachments, choroidal detachment, bleeding, inadvertent breaks, posterior vitreous detachment, and the presence of endophthalmitis.

- *Optical coherence tomography (OCT)* of posterior and anterior segment: allows evaluation of cystoid macular edema, macular vitreoretinal traction, as well as vitreous incarceration at the incision sites and adherence of the iris or the pars plicata.
- *Eye biometry* in aphakic patients can help depending on the degree of corneal edema and opacity media. Ultrasonic or optical biometers can be used. The contralateral eye should be evaluated in cases of similar vision and refraction.

Surgical Techniques and Options

Surgical Procedure: Management of Soft Material, Medium Soft, Hard, and Very Hard

The procedure of choice is a 3-port pars plana vitrectomy (Fig. 5). The goal of the vitrectomy is to remove the remains of retained lens while avoiding vitreous traction and retinal lesions.

First, the corneal wound should be sutured (Fig. 6) (if not previously done) and after that the choice of sclerotomies is made:

- 20G sclerotomy if the hardness of the lens material makes use of ultrasonic phacofragmentator predictable.
- 23G sclerotomy: when the material is not very consistent, it can be extracted by transconjunctival vitrectomy with 23G trocars. New ultrasonic 23G phacofragmentators are being developed, which will allow this technique under this caliber.
- Hybrid surgery can be done using smaller caliber ports (23 or 25G) and transforming one of the ports to 20G to perform ultrasonic phacofragmentation [2, 30].

Intravitreal Maneuvers, Including the Use of Perfluorocarbon Liquids

Both lenticular cortical remnants left in the anterior segment and vitreous incarcerated in the incisions and the iris should be cleaned and released [17, 31], preserving the rest of the anterior capsular support which will serve as support for the future implantation of the intraocular lens.

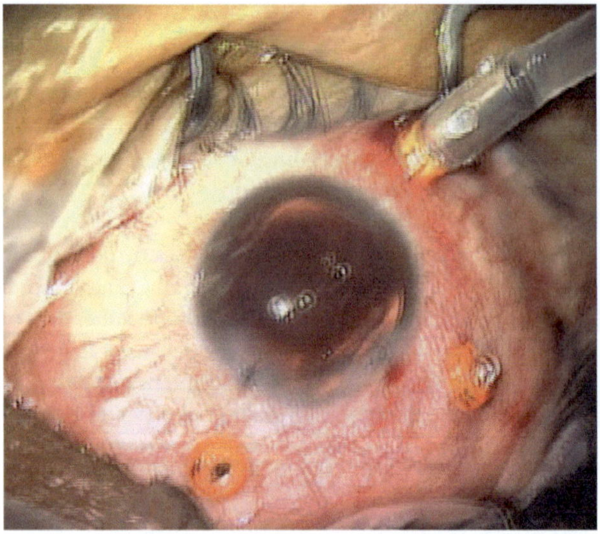

Fig. 5 The procedure of choice will be 3-port pars plana vitrectomy

Next, a thorough central and peripheral vitrectomy must be performed while avoiding vitreoretinal traction generated by the instrument [11, 32, 33] (Figs. 7 and 8).

The use of perfluorocarbon liquid bubble serves as retinal protection against ultrasound energy and mechanical trauma that may be produced by lens remains striking the retina during emulsification [34]. Filling over half of the vitreous cavity is not recommended as this may cause fragments to be retained in the vitreous base. One difficulty in the use of perfluorocarbons is the tendency of the small fragments to settle on the periphery of the meniscus of the perfluorocarbon bubble. Thus, the use of the perfluorocarbon liquid bubble may be advisable in cases of fragments of higher density [32, 35] (Fig. 9).

The next step is phacofragmentation and aspiration of lens remains; when it comes to small remains and soft cores, the vitrectome should be used with a low cutting frequency. The endoillumination probe may also be used to push small fragments to the mouth of vitrectome [31–33].

Phacofragmentation parameters	
Constellation (Alcon)	Stellaris (Bausch & Lomb)
U/S: 50 %	U/S: 0–20 %
Vacuum: 300 mmHg	Vacuum: 200–300 mmHg
Pulsed mode: ten pulses/second	Continuous mode

Both phacofragmentation and core “impalement” maneuvers should be avoided to prevent damage to the surface of the retina [2].

When the remains are abundant and the core is compact and solid, the phacofragmentator can be used for fast, safe, and effective extraction [32, 33] (Fig. 10).

For optimum and safe use of the phacofragmentator, changes in the fluid parameters should be taken into account. High suction capacity should increase pressure infusion. Furthermore, to avoid chatter or repulsion of fragments, it is better to work

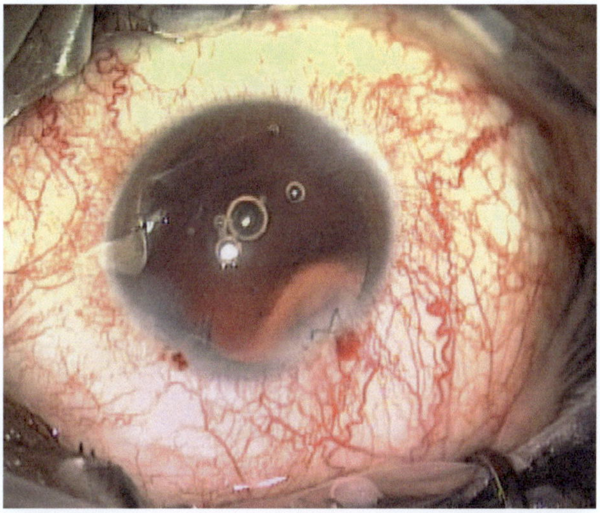

Fig. 6 The corneal wound should be sutured to maintain intraocular pressure

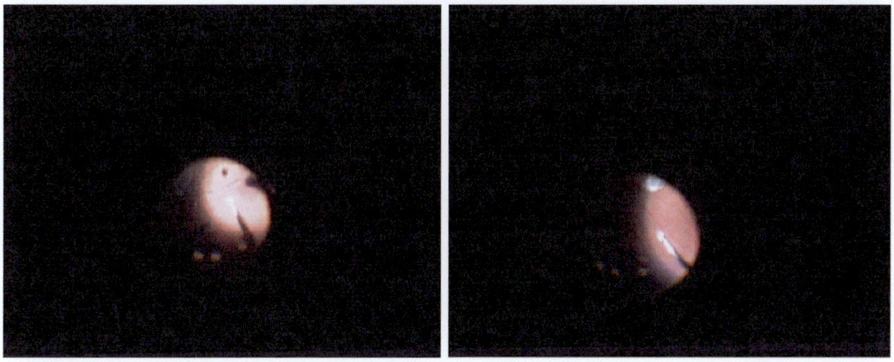

Figs. 7 and 8 Central and peripheral vitrectomy must be performed avoiding vitreoretinal traction generated by the instrument

with the phacofragmentator in linear mode and use low-power phacofragmentation to engage the fragments better.

Pulsed mode should be used to avoid large fragment impalement on the phacofragmentator mouth [31–33] (Figs. 11, 12, and 13).

After removal of all remains, an examination of the peripheral retina must be carried out to detect breaks with scleral indentation in all cases, since traction/energy from the phacofragmentator can generate peripheral retinal breaks.

Implantation of the IOL

It should be noted that in some cases, an IOL implant may not be desirable, and rehabilitation with contact lens should be considered. This happens in other lens

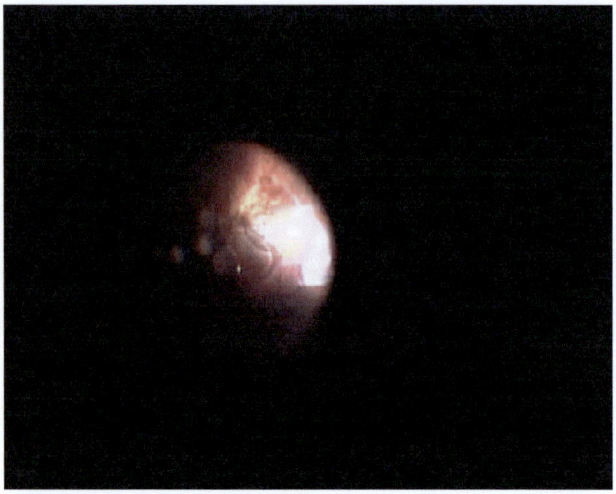

Fig. 9 The use of the perfluorocarbon liquid bubble may be advisable in cases with higher-density fragments

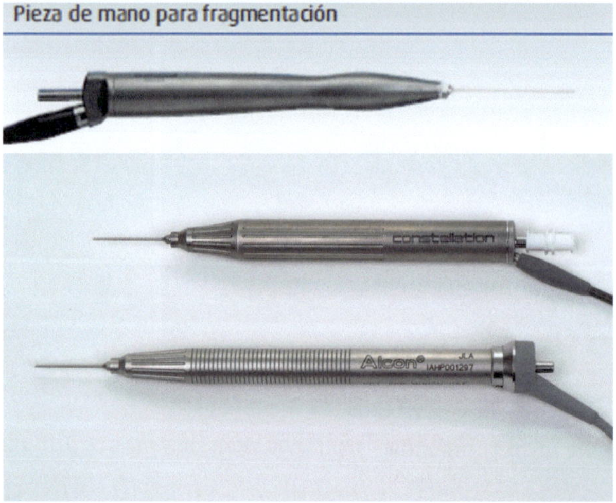

Fig. 10 Different models of phacofragmentators

dislocations that occur in patients with Marfan syndrome, since alterations in the vitreous base can often complicate the suturing of the IOL in the sulcus. In addition, the IOL implant in the anterior chamber may be complicated by glaucoma, a leading cause of blindness in these patients.

In other cases the condition of the remaining capsule must be assessed to decide on the implantation and determine which IOL is to be implanted based on the recommended site.

The IOL must only be placed into the capsular bag that has enough stability. In the posterior chamber, the IOL could also be placed in the sulcus (either on anterior capsule if there is enough support or sutured to the iris). Another alternative could be a lens in the anterior chamber (angular support or on the iris) (Fig. 14).

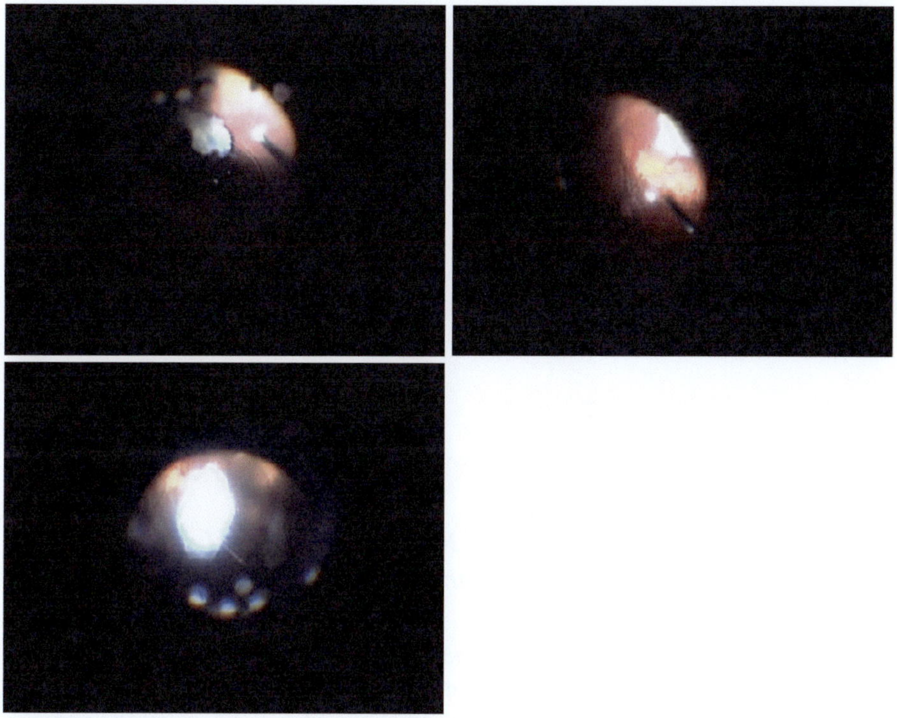

Figs. 11, 12 and 13 The use of phacofragmentator must be done carefully and without approaching the retina to avoid producing damage to it

The surgeon has to be very particular in assessing the remaining capsule, because when dealing with vitrectomized eyes, they do not have the support of the vitreous gel.

The recommendations are as follows:

If there is at least 270° of full anterior capsule, [35, 36] the implantation of an IOL in the sulcus with the following characteristics can be performed: a diameter between haptics greater than 13 mm, hydrophobic, J-shaped haptics, and preferably polypropylene and a three-piece IOL. IOLs should be avoided if under 13 mm, hydrophilic, plate-type design, and/or unique to capsular bag [2].

If there are less than 270 ° of full anterior capsule, there are several options:

- Anterior chamber IOL (specific model and appropriate dioptric power).
- IOL (Artisan type) with anchor iris (specific model and appropriate diopter power).
- Sulcus sutured IOL.
- Three-piece IOL.
- Iris sutured IOL (behind iris): IOL with diameter between haptics >13 mm, hydrophobic, with J-shaped haptics of polypropylene. The iris sutures are placed at 12 and 6 h [2].

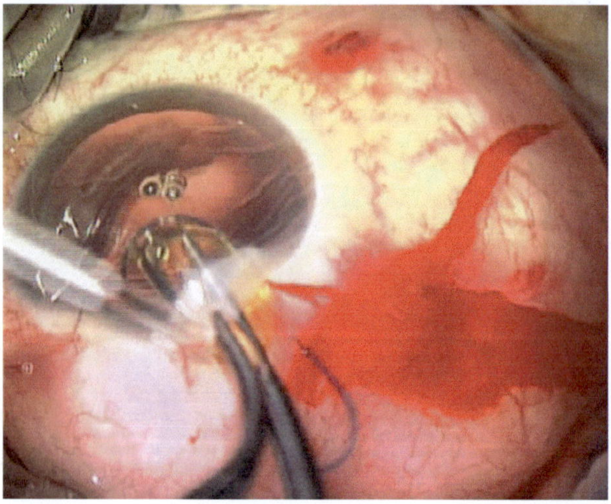

Fig. 14 The IOL only must be placed into the capsular bag when it shows sufficient stability

Outcomes and Complications of Fragment Removal in the Vitreous Following Cataract Surgery

Visual prognosis of patients who have undergone pars plana vitrectomy for removal of lens remains is quite good and has improved since the first published studies. Between 44 and 82 % of patients operated on achieved a BCVA equal to or greater than 0.5 (LogMAR) [6, 12, 17, 37].

The improvement in visual outcomes can be attributed both to the optimization of the surgical technique in complicated cataract surgery and the benefit provided by the PPV for these patients (Fig. 15).

In some cases, the BCVA will be reduced due to the occurrence of a number of complications that can arise before or after the PPV [38].

Major complications of patients who have undergone a PPV for intravitreal lens fragments are cystoid macular edema, glaucoma, and retinal detachment.

Cystoid macular edema is the most common cause of visual loss in patients who have undergone PPV for extraction of intravitreal lens fragments [17]. This complication usually occurs in the first 6 months after the PPV; therefore, adequate monitoring for early detection and initiation of a fast and aggressive treatment is necessary [39].

The appearance of an inflammatory secondary glaucoma, defined as persistent IOP ≥30 mmHg, occurs between 3 and 25 % of cases after PPV [25–27]. Early intervention after complicated cataract surgery could reduce the incidence of this complication.

Retinal detachment can complicate 4–12 % of cases undergoing PPV for the extraction of intravitreal lens fragments [17, 27, 37, 38, 40–42].

Although most retinal detachments can be repaired successfully, the final visual acuity may be compromised. A recent study suggests performing a prophylactic 360° laser photocoagulation at the time of vitrectomy to reduce the incidence of retinal detachment in these cases [2, 29].

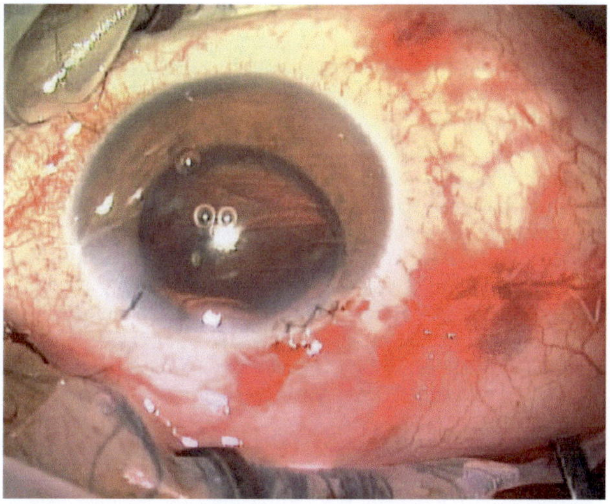

Fig. 15 After observing that the IOL has enough stability, the corneal wound is sutured

Practical Recommendations/Guidelines for the Surgeon in Trouble

- Generally, with exception of complications requiring early intervention, the vitrectomy should be done within the week following the failed phacoemulsification.
- Both lenticular cortical remnants left in the anterior segment and vitreous incarcerated in the incisions and the iris should be cleaned and released, preserving the rest of the anterior capsular support.
- A thorough central and peripheral vitrectomy must be performed to prevent vitreoretinal traction that could be produced by the phacofragmentator.
- The use of perfluorocarbon may be advisable in cases of fragments of higher density.
- A thorough exam of the peripheral retina must be carried out to detect breaks with scleral indentation in all cases.
- When implanting an IOL, the capsular remnant available must be properly assessed, as vitrectomized eyes do not have the posterior support of the vitreous gel.

Conflict of Interest The authors have no commercial or financial interest in the technical or pharmaceutical products described in this chapter.

References

1. Rofagha S, Bhisitkul RB. Management of retained lens fragments in complicated cataract surgery. Curr Opin Ophthalmol. 2011;22(2):137–40.
2. Manejo de la luxación de material cristaliniano y lentes intraoculares en la cavidad vítrea "Guías de Práctica Clínica de la SERV". 2012. Disponible en www.serv.es.

3. Kraff CR, Kraff MC. Cirugía de la catarata. In: Krupin T, Kolker AE, Rosenberg LF, editors. Complicaciones en oftalmología quirúrgica. Madrid: Harcourt; 2000. p. 57–80.
4. Moisseiev E, Kinori M, Glovinsky Y, et al. Retained lens fragments: nucleus fragments are associated with worse prognosis than cortex or epinucleus fragments. Eur J Ophthalmol. 2011;21(6):741–7.
5. Blodi BA, Flynn Jr HW, Blodi CF, Folk JC, Daily MJ. Retained nuclei after cataract surgery. Ophthalmology. 1992;99:41–4.
6. Oruc S, Kaplan HJ. Outcome of vitrectomy for retained lens fragments after phacoemulsification. Ocul Immunol Inflamm. 2001;9:41–7.
7. Kim JE, Flynn Jr HW, Smiddy WE, et al. Retained lens fragments after phacoemulsification. Ophthalmology. 1994;101:1827–32.
8. Kim JE, Flynn Jr HW, Rubsamen PE, et al. Endophthalmitis in patients with retained lens fragments after phacoemulsification. Ophthalmology. 1996;103(4):575–8.
9. Ho LY, Doft BH, Wang L, Bunker CH. Clinical predictors and outcomes of pars plana vitrectomy for retained lens material after cataract extraction. Am J Ophthalmol. 2009;147: 587–94.
10. Yang CS, Lee FL, Hsu WM, Liu JH. Management of retained intravitreal lens fragments after phacoemulsification surgery. Ophthalmologica. 2002;216(3):192–7.
11. Wilkinson CP, Green WR. Vitrectomy for retained lens material after cataract extraction. Ophthalmology. 2001;108:1633–7.
12. Kageyama T, Ayaki M, Ogasawara M, Asahiro C, Yaguchi S. Results of vitrectomy performed at the time of phacoemulsification complicated by intravitreal lens fragments. Br J Ophthalmol. 2001;85(9):1038–40.
13. Kwok AKH, Li KKW, Lai TYY, Lam DSC. Pars plana vitrectomy in the management of retained intravitreal lens fragments after cataract surgery. Clin Experiment Ophthalmol. 2002;30:399–403.
14. Merani R, Hunyor AP, Playfair J, Chang A, et al. Pars plana vitrectomy for the management of retained lens material after cataract surgery. Am J Ophthalmol. 2007;144:364–70.
15. Stewart MW. Managing retained lens fragments: raising the bar. Am J Ophthalmol. 2009;144: 569–70.
16. Soliman Mahdy M, Eid MZ, Shalaby KA, Hegazy HM. Intravitreal phacoemulsification with pars plana vitrectomy for management of posteriorly dislocated nucleus or lens fragments. Eur J Ophthalmol. 2010;20(1):115–9.
17. Scott IU, Flynn Jr HW, Smiddy WE, et al. Clinical features and outcomes of pars plana vitrectomy in patients with retained lens fragments. Ophthalmology. 2003;110(8):1567–72.
18. Lai TY, Kwok AK, Yeung YS, Kwan KY, Woo DC, Yuen KS, Loo AV. Immediate pars plana vitrectomy for dislocated intravitreal lens fragments during cataract surgery. Eye (Lond). 2005;19(11):1157–62.
19. Chen CL, Wang TY, Cheng JH, Tai MC, Lu DW, Chen JT. Immediate pars plana vitrectomy improves outcome in retained intravitreal lens fragments after phacoemulsification. Ophthalmologica. 2008;222(4):277–83.
20. Stewart MW. Management of retained lens fragments: can we improve? Am J Ophthalmol. 2007;144:445–6.
21. Von Lany H, Mahmood S, James CRH, Cole MD, Charles SJ, Foot B, Gouws P, Shaw S. Displacement of nuclear fragments into the vitreous complicating phacoemulsification surgery in the UK: clinical features, outcomes and management. Br J Ophthalmol. 2008;92:493–5.
22. Colyer MH, Berinstein DM, Khan NJ, Weichel ED, Lai MM, Deegan WF, Katira RC, Phillips WB, Sanders RJ, Garfinkel RA. Same-day versus delayed vitrectomy with lensectomy for the management of retained lens fragments. Retina. 2011;31(8):1534–40.
23. Smiddy WE, Flynn Jr HW, Kim JE. Retinal detachment in patients with retained lens fragments or dislocated posterior chamber intraocular lenses. Ophthalmic Surg Lasers. 1996;27(10):856–61.

24. Borne MJ, Tasman W, Regillo C, et al. Outcomes of vitrectomy for retained lens fragments. Ophthalmology. 1996;103:971–6.
25. Vilar NF, Flynn Jr HW, Smiddy WE, et al. Removal of retained lens fragments after phacoemulsification reverses secondary glaucoma and restores visual acuity. Ophthalmology. 1997;104:787–91; discussion 791–792.
26. Margherio RR, Margherio AR, Pendergast SD, et al. Vitrectomy for retained lens fragments after phacoemulsification. Ophthalmology. 1997;104:1426–32.
27. Al-Khaier A, Wong D, Lois N, et al. Determinants of visual outcome after pars plana vitrectomy for posteriorly dislocated lens fragments in phacoemulsification. J Cataract Refract Surg. 2001;27:1199–206.
28. Moore JK, Scott IU, Flynn Jr HW, Smiddy WE, Murray TG, Kim JE, Vilar NF, Pereira MB, Jorge R. Retinal detachment in eyes undergoing pars plana vitrectomy for removal of retained lens fragments. Ophthalmology. 2003;110(4):709–13.
29. Morris RE, Shere JL, Witherspoon CD, et al. Intraoperative retinal detachment prophylaxis in vitrectomy for retained cataract fragments. J Cataract Refract Surg. 2009;35(3):491–5.
30. Cho M, Chan RP. 23-gauge pars plana vitrectomy for management of posteriorly dislocated crystalline lens. Clin Ophthalmol. 2011;5:1737–43.
31. Monshizadeh R, Samiy N, Haimovici R. Management of retained intravitreal lens fragments alter cataract surgery. Surv Ophthalmol. 1999;43:397–404.
32. Wong D, Briggs MC, Hickey-Dwyer MU, et al. Removal of lens fragments from the vitreous cavity. Eye (Lond). 1997;11:37–42.
33. Adán A. Tratamiento quirúrgico de las complicaciones vitreorretinianas en la cirugía del segmento anterior. In: Corcóstegui B, Adán A, García-Arumí J, Mateo C, Nieto I, editors. Cirugía vitreorretiniana: indicaciones y técnicas. Monografía de la Sociedad Española de Oftalmología. Madrid: MacLine; 1999. p. 105–20.
34. Kim IK, Miller JW. Management of dislocated lens material. Semin Ophthalmol. 2002;17(3–4):162–6.
35. Wagoner MD, Cox TA, Arisayu RG, et al. Intraocular lens implantation in the absence of capsular support. Ophthalmology. 2003;110:840–59.
36. Michaeli A, Assia E. Scleral and iris fixation of posterior chamber lenses in the absence of capsular support. Curr Opin Ophthalmol. 2005;16:57–60.
37. Rossetti A, Doro D. Retained intravitreal lens fragments after phaco-emulsification: complications and visual outcome in vitrectomized and nonvitrectomized eyes. J Cataract Refract Surg. 2002;28(2):310–5.
38. Greven CM, Piccione K. Delayed visual loss after pars plana vitrectomy for retained lens fragments. Retina. 2004;24(3):363–7.
39. Cohen SM, Davis A, Cukrowski C. Cystoid macular edema after pars plana vitrectomy for retained lens fragments. J Cataract Refract Surg. 2006;32(9):1521–6.
40. Romero P, Fernandez J, Mendez I, et al. Management of nucleus loss into the vitreous: long term follow up in 63 patients. Clin Ophthalmol. 2007;1(4):505–12.
41. Hansson LJ, Larsson J. Vitrectomy for retained lens fragments in the vitreous after phacoemulsification. J Cataract Refract Surg. 2002;28(6):1007–11.
42. Smiddy WE, Guererro JL, Pinto R, et al. Retinal detachment rate after vitrectomy for retained lens material after phacoemulsification. Am J Ophthalmol. 2003;135(2):183–7.

Chapter 14
Conclusion and Outlook for the Future

Shlomit Schaal and Henry J. Kaplan

Since macular edema is a major cause of visual disability in many different ocular diseases, we have approached this complication in three major areas in this text – Part 1, Pathophysiology and Diagnosis of cystoid macular edema (CME); Part II, Medical Management of CME; and Part III, Surgical Management of CME. It is clear that understanding the pathophysiology of this disease with its many different causes will result in the future development of therapeutic options that do not exist today.

As Behar-Cohen and colleagues described in Chap. 2, the mechanisms leading to macular edema are difficult to discriminate in the various clinical presentations. Nevertheless, the use of multimodal imaging (i.e., fluorescein angiography (FA), indocyanine green angiography, and spectral domain optical coherence tomography (OCT) allows a better understanding of the exact alterations of retinal structures that result in macular edema. Such an understanding will provide more appropriate and targeted treatments. However, molecular mechanisms responsible for this complication of ocular disease are most difficult to determine since the experimental models in rodents provide limited insight since they do not have a macula. Thus, the molecular mechanisms involved in the vasogenic and cytotoxic causes of macular edema still remain to be resolved. However, our current understanding is very nicely presented in this chapter.

Multimodal imaging became of primary importance in recent years to appreciate, diagnose, and follow the development and the resolution of CME in response to treatment. In Chap. 3, Grewal and Jaffe nicely outline how fluorescein angiography (FA) and fundus autofluorescence are used to evaluate CME, while spectral domain OCT allows evaluation of the location, extension, pattern, and microstructural ana-

S. Schaal, MD, PhD (✉)
Professor and Chair, Department of Ophthalmology and Visual Sciences,
University of Massachusetts School of Medicine, Amherst, MA, USA
e-mail: S.Schaal@umassmed.edu

H.J. Kaplan, MD
Evans Professor and Chair of Ophthalmology and Visual Sciences,
University of Louisville, Louisville, KY, USA
e-mail: hank.kaplan@louisville.edu

S. Schaal, H.J. Kaplan (eds.), *Cystoid Macular Edema*,
DOI 10.1007/978-3-319-39766-5_14

tomical features of CME. FA, although a technique used for decades, still is the only technique that allows identification of areas of leakage, thus providing complimentary yet distinct information for diagnosis of CME and monitoring its response to treatment. Future advances in imaging technology with higher acquisition speed and hardware motion tracking along with improved automated image segmentation analysis protocols will allow us to better characterize CME. Development of novel anatomical biomarkers can offer prognostic implications and monitor response to treatment. Newer imaging technologies including noninvasive OCT angiography hold promise to help better elucidate the pathology of CME.

In Chap. 4 Escott and Goldstein discussed the medical management of CME in uveitis. Since macular edema is the leading cause of vision loss in uveitis, its treatment should be initiated early and continued until complete resolution so that there is no permanent retinal damage and loss of central vision. Corticosteroids have been the mainstay of therapy and can be given topically, by periocular injection, by intravitreal injection, via an implantable depot device, or orally. Although the risks of cataract and glaucoma can limit the ongoing use of corticosteroids and require other immunomodulatory agents, it still remains a mainstay of treatment. The authors discussed the use of intravitreal anti-VEGF agents, intravitreal methotrexate, subcutaneous interferon alpha, and systemic antitumor necrosis factor agents in the treatment of this complication in uveitis. They emphasize that the decision about which agent to use has to be individualized and can present therapeutic challenges.

The medical management of CME in diabetes is discussed in Chap. 5 by Turner and Del Priore. They emphasize that the medical management of diabetic macular edema (DME) has evolved since the first reports of the Early Treatment of Diabetic Retinopathy Study (ETDRS) showed a 50% reduction in vision with focal/grid laser. The more sophisticated understanding of the factors involved in the pathophysiology of this complication has resulted in the recognition that anti-VEGF agents are superior to laser for the treatment of DME. This is particularly true in patients with center-involving DME with vision loss. At the present time, the role of intraocular corticosteroids is still not clear although it is common clinical practice to use intraocular corticosteroids in patients who are poorly responsive to anti-VEGF treatment, as well as those patients who are pseudophakic and have no evidence of glaucomatous optic neuropathy. Several factors are involved in the choice of treatment for the management of DME including cost, number of treatments, as well as response to therapy.

Khoshnevis and Sebag discussed the role of vitreo-macular traction (VMT) in the development and management of macular edema in Chap. 6. They discuss how anomalous PVD is the fundamental cause of vitreo-maculopathies associated with macular edema presenting as both vitreo-macular traction, as well as macular pucker. Additionally, vitreo-macular adhesion is an important contributor to macular edema associated with diabetic retinopathy, retinal vein occlusion, and even exudative age-related macular degeneration. Consequently, vitreous surgery has a definite role in the resolution of macular edema in the presence of suspected vitreo-maculopathy. The role of pharmacologic vitreolysis in the management of this complication is still to be determined although there now is a therapeutic option with enzymatic digestion of vitreo-macular adhesion. It is uncertain whether prophylactic pharmacologic vitreolysis will actually prevent the development of macular edema in either primary vitreo-maculopathies or associated comorbid disorders.

Buehl and Schmidt-Erfurth in Chap. 7 have demonstrated that intravitreal therapy with anti-VEGF medication or corticosteroids is currently the most effective treatment option for macular edema associated with retinal vein occlusion. Most specialists currently favor an as-needed or treatment-extended regimen after the initial, monthly anti-VEGF loading dose. However, studies have yet to compare the long-term effectiveness and safety of repeated intravitreal injections with these agents. Similar to the treatment of exudative age-related macular degeneration, the use of aflibercept may allow for longer treatment intervals compared to ranibizumab or bevacizumab. In chronic cases and patients who are nonresponsive to anti-VEGF treatment, the continuous release of corticosteroid medication as with the sustained-release dexamethasone implant may preclude the need for multiple repeated injections of other medications. Undoubtedly, the complications of cataract progression and increased intraocular pressure require judgment by the physician as to the most appropriate use of such sustained-release devices. In the future, prospective trials are needed to compare long-term efficacy in the adverse effects of both anti-VEGF and corticosteroid therapy. The evidence for combination therapy in the treatment of retinal vein occlusion is still needed.

Al-Latayfeh in Chap. 8 discusses the development of CME with retained lens fragments after cataract surgery, since CME is a major complication in this clinical scenario. Although the introduction of modern phacoemulsification techniques resulted initially in an increased incidence of posterior lens fragment dislocation, this trend has certainly resolved. The management of CME with retained lens fragments includes aggressive medical therapy with topical and oral non-steroidal anti-inflammatory drugs (NSAIDs), as well as corticosteroids. If severe intraocular inflammation doesn't resolve quickly, pars plana vitrectomy with removal of residual lens material should definitely be considered.

Grigalunas and T. Merrill elucidate in Chap. 9 the surgical management of CME associated with uveitis. Uveitis is a significant cause of vision loss in young people, and the most common cause of vision loss in these patients is CME. Although the initial management of uveitic CME is primarily medical, when maximum tolerated medical therapy is inadequate, surgical approaches may provide an alternative or adjunctive means of controlling uveitis and uveitic CME. Following vitrectomy in uveitis patients, there is an overall trend in the literature toward decreased CME, improved visual acuity, and reduction of medications. A large, prospective, randomized clinical trial is needed to confirm these findings. The surgical implantation of FLAC implant has proven to be effective in resolving uveitic CME in a majority of cases. The risks associated with implantation and long-term steroid exposure in the implanted eye are significant and must be deliberated in each case. However, for many patients, FLAC implantation provides a viable alternative to systemic therapy for ME in chronic uveitis.

In Chap. 10, Talcott and Eliott describe the surgical management of CME secondary to diabetes. In recent years, because medical therapeutic options for the management of diabetic CME have expanded, surgical options may be deferred or overlooked. It is important to always keep in mind that the eyes with observable vitreous and/or epiretinal traction in addition to diabetic macular changes are most likely to improve after vitrectomy. The eyes with refractory edema and no observable traction, however, are less likely to improve with surgery. Unfortunately, improvement in retinal thickening is often more impressive than improvement in vision even in these select cases. However, vitrectomy and other surgical interventions may be beneficial for select cases of diabetic macular edema, especially when surgical intervention is undertaken early, before photoreceptor damage has occurred.

The surgical approach to CME with vitreo-macular traction (VMT) syndrome is further discussed in Chap. 11 by Maia, Bottós, Elizalde, Badaro, and Arevalo. VMT syndrome is implicated in the pathophysiology of a number of macular disorders, with variable anatomical and function outcomes which underscore the complexity of the underlying disease. These macular changes are intimately related to the VMT configuration, which led to proposals for classification of this syndrome, based on OCT findings. The size and strength of the remaining vitreo-macular attachment may define the specific maculopathy. Focal VMT usually leads to MH formation, tractional CME, and foveal retinal detachment, while broad VMT is widely associated with ERM, diffuse retinal thickening, and poorer recovery of foveal depression.

Hondur and Tezel discuss in Chap. 12 novel surgical approaches to manage CME associated with vascular occlusions. Although venous vascular occlusions are commonly approached conservatively, using injectable pharmacotherapy, there is continuous compiling evidence that surgical intervention may be appropriate in selected cases. Pilot studies that employed surgical interventions in arterial retinal vascular occlusions carry the promise of providing an alternative approach to a disease that commonly results in blindness.

And finally, Peral, Alió, and Quintás describe in Chap. 13 the surgical management of retained lens fragments during or following phacoemulsification surgery. Along with the academic discussion, the authors provide practical and current guidelines for the management of CME related with these surgical complications.

In this comprehensive text, we hope that readers will find guidance to the pathophysiology, diagnosis, medical, and surgical management of CME that results from various causes. As medicine is an ever-changing and ever-progressing art and science, we hope and anticipate that current guidelines will have some modifications and variations with time.

Index

S. Schaal, H.J. Kaplan (eds.), *Cystoid Macular Edema*,
DOI 10.1007/978-3-319-39766-5

MIX
Papier aus verantwortungsvollen Quellen
Paper from responsible sources
FSC® C105338

If you have any concerns about our products,
you can contact us on
ProductSafety@springernature.com

In case Publisher is established outside the EU,
the EU authorized representative is:
Springer Nature Customer Service Center GmbH
Europaplatz 3, 69115 Heidelberg, Germany

Printed by Libri Plureos GmbH
in Hamburg, Germany